Seminars in Liaison Psychiatry

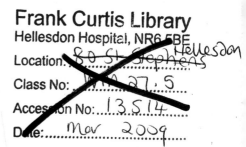

College Seminars Series

Series Editors

Professor Hugh Freeman, Honorary Professor, University of Salford, and Honorary Consultant Psychiatrist, Salford Health Authority

Dr Ian Pullen, Consultant Psychiatrist, Royal Edinburgh Hospital

Dr George Stein, Consultant Psychiatrist, Farnborough Hospital, and King's College Hospital

Professor Greg Wilkinson, Editor, *British Journal of Psychiatry*, and Professor of Liaison Psychiatry, University of Liverpool

Other books in the series

Seminars in Child and Adolescent Psychiatry. Edited by Dora Black & David Cottrell

Seminars in Basic Neurosciences. Edited by Gethin Morgan & Stuart Butler

Seminars in Psychiatric Genetics. By Peter McGuffin, Michael J. Owen, Michael C. O'Donovan, Anita Thapar & Irving Gottesman

Seminars in Alcohol and Drug Misuse. Edited by Jonathan Chick & Roch Cantwell

Seminars in Psychology and the Social Sciences. Edited by Digby Tantam & Max Birchwood

Seminars in Clinical Psychopharmacology. Edited by David King

Seminars in Practical Forensic Psychiatry. Edited by Derek Chiswick & Rosemarie Cope

Forthcoming titles

Seminars in the Psychiatry of Learning Disabilities. Edited by Oliver Russell

Seminars in General Adult Psychiatry. Edited by George Stein & Greg Wilkinson

Seminars in Psychiatry for the Elderly. Edited by Brice Pitt & Mohsen Naguib

Seminars in Psychosexual Disorders. Edited by R. Haslam

Seminars in Liaison Psychiatry

Edited by
Elspeth Guthrie & Francis Creed

GASKELL

British Library Cataloguing-in-Publication Data
A catalogue record for this book is available from the British Library.

ISBN 0-902241-95-8

Distributed in North America
by American Psychiatric Press, Inc.
ISBN 0-88048-576-0

Gaskell is an imprint of the Royal College of Psychiatrists,
17 Belgrave Square, London SW1X 8PG
The Royal College of Psychiatrists is a registered charity, number 228636

The views presented in this book do not necessarily reflect those of the Royal College of Psychiatrists, and the publishers are not responsible for any error of omission or fact. College Seminars are produced by the Publications Department of the College; they should in no way be construed as providing a syllabus or other material for any College examination.

Printed by Bell & Bain Ltd., Thornliebank, Glasgow

Contents

Contributors

Dr Christopher Bass, The John Radcliffe Hospital, Headington, Oxford OX3 9OU

Dr Susan M. Benbow, Consultant Old Age Psychiatrist, Central Manchester and West Cheshire NHS Trusts, SCOPE, Carisbrooke Resource Centre, Wenlock Way, Gorton, Manchester M12 5LF

Professor Francis Creed, School of Psychiatry and Behavioural Sciences, Rawnsley Building, Manchester Royal Infirmary, Oxford Road, Manchester M13 9WL

Dr Gerald H. Dawson, Consultant Old Age Psychiatrist, South Durham NHS Trust, Community Mental Health Elderly Services, Hundens Lane, Darlington

Dr Elspeth Guthrie, Senior Lecturer in Psychiatry, Rawnsley Building, Manchester Royal Infirmary, Oxford Road, Manchester M13 9WL

Peter Haddad, Department of Psychiatry, Withington Hospital, Nell Lane, West Didsbury, Manchester M20 8LR

Dr Bryan Lask, Consultant Psychiatrist, Hospital for Sick Children, Great Ormond Street, London WC1N 3JH

Dr G. Peter Maguire, Senior Lecturer in Psychiatry, Christie Hospital, Wilmslow Road, Withington, Manchester M20 4BX

Dr Richard Mayou, University of Oxford, Department of Psychiatry, The Warneford Hospital, Oxford OX3 7JX

Kate Morgan, Hospital for Sick Children, Great Ormond Street, London WC1N 3JH

Dr Richard K. Morriss, Senior Lecturer, University Department of Community Psychiatry, Royal Preston Hospital, Sharoe Green Lane, Preston PR2 4QF

Dr Michael Murphy, Consultant Psychiatrist, Queen Mary's University Hospital, Roehampton, London SW15

Dr Robert C. Peveler, University Department of Psychiatry, Royal South Hants Hospital, Graham Road, Southampton SO9 4PE

Dr Michael Sharpe, Tutor in Psychiatry, University Department of Psychiatry, The Warneford Hospital, Oxford OX3 7JX

Foreword

Series Editors

The publication of *College Seminars*, a series of textbooks covering the breadth of psychiatry, is very much in line with the Royal College of Psychiatrists' established role in education and in setting professional standards.

College Seminars are intended to help junior doctors during their training years. We hope that trainees will find these books useful, on the ward as well as in preparation for the MRCPsych examination. Separate volumes will cover clinical psychiatry, each of its subspecialities, and also the relevant non-clinical academic disciplines of psychology and sociology.

College Seminars will make a contribution to the continuing professional development of established clinicians.

Psychiatry is concerned primarily with people, and to a lesser extent with disease processes and pathology. The core of the subject is rich in ideas and schools of thought, and no single approach or solution can embrace the variety of problems a psychiatrist meets. For this reason, we have endeavoured to adopt an eclectic approach to practical management throughout the series.

The College can draw on the collective wisdom of many individuals in clinical and academic psychiatry. More than a hundred people have contributed to this series; this reflects how diverse and complex psychiatry has become.

Frequent new editions of books appearing in the series are envisaged, which should allow *College Seminars* to be responsive to readers' suggestions and needs.

Hugh Freeman
Ian Pullen
George Stein
Greg Wilkinson

Preface

This book is intended to help trainee psychiatrists become acquainted with the basic approach of liaison psychiatrists. It is not a comprehensive textbook of liaison psychiatry, but includes chapters concerning the basic clinical approach to psychiatric assessment and treatment in the general hospital setting.

It is recognised that training in liaison psychiatry has been limited in the past. This book is not intended as a substitute for supervised clinical practice but should guide general psychiatrists who find themselves in the unfamiliar setting of the general medical or surgical units.

The book deals with the topics of somatisation and psychological reactions to physical illness in special detail as these are not covered in other textbooks. The chapters on research and treatment are deliberately detailed as they are not well covered in other books. On the other hand, the assessment and treatment of organic psychiatric syndromes are well covered in other specific texts, to which trainees are referred.

It is hoped that this textbook will provide a much needed practical approach for psychiatrists unfamiliar with working in the general hospital setting. It should complement other recent textbooks in the area.

1 International overview of consultation–liaison psychiatry

Richard Morriss & Richard Mayou

Historical development • The status of consultation–liaison psychiatry in Britain • Different patterns of consultation–liaison psychiatry • Consultation–liaison in practice • Coordination of consultation–liaison psychiatry within the general hospital

Liaison psychiatry, or consultation–liaison psychiatry (CL) as it is more generally known in other countries, is concerned with the clinical service, teaching and research in settings where psychiatry and the rest of medicine meet (Lipowski, 1983). Since it is based within general hospitals, it requires both a good knowledge of medicine and special skills in the psychiatric care of the particular physical disorders and symptoms of medical patients. Increasing awareness of the special clinical and administrative skills that are needed and of advances in research has led to claims that CL is a distinct sub-speciality of psychiatry (Robinowitz & Nadelson, 1991), a claim resisted by some general psychiatrists. We review the historical origins of CL, the contrasting development in North America, Britain and the rest of Europe, the different models of care, and the principles of setting up a new CL service in Britain.

Historical development

There is a long history of the management of psychiatric problems within general hospitals (Mayou, 1989). During the 20th century, specialist psychiatry has had an increasing presence with the establishment of out-patient clinics and in-patient units, both in America and Europe. From the beginning, such units were mainly concerned with patients suffering from neurotic or organic disorders rather than with chronic psychotic problems treated in asylums. The presence of psychiatrists within general hospitals encouraged medical and surgical colleagues to ask psychiatrists to advise on the management of their patients with psychiatric problems, and also to teach their staff and medical students.

The informal links, together with experience of treating battle victims in both World Wars and the influence of a few pioneering physicians and psychiatrists, promoted the development of what has become known as consultation–liaison psychiatry (Mayou, 1989; Schwab, 1989).

Specifically planned CL services began around 60 years ago in North America with the aims of improving medical education and providing a clinical service (Lipowski, 1986). In Britain, the rest of Europe and Australasia, development has been much slower.

Development of consultation–liaison psychiatry in the US

The psychosomatic medicine movement associated with the dramatic growth of psychoanalysis in the 1930s stimulated psychiatric and medical interest in the role of emotional factors in the aetiology and course of physical illness. This approach encouraged the consideration of personality and lifestyle as important factors in the education of patients to make medical treatment more effective. However, research failed to support the psychosomatic hypothesis that psychological factors caused many physical illnesses and this resulted in disillusionment in the 1950s and 1960s.

The wider general hospital psychiatry movement has had a more lasting influence. A key factor in the 1930s was the initiative and the financial contribution of the Rockefeller Foundation to set up five general hospital psychiatry centres in the US. Billings who worked at one of these centres, the Colorado General Hospital, coined the term 'liaison psychiatry' in 1939. This service was notable for the use of the multidisciplinary team (psychiatrists and social workers) and because it was a consultation service without separate psychiatric beds. General hospital psychiatrists were seen as ideal teachers of medical students because of their psychiatric training and the setting in which they worked.

The number of CL services in the US increased tenfold between 1939 and 1984. The main impetus for expansion came during the 1960s and '70s from the National Institute of Mental Health (NIMH), who provided federal funding to set up CL services. The aims were principally educational, teaching a holistic approach to medicine to medical students and other health care professionals, training primary health care workers to identify and manage psychiatric disorders, and establishing close working links between medicine and psychiatry. The larger services developed innovative consultation and liaison links with specialist clinical services and set up research programmes.

Consultation–liaison psychiatry is now well established, although proposals for sub-speciality status are still being debated. However, the American Board of Psychiatry and Neurology now requires CL experience for psychiatric resident accreditation (recognition of training). The majority of teaching hospitals and large general hospitals have an on-site CL service, but many are poorly staffed. Many smaller general hospitals tend to rely on contacts with private psychiatrists. A recent survey suggests that a considerable number of psychiatrists now spend a major proportion of their working time in CL psychiatry (Noyes *et al*, 1992). However, at present funding is difficult, especially for liaison, and CL psychiatry is no longer expanding.

An American teaching hospital CL service

There are many models of service provision and methods of funding (Lipowski, 1992; Noyes *et al*, 1992). The Yale University hospital is a good example, and will be described in detail as no such service exists in the UK. The service provides 600 new consultations per year for out-patients and serves a 850-bed general hospital (Leigh, 1987). Under an overall director who is a psychiatrist, it is divided into consultation–liaison and emergency services. The CL service is staffed by a director (a senior psychiatrist), five other psychiatrists, three social workers, two nurse specialists, three trainee psychologists, three medical students and three nursing students. The emergency service has a director (a senior psychiatrist), junior psychiatrists (a part of the training of all psychiatrists at Yale) and two nurse specialists. All initial consultations are performed by psychiatrists. New consultations and periodical follow-ups are presented in a daily team meeting to a senior psychiatrist who assigns follow-up for new consultations to psychiatrists, nurses or social workers depending on the needs of the patient. Liaison work consists of joint rounds with medical/surgical teams (cardiology, surgical trauma, rehabilitation, renal unit and neurology), conferences with staff, informal consultations and education for staff on individual units. In addition, out-patient clinics for oncology and primary care are arranged. The CL service teaches medical students and trainee psychiatrists through a behavioural sciences course emphasising a consideration of biological, physical and social factors in all patients.

Development of consultation–liaison psychiatry in Britain

The first psychiatric out-patient clinics and observation wards for the assessment of acute mental illness were established in a few general hospitals before the First World War. Over a period of 40 years there was a slow steady growth in the number of clinics, but there was little contact between psychiatrists and other medical colleagues. With the establishment of the National Health Service in 1948, out-patient services in general hospitals expanded and in-patient units were established, partly because they were seen as a more cost-effective alternative to the traditional asylum. Some psychiatrists, especially those based in the general hospital (clinics or wards) started to provide informal consultation services to their surgical and medical colleagues (Mayou, 1989).

A major factor in setting up specific services was the abolition of suicide as a criminal offence in 1961 and the recommendation by the Ministry of Health that all cases of attempted suicide were to be assessed by a psychiatrist before being discharged from hospital. Throughout the 1960s and '70s there was a rapid rise in the number of patients who attempted suicide and this resulted in psychiatrists having more regular contact with general hospital emergency departments and wards.

Numerous reports were published at this time describing consultation services (reviewed by Mayou, 1989; Lloyd, 1991). One of the most influential was that established by Sir Dennis Hill in 1961 at the Middlesex Hospital, London. Based on American models, it emphasised liaison by senior psychiatrists who had attachments to individual medical units. Despite those pioneering units, most CL services have remained small and principally concerned with consultation rather than liaison, with an emphasis on assessment of self-poisoning patients.

Development in the rest of Europe

Consultation services and CL units have been set up in most European countries over the last 40 years, especially in The Netherlands and Spain. In contrast, Germany has a well-established tradition of the non-psychiatric speciality of psychosomatic medicine (see below). As in Britain, the American example has been important but overall there are few specialist CL units outside academic centres and services are haphazard.

In 1985, a report by the Conference of European Health Ministers (Regional Office of World Health Organization, 1985) concluded that current facilities for mental health services in general hospitals are generally unsatisfactory and several governments have recently recommended that CL services be established in most general hospitals. In 1987, the European Consultation–Liaison Workgroup (ECLW) was established to exchange knowledge, promote collaborative research and also to inform governments about the status of liaison psychiatry. Details of European services have been described by Mayou *et al* (1991) and two examples are mentioned here.

The Netherlands

The Netherlands have particularly well-developed CL services. Approximately half of the general hospitals have psychiatric units and one-fifth have a specialist CL psychiatrist. In most services liaison nurses have an important role in consultation and follow-up. An example is at the 933-bed teaching hospital at Leyden (Hengeveld *et al*, 1984). All consultations are performed by two senior and two junior psychiatrists generally on the same day as a telephone request from the physician. Further management is arranged with the hospital's psychiatric or social work services. The National Liaison Psychiatry Group has been very active in promoting collaborative clinical research. A government report (Nationale Raad de Volksgeszondheid, 1990) recommended that all general hospitals should have a psychiatrist whose primary role is CL, and provided detailed guidelines for staffing and other resources.

Germany

Germany is unique in that there are three separate services working at the interface of psychiatry and medicine in general hospitals: psychiatry, psychosomatic medicine and medical psychology. Consultation–liaison psychiatry is poorly developed.

The psychosomatic medicine service is provided by specialists who train in psychotherapy and general medicine or psychiatry. A specialist certificate in psychosomatic medicine with a specific training programme is being arranged. There are 36 psychosomatic units in teaching and general hospitals (half with in-patient beds) and a number of special psychosomatic hospitals. They treat patients with neurotic or personality disorders, eating disorders, psychosomatic illness, and problems of coping and compliance. Treatment is predominantly with dynamic psychotherapy and is often multidisciplinary with psychology and social work input. Specific liaison services to medical specialities and joint case conferences with medical units are a feature of psychosomatic medicine services. The German government has recently strongly recommended setting up CL services in the many hospitals which do not have psychiatry or psychosomatic medicine wards.

Differences in the development of CL between the US, the UK and the rest of Europe

Consultation–liaison psychiatry is no longer expanding in the US and in some cases CL services are being cut back. The reported use of CL services varies considerably and has generally been reported in terms of a median consultation rate: number of general hospital patients referred to CL services divided by the total number of general hospital patients. This varies from 3.4% in North America and 2.1% in The Netherlands to only 1.4% in Britain (Hengeveld *et al*, 1984). The differences in organisation and clinical practice between the US and Europe are attributable to the federally-funded expansion of CL in the US and the fact that there are fewer psychiatrists, psychologists, social workers and liaison nurses in all European countries (Lloyd, 1991).

A fundamental difference lies in the health care systems with many European countries, especially Britain, having well developed primary health care which provides considerable psychiatric treatment, including that for somatisation (Bridges & Goldberg, 1985). In Europe, hospital doctors often choose to refer patients with psychiatric problems back to their own GP rather than to a liaison psychiatrist. In contrast, in the US many patients consult hospital specialists for their primary care.

Evaluation

On both sides of the Atlantic there is increasing emphasis on the cost and benefits of CL psychiatry – the claim that CL improves outcome and reduces the use of medical resources needs to be tested. Some evaluations of consultation service have been disappointing (Goldberg, 1992). Negative findings are partly due to major methodological problems (see Chapter 10) but also to the difficulty in ensuring physician and surgeon concordance with CL advice (Huyse *et al*, 1990*b*). Some studies of specific liaison attachments have shown financial savings on a scale which would pay for the services of a small multidisciplinary CL team (Levitan & Kornfeld, 1981; Strain *et al*, 1991*a*). The further growth of CL psychiatry in the US and Europe will depend, not only on demonstrated improvements in the quality of care of general hospital patients, but also on the cost-effectiveness of CL.

The status of consultation–liaison psychiatry in Britain

The development of CL services in the UK has been haphazard and is often given little priority. There are fewer than 20 full-time CL consultant psychiatrists in the UK (Mayou *et al*, 1991). A national survey of CL services (Mayou *et al*, 1990) examined 52 health districts in the UK: 27 had an identifiable CL service, 22 employed a multidisciplinary CL team and 23 had specialist liaison psychiatry attachments to individual general hospital departments. Very few districts keep systematic records of general hospital referrals, and were unable to provide details of patients seen, even though Gater & Goldberg (1991) have reported that 33% of all new psychiatric referrals reach the psychiatric service via the general hospital. CL is largely provided by duty doctors or sector teams in some districts.

In many services in the UK, CL is still limited to the assessment of attempted suicide; 36 of 52 health districts have some attempted suicide assessment arrangements (Mayou *et al*, 1990). The Department of Health recommends that all patients who have attempted suicide should have a mental state assessment by trained doctors or non-medical staff who then decide on the need for psychiatric referral. Research has shown that specially trained and supervised junior physicians (Gardner *et al*, 1977), social workers (Newson-Smith & Hirsch, 1979) or nurses (Catalan *et al*, 1980) can successfully identify patients who are psychiatrically ill or at high risk of further suicide attempts, but, in many health districts, junior doctors or non-medical staff have little or no training, supervision or prompt back-up from consultant psychiatrists. Recent guidelines from the Royal College of Psychiatrists (1994) should lead to an improvement in these services.

Mayou *et al's* survey of 52 health districts in the UK (1990) revealed that most psychiatrists expressed dissatisfaction with the CL services. Reasons for this dissatisfaction include:

(1) Lack of organisation and cooperation in emergency and consultation services to the general hospitals.
(2) Inadequate supervision of junior staff.
(3) The difficulties caused by the sectorised services and service provision by emergency teams.
(4) Poor professional staffing together with minimal administrative resources.

It is clear that CL psychiatry has had to compete for resources with community psychiatry and in most districts the latter is likely to gain priority (Kingdon, 1989). Recent health service reforms present a challenge and an opportunity to CL services, which are now purchased, in part, by general hospitals. There have been two major reviews of CL services in the UK – one produced by the Royal College Group (Benjamin *et al*, 1994) and the other by a joint working party of the Royal Colleges of Physicians and Psychiatrists (RCP/RCPsych, 1995).

The joint Royal Colleges Report

The aims of this report are: (a) to improve the ability of general hospital staff to detect disorders and to increase their skills and confidence in managing them, and (b) to encourage purchasers to establish comprehensive liaison services in all provider units. These measures are expected to lead to an environment in which each patient's psychological and physical needs receive appropriate attention.

Recognition and measurement of psychological disorders in the general hospital is generally poor despite their frequency. This arises because many interviews fail to elicit psychological problems, because modern medicine is orientated towards technological investigations, which may divert attention away from psychological problems, and because many staff have not received adequate training or encouragement to focus their attention on the psychological aspects of patient care. Such training and encouragement requires the support of a liaison psychiatry team (psychiatrist, liaison nurses, social worker and psychologist) who must be readily available and appropriately skilled to provide rapid and comprehensive treatment when necessary.

A liaison psychiatry service, which improves treatment of psychological disorders in the general hospital, should:

(1) Reduce the investigations performed for physical symptoms that actually reflect underlying distress.
(2) Reduce length of hospital stay.

(3) Relieve symptoms of distress and improve the quality of life of patients with serious physical illness.

(4) Contribute to achieving the *Health of the Nation* targets of reduction in rates of suicide and problem-drinking (Department of Health, 1993).

The Joint Working Party Report makes the following recommendations:

(1) All in-patient and out-patient departments, including Accident and Emergency, must have private, quiet and safe facilities so that routine interviews can include a discussion of psychological problems.

(2) All patients should be routinely asked direct questions about their mood, possible alcohol or drug misuse and, where appropriate, suicidal ideas. The results of these questions must be clearly recorded in the notes and brought to the attention of the senior medical staff and the GP.

(3) Medical staff should know how to treat the common psychological disorders, including the development of a management plan for patients with medically unexplained symptoms, and understand how and when to refer a patient to the liaison psychiatry service.

(4) Psychological assessment and appropriate treatment should be available for patients with unexplained physical symptoms, either

---

Box 1.1 The minimum staffing and practical requirements for a new liaison psychiatry service

A consultant who has a clearly defined clinical responsibility for referrals from the general hospital

A system for collecting referrals which is accessible and well-known to general hospital departments

Adequate secretarial support and storage for notes

A well-organised medical record system, preferably with standardised records of liaison psychiatry consultations for audit

Interview rooms, a small reference library and teaching aids, for example for showing acetates

Junior medical staff for consultation work in normal working hours and to provide emergency cover out of hours

The support of psychiatric colleagues (to cover during sickness and holidays, share resources, access to psychiatric in-patient facilities)

The support of general hospital consultants and managers (to ensure the adequate finance and effective use of the CL team)

Access to social work and community psychiatric nurse facilities (preferably access to a psychologist, physiotherapist and dietitian)

within the hospital or from the primary care team. If such symptoms are numerous and persistent, a specific plan of management should be drawn up that includes limitation of hospital investigations and admissions.

(5) A counselling service for alcohol problems should be readily available for in- and out-patients.

(6) The service for deliberate self-harm in each provider unit should be developed so that it conforms to the minimum standards set by the Royal College of Psychiatrists' Consensus Statement (1994).

(7) Purchasers should ensure that they purchase acute medical services in provider units, which include a liaison psychiatry service. The exact model of such a service will vary according to local circumstances but it must be consultant-led (at least five sessions per week of specified consultant psychiatrist time), must include the range of skills required for such work and include a record-keeping system that allows regular audit of the service. Although managed within the mental health unit, the costs of this service should be included within the costs of each medical directorate service.

(8) The training of liaison psychiatrists, physicians and nurses should be improved so that their interviews allow discussion of psychological problems and they have a full understanding of the importance of detection and management of psychological disorders throughout the general hospital. Such training should start at the undergraduate stage and be continued throughout general professional training and be offered as one aspect of continued professional development.

The minimum staffing and practical requirements for a CL psychiatry service are shown in Box 1.1. However, larger hospitals should have a multidisciplinary team (RCP/RCPsych, 1995).

Appropriate level of liaison psychiatry service

At large general hospitals there may be a role for specialist in-patient CL psychiatry services, e.g. Leeds General Infirmary (House, 1994). Such in-patient facilities, staffed by nurses with a general medical and psychiatric background, cater for patients who are both medically and psychiatrically ill (e.g. diabetes and anorexia nervosa). The psychiatric in-patient unit of a district general hospital may be able to offer such care, but most are reluctant to accept physically ill patients. District general hospital psychiatric units are preferable to distant mental hospitals where there may be limited access to specialist medical care and facilities.

It is essential to have a realistic estimate of the demand for CL services. Ideally this should be estimated from the previous year's referral rates but if this information is not available, estimated prospectively from an audit of referrals to the CL service over several months. Patterns of referral are likely to change as the hospital staff become more aware of the CL service (Sensky, 1986; House & Jones, 1987; Creed *et al*, 1993).

A comprehensive British teaching hospital CL service

It is important that trainees, working in a hospital without a fully developed CL service, are aware of the extent of a comprehensive service. Oxford has a full CL service based at the John Radcliffe Hospital for all the Oxford general hospitals, and a separate liaison service run by a part-time consultant psychiatrist for patients with HIV disease or terminal illness and psychological problems at the Churchill Hospital. Children aged under 12 are seen by child psychiatrists independently of the CL service. The John Radcliffe Hospital service, which is run full-time by a NHS consultant liaison psychiatrist, with input from an academic consultant, is divided into an attempted suicide/casualty service and a CL service for other general hospital referrals. Other medical staff include a senior registrar, registrar and GP trainee. Details of all the referrals are recorded in the CL department by staff on a specially designed audit form.

All in-patients who have attempted suicide in Oxford are admitted to the John Radcliffe Hospital and are assessed within 24 hours by specially trained counsellors (nurses or social workers) or junior doctors. Every day (including weekends) the initial assessments are presented to a senior psychiatrist (senior registrars or the consultant in charge of the CL service) who recommends further management, some of which is undertaken by the counsellors. The senior psychiatrist will directly assess the patient's mental state when there appears to be a high risk of further attempted suicide, suspected psychiatric disorder or uncertainty concerning the initial assessment. All assessments are recorded on standardised forms and entered into computers for audit and as a register of all attempted suicides. All referrals from casualty are also seen by one of the counsellors (supervised by a senior psychiatrist) during working hours. Outside these working hours, urgent referrals from casualty or the wards are seen by on-call junior doctors working in psychiatry.

All other ward consultations (including all patients over 65 years) are seen by a member of the medical staff, usually within 48 hours of referral. Junior staff present their assessments to the unit's consultants or senior registrars for supervision. A liaison service is provided by a psychiatrically trained nurse counsellor to the haematology unit. Alcohol problems are assessed by a trained social worker based in the CL service and a consultant psychiatrist specialising in alcohol misuse visits the John Radcliffe Hospital on a weekly basis. Out-patient services are provided by senior CL psychiatrists who have a special interest in abnormal illness behaviour, somatisation disorders and functional disorders, such as hyperventilation and chronic fatigue syndrome. A psychologist and a psychotherapist provide supervision to CL staff for cognitive–behavioural or dynamic psychotherapy. A child psychiatrist supervises the management of referrals of children over the age of 12 years. Psychiatrists for the elderly see cognitively-impaired or physically disabled patients over 65 years of age with mental disorder on a consultation basis if they are referred following an initial assessment by the CL service.

Different patterns of consultation–liaison psychiatry

The principal methods of work with general hospital in-patients are consultation with individual patients and liaison with medical teams. Although there has been much controversy about the merits of these approaches, most psychiatrists try to combine both methods (Creed *et al,* 1993).

The consultation model

This refers to the individual psychiatrist–patient consultation. The consultation is usually performed by a CL psychiatrist or junior doctor working for the CL service. In some instances another member of the multidisciplinary team (e.g. a nurse) makes the initial assessment. This should be supervised by a senior CL psychiatrist.

Lipowski (1986) and other writers have described four models of consultation:

(1) A patient-orientated consultation in which the referred patient is the direct focus of consultant's enquiry, for example, whether psychiatric disorders are responsible for a somatic symptom, such as abdominal or chest pain. The consultation should comprise a diagnostic interview with the patient and his carers including an evaluation of the patient's personality, reactions to present and past physical illness and relevant psychosocial data.

(2) A crisis-orientated consultation e.g. delirious patient, or one who abruptly refuses such life-saving treatment as blood transfusion or renal dialysis. A brief assessment is made of the patient's problem and coping style. The emphasis is on supporting the patient during the initial crisis followed by active attempts at problem solving by the patient.

(3) A consultee-orientated consultation which is focused on the consultee's particular problem with a given patient, e.g. disagreement among staff regarding management of a terminally ill patient.

(4) A situation-orientated consultation which is concerned with the interaction between the patient, family and clinical team, e.g. an anorectic, diabetic patient, whose parents insist treatment should

be forcibly administered, when the clinical team find this unacceptable/impractical and the patient insists on her own discharge.

There are many accounts of patterns of consultation referrals, but these have suffered from widely varying terminologies which have made comparisons difficult. Hengeveld *et al* (1984) have reviewed the literature and shown considerable similarities in patterns of consultation. More women than men are referred and the difference is not explained by referrals from obstetric and gynaecology departments. General medicine and medical specialities make over 70% of referrals to a consultation service with a consultation rate (number of patients referred as a percentage of the total number of admissions) four times that of surgery or obstetrics and gynaecology.

Approximately 13% of liaison consultations are admitted to in-patient psychiatric facilities, 32% are seen again in psychiatric out-patients, 7% are referred to social workers and 48% have no formal psychosocial follow-up after discharge from the general hospital. Huyse and others have demonstrated the value of using properly defined terminology, and meticulous record keeping to describe the reasons for referral, diagnosis system, and management (e.g. Huyse *et al*, 1990*a*).

There are a number of disadvantages to the consultation model. It is reactive rather than proactive, and contact with other hospital doctors is limited. It always relies on both the ability (which is sometimes poor) of busy non-psychiatric staff to detect psychiatric morbidity, and the willingness of general hospital doctors to refer patients to the psychiatrist. There are few opportunities for building up rapport, an exchange of ideas or for informal education about specific psychiatric disorder within a particular hospital unit. Physicians may request CL advice but often not act upon it (Huyse *et al*, 1990*b*). Sometimes the non-psychiatric specialist is unaware of the ways in which psychiatrists can help with the management of a difficult patient.

The liaison model

In the liaison model, the psychiatrist becomes an integrated member of a particular medical or surgical team. There is regular contact between the psychiatrist and the general hospital staff and patients, for example regular attendance at ward rounds, out-patient clinics. The psychiatrist does not wait for referrals be to made, but is readily at hand for advice on assessment and management. Often psychiatrists identify areas where they can be of use when the members of the medical team cannot identify the relevance of psychiatry to the case. The psychiatrist not only advises on the management of a patient's symptoms, but also on staff problems in their relationships with the patient and each other during clinical work. Approaches to liaison vary from the psychiatrist becoming a member of the medical team, to a collaborative working relationship in which the psychiatrist provides general support and advice alongside consultation.

Opponents of liaison psychiatry have argued that intensive liaison is time consuming, costly and unwelcome to many physicians who view it as an intrusion and a nuisance. However, it has increasingly been recognised that liaison psychiatry is particularly appropriate to a number of types of unit in which patients are at high risk of psychiatric disorder, e.g. oncology. This may sometimes involve screening all patients with particular types of medical problem, for example, prior to transplant surgery. It is also evident that there is no clear distinction between consultation and liaison. Good consultation involves close working relationships with wards and other units, and the development of increasingly sophisticated and effective referral patterns (Sensky, 1986; House & Jones, 1987).

Consultation–liaison in practice

In practice, most large consultation–liaison units provide a consultation service which is available to the whole hospital, and liaison with a number of medical or surgical units. Staffing is generally multidisciplinary, and there is a considerable emphasis on the coordination of CL with all other forms of psychiatric, psychological and social input to general hospital patients.

Out-patient services

Accounts of CL services have largely concentrated on in-patient referrals. There has been recent overdue, but welcome, interest on the management of a much larger proportion of general hospital patients who are out-patient attenders. CL out-patient clinics develop special expertise in managing psychiatric problems associated with physical illness and in the assessment of treatment of functional somatic symptoms (Creed *et al*, 1993). It is often preferable for such patients to be seen in a specialist CL clinic rather than by sector general psychiatry teams. Specialist out-patient clinics, which are multidisciplinary, are now being developed for chronic fatigue and pain, and there are combined psycho-geriatric clinics. As yet there have been no systematic assessments of such out-patient clinics, although two have recently been described (House, 1994; Blewett & Jenkins, 1994).

Emergency departments

Although deliberate self-harm is usually the commonest form of psychiatric emergency to be referred for a CL opinion, urgent opinions may be requested on a wide range of other acute psychiatric problems including alcohol and drug misuse. There are strong arguments for developing multidisciplinary liaison presence within the accident and emergency department so that psychiatric, substance misuse and behavioural problems can be recognised and managed more effectively.

The multidisciplinary CL team

Most large CL units have a multidisciplinary staff, including senior psychiatrists, trainee psychiatrists, GP trainees, social workers, liaison nurses, occupational therapists or psychologists (House, 1994; RCP/ RCPsych, 1995). A considerable advantage of the team approach is that its different members can foster links with colleagues outside the general hospital, for example a social worker will know how to get the best use of resources from social services. In addition, liaison nurses are often made aware of problems by general hospital nursing staff which would not be referred to a psychiatrist, such as situational disturbances, patients suffering from atypical bereavement, problems within the family and staff difficulties (Stickney & Hall, 1981; Hicks, 1989).

Liaison nursing has been a rapidly expanding area of nursing in America and is becoming an important feature of British CL psychiatry (Egan-Morriss *et al*, 1994). Liaison nurses are often able to understand, assess, and communicate the problems faced by general hospital nurses better than psychiatrists, and to devote more time to the individual patient and family care. It is essential that liaison nurses receive practical training in the recognition and management of cognitive and psychiatric syndromes. Community psychiatric nurses (CPNs) can have an important role in CL, both in the management of out-patients and in follow-up care. Some patients require more prolonged specialist care which is not easily provided by busy community services with no special expertise in this area of training.

The primary role of social workers in the multidisciplinary team has been in the evaluation of the family and the patient's social circumstances and the planning of psychosocial aftercare for patients and their families within the community. However, their role has been expanded to include counselling and psychotherapy, especially involving the family (Stollar & Knight, 1982).

Working with other hospital services

There are number of hospital services outside psychiatry which deal with psychiatric problems and which need to be coordinated with the CL service.

(1) Medical social workers are a useful resource. They see many patients with psychiatric problems. A number of American reports have

described services in which social work and psychiatric services have been combined or closely coordinated (Strain *et al*, 1991*b*).

(2) Behavioural medicine has become an important psychologist-led movement in the USA (Lipowski, 1981). It is concerned with the principle of behavioural psychology applied to general medicine and health. In Britain, many general hospital clinical psychologists also work independently from the CL unit, being employed by the medical unit, and have little contact with it. They have a particular role to play in the behavioural or cognitive assessment of patients and the teaching and supervision of psychological treatments, especially cognitive–behavioural therapy.

(3) Specialist nurses (e.g. stoma therapist, cancer and diabetic nurses) appointed by medical and surgical units make a growing contribution to the care of a wide range of acute and chronic medical problems. They have little formal or informal contact with psychiatry and it is essential that CL units attempt to offer supervision and training as well as clinical back-up for psychiatric assessment and specialist treatment (Maguire & Hopwood, 1994).

(4) Occupational therapists often have training in individual and group psychological treatments in addition to skills in the assessment of daily living skills and rehabilitation of patients with psychological and/or physical problems. Dietitians and physiotherapists may respectively play a useful role with individual patients who have eating disorders, or require skilled rehabilitation because of abnormal illness behaviour or physical illness.

Coordination of consultation–liaison psychiatry within the general hospital

If the CL psychiatrist is to ensure the best possible service for psychiatric problems in the general hospital he must fulfil, in part, a coordinating role. This includes collaboration of the various disciplines mentioned above and local psychiatric sector teams, together with psychiatrists caring for the elderly, children and substance misuse patients. It is necessary to define which are seen by the CL service (and referred to the specialist psychiatric services if necessary) and which are assessed by the specialist psychiatric services alone. The details of liaison for alcohol/drug problems, child and adolescent and the elderly are dealt with in Chapters 4, 7 and 8.

The elderly

In Britain, psychiatrists for the elderly often extensively liaise with geriatricians and sometimes other hospital departments, e.g. orthopaedics (see Chapter 8). The extent of this liaison varies considerably; many areas rely on close informal contacts between the geriatricians and the psychiatrists for the elderly, while others have special arrangements, such as the assessment of all attempted suicide cases over 65 years of age by psychiatrists for the elderly, a joint weekly case conference with geriatricians, joint attendance at some out-patient clinics and ward rounds. The main reason for such close ties is that physical illness and mental illness are much more commonly associated in the elderly than at other ages. Even where there are prior arrangements between the geriatricians and psychiatrists for the elderly, liaison psychiatrists will be asked to see the elderly mentally ill because so many are treated by general hospital staff who are not geriatricians.

Children and adolescents

CL plays a large part in the work of most child and adolescent psychiatrists; a survey of the National Liaison Psychiatry Group by Mayou & Lloyd (1985) found that over one-quarter of its members worked in child psychiatry. Paediatricians and child psychiatry services may have informal links at consultant level, joint case conferences or joint out-patient clinics. However, in some areas of CL psychiatry the multidisciplinary team will be expected to assess and manage adolescent psychiatry problems (see Chapter 7). In other areas, child psychiatrists may assess deliberate self-harm patients under the age of 16 and other adolescent patients who present to the general hospital with psychiatric problems.

Substance misuse

Substance misuse services may set up their own liaison links with certain general hospital units, e.g. emergency departments, liver specialists, genitourinary medicine. Because of the growing problems of the high prevalence of problem drinking in general hospital patients (e.g. Jarman & Kellett, 1979) and the association between deliberate self-harm and substance misuse, the CL team needs considerable expertise in the assessment and management of patients who misuse alcohol and illicit drugs (see Chapter 4).

The role of education of consultation–liaison psychiatrists

A major function of liaison psychiatry is to educate non-psychiatric clinicians and nurses with the aims of sensitising them to psychosocial aspects of patient care, and the early detection or prevention of psychiatric problems in their physically ill patients (RCP/RCPsych, 1995). General hospital staff can improve their communication techniques, and learn the appropriate use of simple psychiatric skills to enhance the quality of patient care from a psychosocial perspective. The aim is therefore to be proactive rather than reactive to patient and staff difficulties. As a result, the number of referrals to the CL psychiatrist are increased but the psychiatrist may not need to see every patient.

In addition, CL psychiatry units have a valuable role for the education of psychiatric or GP trainees (since psychiatric disorders in general practice are closer to those seen in the general hospital than on general adult psychiatry units) and non-psychiatric staff. Teaching hospitals should be able to provide some specialist CL psychiatry attachments for training and service provision. CL psychiatrists in teaching and large district general hospitals should also teach psychiatry to medical students, junior doctors in non-psychiatric specialities and psychiatric trainees. Such trainees may be involved in audit and research. Recommendations concerning undergraduate and postgraduate training relevant to liaison psychiatry, including those for psychiatric trainees, have been published (Bell, 1994; Guthrie & Creed, 1994).

Summary

Consultation–liaison psychiatry has developed over the last 60 years in North America due to the needs of medical education, and over the last 30 years in Britain because of influential individual psychiatrists and the assessment of attempted suicide. Throughout Europe and America, CL psychiatry services have developed haphazardly and vary considerably in their scope. The differences in CL psychiatry between Britain and America reflect the later development, the provision of comprehensive primary health care and the sectorisation of psychiatric services in Britain. A number of different models of CL psychiatry care have been devised. The further development of CL services may depend on the demonstration of useful benefits in the quality of life of patients or their cost-effectiveness (Creed, 1991*a,b*). CL services can take many forms but their effectiveness depends on adequate support from colleagues, staff, and administrative procedures.

Further reading

Lipowski, Z. J. (1982) Modern meaning of the terms 'psychosomatic' and 'liaison psychiatry'. In *Medicine and Psychiatry – A Practical Approach* (ed F. H. Creed & J. M. Pfeffer). London: Pitman.

References

Bell, G. (1994) Undergraduate teaching. In *Liaison Psychiatry. Defining Needs and Planning Services* (eds S. Benjamin, A. House & P. Jenkins), pp. 95–98. London: Gaskell.

Benjamin, S., House, A. & Jenkins, P. (1994) *Liaison Psychiatry. Defining Needs and Planning Services*. London: Gaskell.

Blewett, A. & Jenkins, P. (1994) Setting up a consultation–liaison psychiatry service in South Gwent. In *Liaison Psychiatry. Defining Needs and Planning Services* (eds S. Benjamin, A. House & P. Jenkins), pp. 47–57. London: Gaskell.

Bridges, K. W. & Goldberg, D. P. (1985) Somatic presentation of DSM–III psychiatric disorders in primary care. *Journal of Psychosomatic Research*, **29**, 563–569.

Catalan, J., Marsack, P., Hawton, K. E., *et al* (1980) Comparison of doctors and nurses in the assessment of deliberate self-poisoning patients. *Psychological Medicine*, **10**, 483–491.

Creed, F. H. (1991*a*) The future of liaison psychiatry in the UK. *International Review of Psychiatry: Liaison Psychiatry*, **4**, 99–107.

—— (1991*b*) Liaison psychiatry for the twenty-first century: a review. *Journal of Royal Society of Medicine*, **84**, 414–417.

——, Guthrie, E., Black, D., *et al* (1993) Psychiatric referrals within the general hospital – comparison with general practitioner referrals. *British Journal of Psychiatry*, **162**, 204–211.

Department of Health (1993) *The Health of the Nation: Key Area Handbooks, Mental Illness*. London: HMSO.

Egan-Morriss, E., Morriss, R. & House, A. (1994) The role of the nurse in consultation–liaison psychiatry. In *Liaison Psychiatry. Defining Needs and Planning Services* (eds S. Benjamin, A. House & P. Jenkins), pp. 34–44. London: Gaskell.

Gardner, R., Hanka, R., O'Brien, V. C., *et al* (1977) Psychological and social evaluation in cases of deliberate self-poisoning admitted to a general hospital. *British Medical Journal*, ii, 1567–1570.

Gater, R. & Goldberg, D. P. (1991) Pathways to psychiatric care in south Manchester. *British Journal of Psychiatry*, **159**, 90–96.

Goldberg, D. (1992) The treatment of mental disorders in general medicine settings. *General Hospital Psychiatry*, **14**, 1–3.

Guthrie, E. & Creed, F. (1994) Postgraduate training. In *Liaison Psychiatry. Defining Needs and Planning Services* (eds S. Benjamin, A. House & P. Jenkins), pp. 99–116. London: Gaskell.

Hengeveld, M. W., Rooymans, H. G. M. & Vecht-Van Der Bergh, R. (1984) Psychiatric consultations in a Dutch university hospital: a report on 1814 referrals, compared with a literature review. *General Hospital Psychiatry*, **6**, 271–279.

Hicks, S. (1989) The psychiatric nurse in liaison psychiatry. *Australian and New Zealand Journal of Psychiatry*, **86**, 481–499.

House, A. (1994) Liaison psychiatry in a large teaching hospital. In *Liaison Psychiatry. Defining Needs and Planning Services* (eds S. Benjamin, A. House & P. Jenkins), pp. 58–64. London: Gaskell.

—— & Jones, S. J. (1987) The effects of establishing a psychiatric consultation–liaison service: Changes in patterns of referral and care. *Health Trends*, **19**, 10–12.

Huyse, F. J., Strain, J. J. & Hammer, J. S. (1990*a*) Interventions in consultation–liaison psychiatry. I. Patterns of recommendations. *General Hospital Psychiatry*, **12**, 213–220.

——, —— & —— (1990*b*) Interventions in consultation–liaison psychiatry. II. Concordance. *General Hospital Psychiatry*, **12**, 221–231.

Jarman, C. M. B. & Kellett, J. M. (1979) Alcoholism in the general hospital. *British Medical Journal, ii*, 469–472.

Kingdon, D. (1989) Mental health services: results of a survey of English district plans. *Psychiatric Bulletin*, **13**, 77–78.

Leigh, H. (1987) Multidisciplinary teams in consultation–liaison psychiatry: the Yale model. *Psychotherapy and Psychosomatics*, **48**, 83–89.

Levitan, S. J. & Kornfeld, D. S. (1981) Clinical and cost-benefits of liaison psychiatry. *American Journal of Psychiatry*, **138**, 790–793.

Lipowski, Z. J. (1981) Liaison psychiatry, liaison nursing and behavioural medicine. *Comprehensive Psychiatry*, **22**, 554–561.

—— (1983) Current trends in consultation–liaison psychiatry. *Canadian Journal of Psychiatry*, **28**, 329–338.

—— (1986) Consultation–liaison psychiatry: the first half century. *General Hospital Psychiatry*, **8**, 305–315.

—— (1992) Consultation–liaison psychiatry at century's end. *Psychosomatics*, **33**, 128–133.

Lloyd, G. G. (1991) *Textbook of General Hospital Psychiatry*. Edinburgh: Churchill Livingstone.

Maguire, P. & Hopwood, P. (1994) Providing a psychiatric service to a large cancer hospital. In *Liaison Psychiatry. Defining Needs and Planning Services* (eds S. Benjamin, A. House & P. Jenkins), pp. 65–69. London: Gaskell.

Mayou, R. A. (1989) The history of general hospital psychiatry. *British Journal of Psychiatry*, **155**, 764–776.

—— & Lloyd, G. (1985) A survey of liaison psychiatry in the United Kingdom and Eire. *Bulletin of the Royal College of Psychiatrists*, **11**, 214–218.

——, Anderson, H., Feinmann, C., *et al* (1990) The present state of consultation and liaison psychiatry. *Psychiatric Bulletin*, **3**, 321–325.

——, Huyse, F. & The European Consultation–Liaison Workgroup (1991) Consultation–liaison psychiatry in Western Europe. *General Hospital Psychiatry*, **13**, 188–208.

Nationale Raad voor de Volksgeszondheid (1990) *Advies: Psychiatrische Hulpverlening in het Algemeen Ziekenhuis*. Codenummer 4142–110. Rotterdam.

Newson-Smith, J. G. B. & Hirsch, S. R. (1979) A comparison of social workers and psychiatrists in evaluating parasuicide. *British Journal of Psychiatry*, **134**, 335–342.

Noyes, R., Wise, T. N. & Hayes, J. R. (1992) Consultation–liaison psychiatrists. How many are there and how are they funded? *Psychosomatics*, **33**, 123–127.

Regional Office of the World Health Organization (1985) *Report on the Prevention of Mental, Psychosocial and Neurological Disorders in the European Regions*. EUR-RC38-10. Copenhagen: WHO.

Robinowitz, C. B. & Nadelson, C. C. (1991) Consultation–liaison psychiatry as a subspeciality. *General Hospital Psychiatry,* **13**, 1–3.

Royal College of Psychiatrists (1994) *The General Hospital Management of Adult Deliberate Self-Harm: A Consensus Statement on Standards for Service Provision.* London: RCPsych.

Royal College of Physicians & Royal College of Psychiatrists (1995) *The Psychological Care of Medical Patients. Recognition and Service Care.* CR 35. London: RCP/RCPsych.

Schwab, J. J. (1989) Consultation–liaison psychiatry: a historical overview. *Psychosomatics,* **30**, 245–254.

Sensky, T. (1986) The general hospital psychiatrist: too many tasks and too few roles? *British Journal of Psychiatry,* **148**, 151–158.

Stollar, T. & Knight, M. (1982) The role of the social worker in liaison psychiatry. In *Medicine and Psychiatry – A Practical Approach* (eds F. Creed & J. M. Pfeffer), pp. 201–209. London: Pitman.

Stickney, S. & Hall, R. (1981) The role of the nurse on a consultation–liaison team. *Psychosomatics,* **22**, 229–235.

Strain, J. J., Lyons, J. S., Hammer, J. S., *et al* (1991*a*) Cost offset from a psychiatric consultation–liaison intervention with elderly hip fracture patients. *American Journal of Psychiatry,* **148**, 1044–1049.

——, Gise, L. H., Fulop, G., *et al* (1991*b*) Patterns of referral from consultation–liaison to social work services. *General Hospital Psychiatry,* **13**, 88–94.

2 Basic skills

Elspeth Guthrie & Francis Creed

*Conducting the consultation • Understanding the referral •
Interviewing skills and mental state assessment • Assessment of
depressive disorder in the physically ill • Detection of psychological
disorders that present with somatic symptoms • Assessment of illness
behaviour • Liaison case summaries*

The basic skills required in consultation–liaison psychiatry are similar to those in other psychiatric settings. In addition, however, the psychiatrist has to develop several new skills:

(1) learning how to conduct complex psychiatric assessments in the alien setting of medical or surgical wards
(2) how to understand and respond to the needs of the referrer, either physician or surgeon, even when no psychiatric disorder is present
(3) particular interview skills are required to initiate and complete a psychiatric assessment and record the appropriate clinical signs in the mental state
(4) assessment of depression in the physically ill
(5) detection of psychological disorders that present with somatic symptoms
(6) assessment of illness behaviour
(7) the psychiatrist should be able to assimilate all the relevant facts into a formulation of the case including both physical and psychological aspects.

Further descriptions of the consultation process have been published (Pfeffer, 1982; Bass, 1995). This chapter aims to be a practical guide to help the new trainee overcome the obstacles of working in this area.

Conducting the consultation

Consultation–liaison referrals can be rather daunting experiences for the inexperienced trainee. The referral letter may contain little information regarding the patient's psychiatric status, the reason for referral may not be clearly stated, and it may be difficult to find somewhere private to interview the patient.

The following example caricatures the difficulties encountered by a trainee who commences assessments in the general hospital without being properly briefed. Other common pitfalls are listed in Box 2.1.

21

Trainee psychiatrist, Dr New, is given a consultation request form by his consultant's secretary and told to assess a patient on a surgical ward. The referrer has requested that Mrs Simmons, a 39-year-old woman, be assessed as she 'burst into tears' on his ward round and is 'query depressed?'.

Dr New arrives on the ward to find that Mrs Simmons is not there as she is having a gastroscopy, but is expected to return soon. After a considerable delay a sickly Mrs Simmons returns to the ward. The notes are unavailable because they are still in the endoscopy unit. Dr New establishes from a student nurse that Mrs Simmons is being investigated for weight loss and abdominal pain. He approaches her bedside and the following conversation ensues:

Dr: Hello Mrs Simmons, I'm Dr New, I'm the psychiatrist.
Mrs Simmons: Psychiatrist? What do you mean? Why are you here?
Dr (tentatively): Didn't the surgeon tell you?
Mrs Simmons: Obviously not. Why do I need to see a psychiatrist?
Dr: Have you been having any trouble with your nerves recently?
Mrs Simmons: It's not in my mind you know, if that's what you think.

The other patients on the ward, who are all listening intently, murmur approval and support for this last statement. Encouraged by the support of her audience, Mrs Simmons clutches her stomach, rolls over in the bed and sighs: Look I'm too ill to see you, I don't need a psychiatrist, please leave me alone.
Dr: Well, if you insist.

Dr New returns to the ward office, and writes on the consultation request form: 'Many thanks for referring this 39-year-old married woman with a history of abdominal pain and weight loss. Unable to take full history as patient uncooperative. No obvious evidence of a depressive illness or retardation. No indication for further psychiatric intervention.' He gives the form to the student nurse to file in the notes. As he returns to the psychiatric department he realises the whole episode has taken him nearly 2 hours.

Box 2.1 Common difficulties encountered when conducting consultation–liaison assessments

Arrive on the ward to find the patient is elsewhere
Discover that a psychiatric referral has not been discussed with the patient who is alarmed and dismayed by the arrival of a psychiatrist
Discover that the patient cannot speak English
Find that there is nowhere private to interview the patient, so either conduct the interview at the patient's bedside or in the bathroom
Discover that the patient is not fully conscious and unable to give a history

In the above example the consultation failed because the trainee psychiatrist had not performed the necessary preparatory work; he had, presumably, not been offered advice and help before undertaking the referral. It is not unheard of for liaison referrals to be allocated to a junior psychiatrist even though he has not been taught the specific skills to perform such a referral. The above illustration highlights the importance of the following general points when conducting a liaison psychiatry consultation (Box 2.2).

Discuss the referral with a senior psychiatrist

A senior psychiatrist should be able to identify from the referral the key issues of the clinical problem and help the trainee to focus on certain areas. This may mean concentrating, during the initial consultation, on one or more of the following:

(1) techniques to overcome resistance to the referral and establishing rapport between patient and psychiatrist
(2) ensuring that there is a full medical history summarised in the notes
(3) examining the charts for recent pyrexia or medication changes that might be associated with delirium
(4) eliciting further information from the medical team because the referral suggests possible tension between staff and patient regarding certain aspects of management.

Ward consultation requests rarely contain all the appropriate information. The trainee should therefore speak to the doctor who wrote the referral to discover the main reason for referral (see below) and often may benefit from a further discussion with the senior psychiatrist prior to seeing the patient.

Discuss the case with the referrer before seeing the patient

Satisfactory referrals depend upon a good relationship between the psychiatrist and the physician. In ideal circumstances a joint meeting with physician and psychiatrist can be very valuable, so the reason for referral can be discussed and the psychiatrist is regarded by the patient as part of the medical/surgical team. Any ambiguities about the patient's diagnosis, treatment, or plans for further investigations can be discussed at the outset. In the absence of such a joint meeting the reason for referral and other details must be discussed by the psychiatrist with at least one member of the medical team.

It is important to establish whether the patient has been told of the proposed psychiatric consultation. If this has not been done the psychiatrist should not attempt the consultation. Sometimes, the physician/surgeon has not told the patient about the psychiatric referral for fear that the patient might refuse or be annoyed. However, a psychiatrist cannot be expected to assess a patient under such conditions.

We advise that the physician should be quite explicit about the reason for referral: the patient may be depressed or anxious, which requires expert help, or there may be additional aspects of management about which specialist advice is requested: for example, a behavioural programme for pain, or anxiety management for breathlessness.

In a few patients, who are highly defensive, it may be counterproductive for the physician to offer an explanation for the psychiatric referral in terms of psychological problems; in such cases it may be more profitable for the physician to introduce the psychiatrist as having expertise in 'treating pain' or 'rehabilitation'. In these cases it is essential that the psychiatrist is told beforehand what explanation has been given to the patient.

Contact the ward to arrange the assessment

The ward staff can ensure that the patient will be on the ward at the appropriate time and will be expecting the psychiatrist's visit. If relevant, the ward can also arrange for one of the patient's relatives to be present. Contacting the ward beforehand not only saves time but makes it easier for the psychiatrist to discuss the referral and gain valuable information from nursing staff before seeing the patient. The staff can usually comment on the patient's behaviour, they can examine the cardex for observations made regarding the patient's sleep pattern, or variation in mood at different times during the day.

Check whether the patient can speak English and give a coherent history

Most hospitals employ interpreters or have a list of volunteers to help patients who do not speak English; it is advisable to check with the referrer or the ward whether the patient speaks English. If not, the psychiatrist should ask the ward to arrange for an interpreter as well as a relative to be present. It is not the psychiatrist's job to take a medical history from a patient who does not speak English. This should have been done prior to referral.

Review the patient's medical notes

The importance of this for patients who somatise their psychological distress is emphasised in Chapter 5. In all cases, however, a thorough review of the patient's notes is necessary to be fully familiar with the patient's previous medical and surgical history prior to interviewing. With thick notes, it is best to start with the letters, which will give an overview

---

Box 2.2 Conducting a consultation–liaison assessment

Discuss the referral with senior psychiatrist prior to assessment
Discuss with referrer:
  (i) reason for referral
  (ii) that patient has been informed of the psychiatric
       consultation
Contact ward to arrange time to conduct assessment
Enquire whether patient speaks English and can give a coherent
    history
Review the patient's medical notes
Interview the patient in private
Discuss the assessment with a senior psychiatrist
Discuss with referrer. Establish ongoing medical responsibility
Liaise with nursing staff – ensure GP is informed by medical
    staff
Leave a brief but clear account of the psychiatric assessment
    in the medical notes

---

of the patient's previous medical history. In such cases the past medical history is best taken from the casenotes by summarising all previous admissions and new out-patient presentations. In addition, comments made in medical correspondence can often be very revealing of the patient's previous mental state and attitude towards symptoms. The patient's current medication should be scrutinised for any drugs that alter mood (Chapter 9). It is reasonable for a consultant liaison psychiatrist to ask the house physician to prepare such a medical summary prior to seeing the patient; the trainee may wish to ask the senior psychiatrist to make this request.

See the patient in private in a proper room

A liaison psychiatry consultation should not be conducted by the patient's bedside on the ward. It is extremely important to ensure that the patient is interviewed in private (see recommendation of RCP/RCPsych, 1995). This may mean making arrangements beforehand with the ward sister to make sure a suitable room is made available.

Discuss the findings with a senior psychiatrist after you have assessed the patient

The Royal College of Psychiatrists suggests that all trainee psychiatrists should have experience of consultation–liaison psychiatry and that this experience should be carefully supervised by a senior psychiatrist (House

& Creed, 1993). Since the referral originates with the consultant physician or surgeon it is reasonable that the psychiatric opinion is that of a consultant psychiatrist.

Discuss your findings with the referrer and establish ongoing medical responsibility

At the end of the interview, it is important that the psychiatrist decides with the physician and ward staff what will happen next (seeing a relative, initiation of drug treatment, further interviews, psychiatric out-patient appointment etc.) and relays this to the patient. This is best done immediately and the psychiatrist should bleep the HO/SHO to discuss any further psychological management. If the patient has been seen late in the afternoon and the referring doctor is unavailable, then contact should be made the following morning.

The psychiatrist should then check that both the nursing staff and the patient have understood the nature of any further treatment the psychiatrist is offering. If medication is being suggested it must be made clear who the prescribing doctor is to be – in general, for medical in-patients this should be the physician.

If the psychiatrist is to be involved in further management of the patient it is important to state which consultant (physician or psychiatrist) will carry the principal medical responsibility. If both are to be involved, how often will the patient be seen in the medical and psychiatric clinics? Patients are often seen by many different doctors during a stay in hospital and it should not be assumed that the patient grasps that further psychiatric treatment will mean attending a different hospital department. This should be explained.

Liaise with nursing staff and the patient's GP

The psychiatrist should also discuss his findings with the nursing staff, and should not assume that the physician/surgeon will pass on information. If the patient is disturbed or agitated the psychiatrist may need to spend a considerable amount of time advising nursing staff about management and should also be willing to provide on-going support. The involvement of a liaison nurse may be invaluable in such a situation.

It is good clinical practice to ensure that the patient's general practitioner is informed of the main findings of the psychiatric consultation. It is often worth contacting the GP directly as he will usually be able to provide valuable additional information about the patient's previous psychiatric and medical history, social circumstances and family background. If psychiatric treatment has been started the GP will require detailed advice regarding the patient's overall management.

Record of psychiatric consultation in the medical notes

A brief account of the main findings and advice about further management should be clearly entered in the medical notes. Detailed personal histories should not be written in the medical notes, as these do not have the same safeguards regarding confidentiality as psychiatric notes. It should be legibly written, dated and signed. If the case has been seen or discussed with the consultant psychiatrist this should be stated. The brief handwritten record in the medical casenotes should be followed up with a typed formal response that can later be filed in the notes and a copy sent to the patient's GP.

Ideal consultation

If the above points are followed the consultation should proceed as follows:

Trainee psychiatrist, Dr New, is given a consultation request form by his consultant's secretary with instructions to discuss the case with his consultant before assessment. His consultant suggests that he contacts the referrer to obtain more information about Mrs Simmons' mental state and the reason for referral. The surgical SHO explains that Mrs Simmons has had abdominal pain for the last 10 months, with poor appetite and weight loss of one stone. She has looked despondent since admission and has complained of being unable to sleep.

Dr New checks whether Mrs Simmons knows that a psychiatric assessment has been requested. The SHO explains that the consultant surgeon did not want to upset Mrs Simmons and thought it would be better if the "psychiatrist dealt with that kind of thing". Dr New explains that he has been advised by his consultant not to carry out the assessment unless Mrs Simmons has been clearly informed beforehand of the nature of his visit. He suggests some ways that the SHO could tactfully explain the psychiatric referral to Mrs Simmons.

Once this is agreed, Dr New rings the ward, asks to speak to the nurse in charge, and arranges a suitable time to see Mrs Simmons. Sister explains that Mrs Simmons is having a gastroscopy, will probably feel drowsy following this, and that it would be best to visit her the following morning. Dr New says that he will come at 11.00 am and stresses that he will need somewhere private to interview Mrs Simmons. There are no interview rooms on the ward, but sister says that she will make sure her office is free at that time. Dr New also takes the opportunity to find out what the nursing staff feel about Mrs Simmons. Sister reports that they are concerned about her; she eats very little, does not interact with the other patients and looks tired and worried. Dr New asks whether the nurses have noticed whether Mrs Simmons wakes early in the morning. Sister says that she does not know, but will check with the night staff.

The next day Dr New arrives on the ward, and after carefully reading the casenotes, warmly greets Mrs Simmons and escorts her to Sister's office. Mrs Simmons has been expecting him. It does not take long to establish that Mrs Simmons has a depressive illness with several biological symptoms. Dr New learns from taking a careful history that the psychological symptoms and abdominal pain began at roughly the same time. The pain is not affected by eating or posture, it is central abdominal and burning in quality. Dr New remembers from the casenotes that there is a family history of bowel cancer, and enquires gently about this. Mrs Simmons begins to cry softly and recounts how her mother died 12 months ago from a stomach tumour. Her mother had complained of pain for several months but had been reluctant to see a doctor as she did not want 'to make a fuss'. She had seen her mother literally waste away and die, and was filled with guilt that she had not insisted earlier that her mother seek help. She was terrified that she also had cancer, but on another level felt that if she did have cancer, it was her own fault.

Dr New spent a further 30 minutes with Mrs Simmons, taking a psychosocial history and encouraging her to express how she felt. He had also noticed from the casenotes that Mrs Simmons had a raised MCV but normal B_{12} and folate, and established that, since her mother's death, Mrs Simmons had been drinking up to a bottle of sherry each day. He explained that he was going to discuss things with his consultant and would return to see Mrs Simmons later in the day.

In discussion with his consultant, Dr New reaches a formulation of the case. Mrs Simmons has a depressive illness in the context of an abnormal grief reaction. An added factor is alcohol misuse which may be contributing to the lowered mood state and, probably, the abdominal pain. Dr New has checked that the gastroscopy is normal and thinks that the pain is most likely to be psychological in origin.

He returns to see Mrs Simmons with his consultant, who explores Mrs Simmons' response to the psychiatric consultation and explains at some length that seeing a psychiatrist did not in any way imply that the pain was not real and severe. The consultant then discusses the possible relationship between Mrs Simmons' abdominal pain and mood state. The time course suggests a link between the two.

They suggest a course of antidepressant medication, in conjunction with regular follow-up in the out-patient department by Dr New, with the aims of bereavement counselling and monitoring improvement of the depression. They establish that Mrs Simmons stopped drinking alcohol on admission and discover that mild withdrawal symptoms have now ceased: they explain why it is important that Mrs Simmons should not drink again. Dr New gives

Mrs Simmons an out-patient appointment and asks if her husband could come with her on the first occasion, so Dr New can clarify the situation with him and explain to him the aim of treatment and how he can help his wife.

Before leaving the ward, they discuss the case with the surgical SHO and nursing staff. Dr New's consultant explains the importance of stopping investigations as the clinical picture is now clear, and emphasises that further tests may only increase Mrs Simmons' fears that she has cancer. The consultant psychiatrist tells the staff that she will personally speak to the consultant surgeon about Mrs Simmons' further management, and asks them to monitor her appetite and weight while she remains on the ward. The consultant also asks Dr New to inform Mrs Simmons' GP of the consultation. The consultation process has taken 2 hours.

Understanding the referral

The most frequent complaints made about psychiatrists in the general hospital are their unavailability; their statement, after seeing the patient, that 'no psychiatric disorder is present' even when the physician feels the patient is disturbed in some way; and not giving clear advice about management. In order to offer help and useful advice, even when there is no psychiatric disorder present, the psychiatrist must understand why the referral has been made.

The great majority of patients with psychological problems in the general hospital are not referred to psychiatrists. This may reflect the fact that the psychiatric disorder has not been recognised by the medical/nursing staff but usually means that the staff do not think the psychological problem worthy of referral (Seltzer, 1989).

When a referral arrives, therefore, the psychiatrist's first question should be: "Why has this patient been referred at this time?" When contacting the referrer, it is helpful to have the following possibilities in mind:

(1) the patient is obviously distressed, for example bursts into tears or otherwise depressed
(2) non-compliance with medication or treatment
(3) patient is disruptive or violent
(4) 'hopeless' case and feelings of staff frustration
(5) staff think the patient would be better managed on a psychiatric ward
(6) medical staff unclear about the cause of symptoms – is it psychiatric?
(7) specific advice required on medication e.g. analgesia, sedation, antidepressants
(8) consultant recently attended a conference – "I heard psychiatrists can treat this sort of complaint"
(9) research interest.

If the patient has an overt psychiatric disorder, e.g. depression or psychosis, the assessment is similar to that in any other setting. If the reason for referral is any of the points 2–6 above, a more general understanding of the patient's reaction to the illness, the hospital and the staff is necessary in addition. It is appropriate to ask who suggested the referral? – was it the consultant, junior medical staff, nurses, patient or a relative?

The psychiatrist can contribute to the general psychological care of the patient because of his familiarity with psychological aspects of illness even in the absence of formal psychiatric disorder. Simply by taking a psychiatric history the psychiatrist takes a longitudinal view of illness, which puts the current episode in the context of a patient's personality, current social situation and previous illness experience. This will help to explain the patient's emotional reaction to illness, which should always be explored during the psychiatric interview.

Non-compliance and disruptive behaviour

Non-compliance may reflect depressive ideation, that the future is hopeless and disability or death is inevitable. More often it reflects frustration or conflict between patient and staff that arises because of the patient's feelings about their illness and/or conflicts in the patient's interpersonal relationships outside of hospital. Similarly, disruptive or violent behaviour may be on the basis of hallucinations, persecutory ideas or irritability accompanying depression; but frustration with illness and hospitalisation are common explanations.

Two clinical examples will help to illustrate where the psychiatrist can help, even in the absence of formal psychiatric disorder.

> A 23-year-old diabetic woman had difficulty accepting her diabetes. The staff had always found her rather difficult but during the months prior to referral she had become openly non-compliant with her insulin and dietary regimes. The reasons for this were poorly understood. She did not have a depressive illness or mood swings that could be categorised as adjustment disorder. During psychiatric assessment it became clear that the onset of diabetes had closely coincided with two traumatic life events – the break up of a close relationship with a boyfriend and the first ever meeting with her genetic mother (she had been adopted). The negative feelings about these events had been transferred to her diabetes and after a course of psychotherapy she resolved many of her feelings regarding the events and took much better care of herself and her diabetic control.
>
> A 43-year-old man was making a poor adjustment to multiple sclerosis and became irritable and at times aggressive to the nursing staff. This behaviour was not understood and could not

be explained by formal psychiatric disorder. During the psychiatric interview it transpired that he had previously rid himself of his tensions and frustrations by hitting a squash or golf ball – both were now denied him by the weakness of his legs. This increased understanding helped the nursing staff cope with his tension more positively; further discussions led to the development of several alternative ways of dissipating his frustrations.

Hopeless case/staff frustration – request for transfer

The psychiatrist should not be resentful of being asked to see a 'trivial problem' – he should try to understand why the referral has been made. It may be an indication of staff conflict or a unit-wide problem, rather than indicating psychological disturbance in a patient. The importance of receiving supervision on liaison referrals from a senior psychiatrist has already been emphasised. If such problems are identified it is the consultant psychiatrist's responsibility to address them at a consultant-to-consultant level.

The following examples indicate the types of situations where staff frustration may result in a liaison referral.

(1) The referral of a patient because of her failure to comply with treatment may in fact represent divided feelings among the staff. A brittle diabetic patient is unlikely to gain control of her illness on a ward where one or two of the nursing staff feel it is wrong or unethical to invade her privacy for purposes of ensuring she does not deviate from the specified diet or insulin regime.

    A terminally ill patient who has been nursed through several previous near fatal episodes of leukaemia but who now refuses chemotherapy and wants to be left alone will cause very strong feelings in nursing and medical staff; the staff may show different, even conflicting, responses to this request – some staff may appear to acquiesce and others aggressively counteract it.

(2) A spate of referrals from the renal unit of apparently minor problems were dealt with by a series of different duty psychiatrists, one of whom discussed this with the liaison psychiatrist. It transpired that a patient on long-term dialysis awaiting transplant had recently committed suicide. This led to increased anxiety among the staff about possible suicidal acts and an increased referral rate.

(3) An urgent and troublesome referral. Sometimes a patient is referred several times by different members of staff – the psychiatrist's secretary may even comment on the anxiety surrounding the referral. The psychiatrist may feel under some pressure to resolve the situation but this may be achieved only by working with the staff rather than attempting to treat the patient, whose behaviour may not easily be changed. The difficulties that have arisen between

the patient and the medical/nursing staff may be repeated between these staff and the psychiatrist unless the latter recognises what is happening, and addresses the conflict in a supportive and understanding manner.

These clinical situations can raise complex issues for staff about the 'worthiness' and 'meaning' of their work. In this context, the psychiatrist must work with the staff to help them resolve their difficulties in order to help the patient. This can only be done when the psychiatrist and staff know and trust each other.

Interviewing skills and mental state assessment

Taking a psychiatric history

Even if the referral process runs smoothly, some patients referred to the liaison psychiatrist are difficult to interview either because they are reluctant to see a psychiatrist or because they have some degree of cognitive impairment. The psychiatrist should use his usual interview techniques but be prepared early in the interview to employ techniques which address these problems. (For further advice about patients who present somatic symptoms see the section below and chapter 5.) For patients who are cognitively impaired, it may only be possible to assess the mental state at the initial interview. Examples are confusion following a stroke or neurosurgery or because the patient is delirious or demented. In such cases the mental state should be recorded in great detail and a history taken from an informant.

In a fully conscious patient, the aims of the first interview are: (a) to overcome any difficulties or reluctance that the patient has to a psychiatric assessment; (b) take a full psychiatric history and record the mental state; (c) explore the relationships between medical symptoms/illness and psychiatric symptoms, and (d) engage the patient in a discussion of psychological issues to increase patient's awareness of psychological factors and facilitate the treatment process which may be continued by medical staff, GP or psychiatrist. The general points about interview techniques are summarised in Box 2.3.

Patient's feelings about being referred to a psychiatrist

This should always be addressed early on in the interview, as the majority of patients have real fears and anxieties about being referred to a psychiatrist. Psychiatry still carries a social stigma and the patient may feel that their symptoms are not being taken seriously by the medical team looking after them. Many patients still believe that being referred to a psychiatrist means that their doctors think that they are either 'mad' or 'making-up' their symptoms. It is important that the psychiatrist checks that the patient has been told of the psychiatric assessment and finds out what the patient understands and feels about this. The patient's understanding of the reason for the referral may be very different to that given to the psychiatrist by the medical staff. There may be considerable negative feelings which may impair history-taking unless discussed openly at the outset.

History of physical symptoms

It is usually best to ask patients about their recent and past physical symptoms before enquiring about psychological symptoms. Even patients who readily admit to depression in association with organic disease may be wary of seeing a psychiatrist, and will be more used to discussing physical as opposed to psychological problems. The psychiatrist builds up trust and gains important information by starting with a detailed and chronological account of the physical symptoms and their treatment. This forms a template of the patient's physical symptoms against which life events and psychological symptoms may later be compared. In addition, during the course of this medical history-taking it is not unusual for patients to experience visible distress. The points at which this occurs should be noted and the psychiatrist should pick up the cues as they provide a natural transition to discussion of psychological issues.

History of psychological symptoms

The psychiatrist should only enquire about the patient's psychological symptoms when a general medical history has been taken and a satisfactory rapport established. The history of anxiety, depression, alcohol and drug misuse etc. should be taken in the usual way, and followed by the family, personal and social history.

Box 2.3 Interview skills in liaison psychiatry

Address patient's feelings about psychiatric referral, facilitate the expression of any negative concerns or worries

Enquire about physical symptoms, detailed history and time course

Pick up verbal and non-verbal emotional cues

Use empathic style

Enquire about psychological symptoms

Link psychological with physical, use a tentative style so patient takes a more active role

---

Basic interview techniques – emotional cues and empathic style

The psychiatrist should be particularly aware of any verbal and non-verbal cues of emotional distress, as medical patients are sometimes worried about disclosing their distress to a psychiatrist in case this confirms that they are 'mad'. Some of the interview techniques required by a liaison psychiatrist are described by Creed & Guthrie (1993). Useful additional questions are:

> So the doctor said you had a small heart attack – what did you feel when he told you? What were your greatest fears at that news?
>
> So you learnt that it was unlikely that there would be a kidney donor for several years. What effect did that news have on you?
>
> What did you feel like saying to the doctor at that time?
>
> When you noticed that you had lost weight, what did you think was the reason?
>
> The doctor said the tests were normal – what did you think then?
>
> So you developed this pain six months ago – what did you think at the time caused the pain? How much did this pain affect your life?

Clinical signs

During the liaison consultation, it is important to record any signs of abnormal mood, behaviour, psychotic symptoms or cognitive defects in the usual way. There are also some particular signs in patients seen in the general hospital and it is particularly important to assess the following:

Appearance and behaviour

State of physical health.   This should be described briefly for all patients with obvious disability, for example difficulty with respiration, motility problem. It is important to describe how the patient walks from his bed to the interview room. This may indicate obvious difficulties of gait and other movements, breathing, coordination, hearing and vision as well as attitudes to the nursing staff and the initial reaction to seeing another doctor.

Level of arousal.   The delirious patient may at times be alert, fearful, even hostile, to those who approach; at other times quite withdrawn and show psychomotor retardation. There may be restless noisy behaviour which has led to cot sides being erected. Behaviour may be determined by hallucinations or delusions.

Evidence of confusion or disorientation.   Unless the patient is grossly disorientated this is often overlooked by medical and nursing staff. The psychiatrist should always perform detailed cognitive testing (see below). Milder forms of confusion may be evident in the patient's wandering attention or inconsistencies in the history. Evidence of confusion may only be apparent at night – for this reason the psychiatrist must consult the nursing staff and their cardex to discover if the patient is disorientated at night though perfectly coherent during daytime and at the time of the psychiatrist's visit.

The day on which confusion started should be determined as precisely as possible, to see if it corresponds to starting a new drug, to pyrexia developing or to the withdrawal of alcohol at admission. It may be necessary to consult the patient's relatives about the earliest sign of confusion; they are often most sensitive to mild disorientation.

Abnormal illness behaviour. Patients may make exaggerated expressions of discomfort, move slowly and adopt an awkward posture. They may appear to be in severe pain at times during the interview but appear comfortable at other times, when distracted by the interviewer. This is suggestive of abnormal illness behaviour. The psychiatrist should observe when pain behaviours become accentuated during the interview, for example when discussing the death of a close relative.

The patient who is excessively concerned about physical illness may frequently interrupt the interview to ask about bodily events, e.g. fast heart beat, twinges of pain or borborygmi, and insist that a further investigation is necessary. The psychiatrist may find himself facing questions about whether a new investigation has been developed to find a cause of the patient's symptoms. The psychiatrist must note such interruptions as part of the mental state examination, they represent a preoccupation or overvalued ideas (see below).

Attitude of patient to interview with psychiatrist and rapport developed. This should be recorded in the usual way, but any persisting difficulties should be noted as they may indicate that the psychiatric history is superficial and specially aimed at avoiding disclosure of personal details or distress.

Speech

The confused patient may wander in speech and appear to be rambling, although not with formal thought disorder. Some patients may constantly return to the topic of their physical symptoms during the conversation. This may reflect a preoccupation with a physical illness or it may reflect the abnormal illness behaviour seen in somatoform disorders. Such patients may also have limited use of emotional language and descriptive vocabulary. When asked to describe a symptom they may say, "it's just a pain, it hurts, I don't know what it's like, it just hurts". A paucity of descriptive language and imagination is a useful clinical sign that must be recorded as it gives an insight into the patient's familiarity with psychological concepts.

Affect

The patient's level of depression or anxiety should always be noted and the usual questions asked. A patient may be obviously anxious or depressed, even tearful at interview but insist that this is solely attributable to the pain and disability of the physical symptoms. This reaction may be a form of denial – the distress may also reflect one or more unhappy aspects of the patient's family or social life, to which the patient is reluctant to admit.

The range and depth of the patient's emotional responses should be recorded. These may be exaggerated in those with hysterical and antisocial personalities, who respond particularly badly to hospitalisation. The responses may be blunted in chronic organic states affecting the brain. The patient with chronic somatisation may seem detached, bland and affectless, either showing 'inappropriate lack of concern' towards the pain or disability, which is central to the condition or showing 'denial of affect' insisting that he is not upset even when appearing close to tears.

Abnormal hostility expressed towards doctors and nurses, occasionally indicates persecutory ideas, projected anger or defensiveness. Hostility or anger can in some cases be justified and the psychiatrist should attempt to assess the appropriateness of the patients' anger towards the medical team.

Thoughts

The psychiatrist must always assess the patient's beliefs regarding his physical symptoms. This may reveal the typical abnormal thoughts or delusions seen in severe depression or schizophrenia. Examples are the patient with schizophrenia who believed that a leg ulcer was caused by neighbours shining rays through the wall, and the depressed patient who was quite convinced that she had no brain (nihilistic delusion) and was requesting a CT scan of her head. In addition, a patient may have overvalued ideas concerning the cause of his symptoms and occasionally may have bizarre hypochondriacal beliefs, which, if challenged, may lead to overt hostility. The psychiatrist can test the degree of conviction with which these beliefs are held by asking "if this investigation is performed and the result turns out to be normal, what will you think?". A response that the investigation must have been inadequate indicates the underlying strength of conviction of the patient's belief.

The patient who is delirious may have clear persecutory delusions, which are often secondary to illusions and visual hallucinations. These may be very much more pronounced at night. They may be accompanied by overt emotional and psychological changes with the patient being obviously agitated and overactive, even to the point of wishing to leave the ward.

Perception

Illusory experiences are common in hospital settings, particularly in patients who are mildy confused. Drip stands, television sets, ventilation ducts etc. are often mistaken for creatures or aliens. True visual hallucinations are common in organic psychosyndromes, and any patient presenting with visual hallucinatory phenomena should be carefully investigated.

Cognitive tests

Cognitive testing in liaison psychiatry is the same as that in general psychiatry but difficulties arise with a patient who has only mild impairment of consciousness. Thus the liaison psychiatrist may examine a patient during the day time who had been overtly disturbed during the previous night. This is the characteristic fluctuation of delirium and a careful history from the nursing staff, including reference to the nursing cardex (for the patient's mental state in the night), is necessary as well as examination of the mental state during daytime.

Even if the patient appears orientated for the day, date, month and the year, minor degrees of temporal disorientation may be indicated by asking the patient to estimate the time of day or the time since the interview commenced. Lishman (1987) states that orientation for time is commonly the first aspect of cognition to suffer in the course of mild impairment of consciousness.

Box 2.4 Diagnostic features of delirium

Impairment of consciousness and attention
Global disturbance of cognition including perceptual distor-
    tions, illusions and hallucinations together with impairment
    of immediate recall and of recent memory but with relatively
    intact remote memory
Psychomotor disturbances with increased or decreased
    activities and unpredictable shifts between these
Disturbance of sleep – wakefulness cycle with daytime
    drowsiness and nocturnal worsening of symptoms often
    leading to gross disturbance of behaviour
Emotional disturbances usually anxiety, fear, irritability or
    depression

Attention and concentration may show fluctuation. It may be difficult to gain the patient's attention or to hold the patient's concentration on a single topic throughout the item being tested. Concentration may easily become fatigued. It is best to use simple tests (i.e. Serial 3s rather than Serial 7s) and days of the week or months of the year in reverse order. If the patient shows clear impairment of attention or concentration it may prove impossible to obtain reliable information from the subsequent memory tests, which need not be carried out.

Tests of memory should be the same as those used in general psychiatry. It is recommended that the psychiatrist uses the same tests so that he becomes familiar with the habitual response to them. A single Stanford-Binet sentence and a name and address both retested after one minute and five minutes are very useful tests.

Long-term memory can be assessed using the patient's knowledge of past events. Any impairment will generally become apparent during the past and previous medical history. Many patients who suffer delirium may have had underlying memory impairment prior to hospitalisation. A patient who misuses alcohol may have Korsakoff's syndrome or alcoholic dementia, upon which is superimposed the clinical picture of delirium tremens if the patient is in a withdrawal state. This means there will be disorientation and other features of delirium (see Box 2.4) as well as longer-term memory impairment. A patient who has sustained a head injury may have selected impairment of memory in relation to the head injury – i.e. retrograde or anterograde amnesia.

It is important to record any confabulation for false memories which occurs in a patient who has a long-standing memory deficit (e.g. secondary to alcohol). Obvious discrepancies, such as profound amnesia for certain times but with normal ability to retain new information, need to be explored and recorded in full as they usually indicate an hysterical amnesia. The psychiatrist would do well to use a standardised assessment e.g. the Mini Mental State (Folstein *et al*, 1975). Further details of extended cognitive testing are found in Lishman (1987).

Assessment of depressive disorder in the physically ill

There are two important aspects of diagnosing depression in liaison psychiatry: distinguishing depressive disorder from adjustment reactions in the physically ill, and defining the relationship between depression and physical illness when both are present.

Distinguishing depressive disorders from adjustment disorders in the physically ill

Adjustment disorders are very common in the physically ill. Deciding whether a depressive disorder is present follows the same lines as

---

Box 2.5 Symptoms of depression in the medically ill

Fearful or depressed appearance*
Social withdrawal or decreased talkativeness*
Psychomotor retardation or agitation*
Depressed mood*
Mood that is non-reactive to environmental events*
Morning depression
Marked diminished interest or pleasure in most activities*
Brooding, self-pity or pessimism*
Feelings of worthlessness or excessive or inappropriate guilt*
Feelings of helplessness
Feeling a burden
Recurrent thoughts of death or suicide*
Thoughts that the illness is a punishment
Frequent crying

*Endicott's criteria (1984) which should be present for at least
   two weeks for a diagnosis of depressive illness.

---

differentiating between a normal bereavement reaction and a diagnosis of depressive disorder – severity and duration of symptoms are important. Feelings of devastation and despondency are short-lived and transient in adjustment disorders. They may become prolonged and even lead to suicidal ideas in those with depressive disorder. Crying may occur at every reminder of the person's illness/disability in depressive disorder; loss of concentration and interest are coupled with a feeling of hopelessness.

The psychiatrist must take a careful history of the development of these symptoms following the initial onset and over recent weeks. It often becomes clear that the depressive symptoms became more pronounced when the illness became more severe or disabling and/or when a concomitant social stress occurred.

It is usually best to measure severity with a depression scale e.g. the Beck Depression Inventory (Beck *et al*, 1961) or the Hospital Anxiety and Depression Scale (Zigmond & Snaith, 1983). The former provides more details of cognitive symptoms and may indicate when cognitive therapy is helpful in addition to antidepressants. The latter is more useful as a screening instrument than for the individual case. Meakin (1992) has reviewed screening instruments in the physically ill. There seems little to choose between them, but each requires validation with a specific illness to provide an accurate assessment of 'caseness'.

The presence of somatic symptoms in the medically ill, for example fatigue, weight loss, insomnia, pain, are generally poor measures of depression as they may result from physical illness not depressive disorder (Cavanagh, 1983). Endicott (1984) proposed that additional psychological symptoms should be substituted for physical symptoms when making a diagnosis of depression in the medically ill (Box 2.5). He suggested that depressed appearance, social withdrawal, brooding and non-reactive mood should replace weight loss, insomnia, fatigue and poor concentration. Box 2.5 lists symptoms, including Endicott's, which should be elicited when making a diagnosis of depression in the physically ill.

It is apparent from the above that the diagnosis of depressive disorder in the physically ill relies on the presence of affective symptoms. The psychiatrist should note, however, that symptoms such as inappropriate guilt, sense of being punished and loss of self-esteem are less likely to occur in the medically ill than in those depressed persons presenting direct to the psychiatrist. Hawton *et al* (1990) found that three affective symptoms provided good discrimination between depressed medical patients and non-depressed medical controls; these were depressed mood, morning depression and hopelessness. Further discussion of mood disorders in the medically ill can be found in House (1988) and Jenkins & Jamil (1994).

Defining the relationship between depression and physical illness

Moffic & Paykel (1975) noted three patterns:

(1) Depressive disorder that was a clear reaction to the physical illness and its treatment. Such depression obviously occurs after the physical illness and will fluctuate according to the phase of severity of the physical illness. This accounts for two-thirds of depression in general medical wards.

(2) Depression which precedes the onset of physical illness. Both the depression and the physical illness may start soon after a severe life event, such as bereavement (Murphy & Brown, 1980). It may become clear that the patient was previously predisposed, through family history, to develop both depression and heart disease.

(3) Depressive disorder which precedes the physical symptoms may actually be responsible for the physical symptoms – either directly or indirectly. Presentation of depression as somatic symptoms (a process known as somatisation) is clinically very important. The following clinical examples indicate where depression indirectly leads to the current presenting physical problem.

> A 51-year-old man with chronic renal failure, undergoing home dialysis, required repeated admissions because his dialysis was failing to maintain adequate renal function. He appeared sad and despondent on the ward, which was attributed by the staff to be

understandable in terms of his poor physical health and social isolation. A psychiatric opinion was requested as he began to cry openly on the ward and it transpired that he had been feeling persistently depressed for several months, with sleep disturbance, lethargy, anhedonia and two stone weight loss. All these symptoms had been attributed to his physical status but their severity and the fact that he felt that life was not worth living indicated a depressive disorder. He confided to the psychiatrist that he had often missed doing his renal exchanges at home because he could no longer see the point, which was the primary reason for the deterioration of his physical state.

In the above example the development of a depressive disorder led to the deterioration of a patient's physical condition; increased efforts to correct the latter became the focus of attention for medical and nursing staff leading to the psychiatric disorder only being detected when it was quite severe.

A 39-year-old man with diabetes and a below-knee amputation complained of feeling low and tired all of the time. Part of his treatment involved long courses of antibiotics which made him nauseous and resulted in weight loss. He had found it hard to accept that he had lost his leg and acted on occasions as if he still had two normal legs. For example, on a busy bus, he had stood-up for the entire length of the journey despite being in considerable pain with the consequence that his stump became ulcerated as it rubbed against his artificial leg. He required further surgery to prevent septicaemia, but when asked to consent to an above knee amputation, he refused. This refusal to accept treatment led to psychiatric referral. On mental state examination he was found to feel hopeless and worthless. He felt that he was no longer worthy to be a father to his children, as he could not play football with them or take them for walks. He felt that no one really cared about him and his family would be better off without him.

The history indicated that this patient had persistently failed to show any form of psychological adjustment to his amputation. This man has a severe depressive illness with persistently lowered mood, hopelessness and suicidal ideation.

In both of these examples the depression developed after the physical illness and can be related to it. However, the situation is complicated, in both cases, by the fact that the depression led to secondary deterioration of physical illness and presentation of somatic symptoms (fatigue, weight and sleep loss and general ill health in the first case, persistent sepsis in the second), which were, indirectly, a result of the depression. Such a cycle of depression and worsening of physical illness through non-compliance with treatment is common when depressive disorder occurs in the medically ill.

Detection of psychological disorders presenting with somatic symptoms (somatisation)

Many consultations come to the psychiatrist requesting an opinion as to whether a somatic symptom could be caused by an underlying psychological problem. Making up one's mind on this issue may be difficult and the trainee is always advised to discuss such cases in detail with the consultant psychiatrist as the physician's decision to continue or stop investigations for organic disease may rest on the psychiatrist's findings. The general phenomenon of somatisation is discussed in detail in Chapter 5.

Many general psychiatrists are unfamiliar with patients who somatise their psychological distress and may be at risk of deciding that such a patient has 'no psychiatric illness' which may be of little help to the physician. This conclusion may be reached because there is no obvious affective disturbance, or the patient has successfully persuaded the psychiatrist that any anxiety or depression is entirely secondary to the physical symptoms. Many patients who somatise their distress also have physical illness (Bridges & Goldberg, 1985; Kroencke & Mangelsdorff, 1989) so particular care is required to distinguish the aetiology of a particular somatic symptom (e.g. atypical chest pain) from other symptoms (e.g. typical angina), as both may occur in the same patient.

During clinical assessment the psychiatrist should use the following six criteria in reviewing evidence that a somatic symptom might have an underlying psychological basis (Cohen, 1982; Creed, 1992).

(1) *Is the presenting bodily symptom accompanied by psychological symptoms or other somatic symptoms typical of anxiety or depression?* An example is the patient who is being investigated for chest pain, for which no organic cause can be found. Evidence suggesting that the chest pain might be associated with anxiety comes from the fact that the chest pain is generally accompanied by headaches, palpitations, frequency of micturition, abdominal churnings etc. These symptoms may amount to a panic attack with the patient's fears centring around the possibility of a heart attack.

The psychiatrist may also elicit that during the time since the patient developed chest pain there has been sleep disturbance, loss of appetite, reduced libido, some impairment of concentration and generally reduced enthusiasm and enjoyment of life. All of these symptoms appear relatively unimportant, compared to the chest pain, and may not have previously been reported; the patient selectively attends to the chest pain and tends to ignore the other symptoms. These are all contributory evidence to the fact that the chest pain may have a psychological basis; but not conclusive evidence as patients with heart disease may also suffer panic attacks.

**Box 2.6 Detection of psychological disorders that present
with somatic symptoms (somatisation)**

Is the presenting bodily symptom accompanied by psycho-
  logical symptoms, or other somatic symptoms typical of
  anxiety or depression?
Is the somatic symptom typical of organic disease?
Previous episode of medically unexplained symptoms
Precipitation by stress and alleviation by the relief of stress
Family or past personal history of psychiatric disorder
The symptoms may respond to psychological treatment when
  they have failed to respond to medical treatment

---

(2) *Is the somatic symptom typical of organic disease?* In addition, it
may become apparent that the chest pain is not brought on by exertion;
it may be brought on by any reminders of heart disease (e.g. through
television or newspapers), of which the patient is afraid. Chest pain is an
example where it may be difficult to decide whether the symptom is
typical or atypical of that caused by heart disease. Other examples may
be clearer. The hallmark of some conversion symptoms is the fact that
they are not typical of organic disease (e.g. hemianesthesia, functional
paralysis with brisk reflexes) (Lishman, 1987).

(3) *Previous episode of medically unexplained symptoms.* The patient
may have experienced previous episodes of medically unexplained
symptoms, usually at a time of stress.

> A 60-year-old man developed a persistent sore throat and, later,
> loin pain, which were thoroughly investigated; these were normal
> but he could not be reassured that he did not have cancer. Detailed
> enquiry revealed that these symptoms had developed after his
> brother's death and that on two previous occasions he had
> experienced physical symptoms which had required investigations:
> severe headaches occurred after his sister had died with a cerebral
> haemorrhage and chest pains followed his mother's death from
> heart disease. Although the patient had some insight into the early
> episodes, his current anxieties about cancer required specific
> treatment (see Hopkins, 1992).

(4) *The symptom may have been precipitated by stress and alleviated by
the relief of stress.* There is extensive experimental evidence linking the
onset of psychological disorders and associated somatic symptoms with
life events (Creed, 1991, 1993). These details may only be obtained in
clinical practice, however, if a careful medical history is taken first and

events clearly dated; a thorough family, personal and social history taken subsequently may reveal coincidence of dates between psychosocial events and variation in the symptom pattern previously established.

> A middle-aged woman suffered from abdominal pain which had commenced at the time of two stressful life events: her daughter's divorce and her own marital problems. Her abdominal symptoms largely remitted for a three month period when it appeared that both these problems had resolved. The pain recurred, however, when she experienced further conflict in her marriage.

(5) *Family or past personal history of psychiatric disorder.*   Even in the absence of current psychiatric symptoms there may be evidence of predisposition to develop psychiatric disorder in the form of a family and past personal history.

> A 26-year-old woman was referred from the endocrinologists because of menstrual problems and abdominal pains that had originally been attributed to possible endometriosis. Although there was no current evidence of psychiatric disorder, nor was there a clear precipitating stressor, her father had been treated in the past for alcoholism and her mother for anxiety and depression. She had been in care herself as a child and had been seen previously by a psychiatrist who had stated that no psychiatric disorder was present. The patient's history, suggested that she might be predisposed to develop depression even though no current depressive symptoms were apparent. When this was discussed with the patient she recognised that the problem may have had an underlying psychological basis and she agreed to further psychological assessment. It transpired that she had been sexually abused by her father and in the previous six months had embarked on her first sexual relationship, which had precipitated the current menstrual and abdominal symptoms; she could not enjoy sex but was afraid to tell her boyfriend as she was frightened he would leave her.

In this case, previous life experience (the abusive relationship with her father) and a recent life event (her first sexual relationship) had resulted in the development of somatic symptoms (atypical menstrual problems).

In a study of patients with chronic pain, Katon *et al* (1984) found that more than half of the patients had a past history of one or more episodes of major depression or alcohol abuse before the onset of their chronic pain. Sixty per cent of the patients had at least one first degree relative with chronic pain, 30% had a family member with affective illness, and 38% had a family member with alcohol abuse. Patients with somatisation disorder have also been found to have family histories of alcoholism and antisocial personality (see Chapter 5). Thus when faced with a patient who has medically unexplained pain the search for predisposing factors is as important as the search for current psychiatric symptoms.

(6) *The symptoms may respond to psychological treatment when they have failed to respond to medical treatment.* Sometimes the liaison psychiatrist is referred a patient with no apparent psychiatric disorder, but who has failed to respond to any form of treatment intervention. Often there is some organic basis for the patient's problems but not enough to explain all the patient's symptoms.

> A 35-year-old man was referred from the neurologist with a history of blackouts and fits. He had an abnormal EEG; temporal lobe epilepsy had been diagnosed and treated, but control was poor. There was no psychiatric illness. During a course of brief psychotherapy he admitted that some of his fits had occurred in the middle of arguments he had with his parents about leaving home. He appeared to be enmeshed in an over-close relationship with his parents and the fits indicated how impractical (and dangerous) it would be for him to leave home. Once his fears about leaving home, and his anger towards his parents were worked through, he was helped to separate from his parents and the frequency of his fits diminished.

In this example the importance of psychological factors in the aetiology of his disabling physical illness is clear but there was no evidence in the original psychiatric assessment that this was the case; the problems with the parents only came out during a more prolonged therapeutic interview.

Summary

When assessing a patient with unexplained medical symptoms, the liaison psychiatrist should review all evidence under each of the above headings – nature of accompanying symptoms; whether such symptoms are typical of organic disease; whether there have been previous episodes of unexplained medical symptoms; whether the symptoms are exacerbated by stress; family and previous personal history of psychiatric disorder, and whether there is previous or current evidence that the symptoms improved with psychological treatment.

Assessment of illness behaviour

For all cases in liaison psychiatry it is worth making an assessment of the patient's attitude towards their illness and their illness behaviours (Mechanic, 1961). These may be quite normal and appropriate to the severity of the illness. On the other hand, they may be abnormal as a result of psychiatric disorder (notably depression) or may be abnormal in the absence of formal psychiatric disorder. In the examples given (p. 41) there was clear evidence of abnormal actions in relation to illness – the diabetic patient denied his disability and exacerbated the stump infection; the patient in renal failure ceased to do his exchanges consistently. In each case a depressive disorder was responsible. In the following example, the appropriate diagnosis would be somatisation disorder (see Chapter 5).

> A 45-year-old man had severe pain for 10 years following a minor accident at work, when he had fallen off a ladder. The only abnormality arising from numerous investigations were minor osteoarthritic changes on X-ray but these were considered inadequate to explain the pain. He had eventually retired on the grounds of ill health and had lived off his disability allowance supplemented by his wife's earnings; she had a part-time job as well as doing all the household management.
>
> This patient had adopted an extremely restricted life style, rarely going out, even though the pain did not prevent him from leaving the house. In the clinic he was observed to be relaxed and apparently pain free at times but appeared to be in severe pain at others, especially while in the doctor's office.
>
> He was excessively angry with the doctors for not having found a cure to his back problems even though they had tried many forms of treatment and physiotherapy. He did not see any relationship between the onset and continuation of his pain and the loss of his mother (his chief carer), and attributed all his symptoms to the accident at work.
>
> There were a number of features of this presentation which indicated abnormal illness behaviour (Box 2.7). His disability was out of proportion for the objective findings. He relentlessly sought treatment from doctors even though he could not accept their explanation that there was no serious physical disease and blamed them for not finding a cure to his problems. He had adopted a life style around the sick role, which was reinforced by his wife and the disability payments.

Understanding abnormal illness behaviour

At the initial assessment the psychiatrist may identify abnormal illness behaviours but these can often only be explained if the psychiatrist has further interviews of a psychotherapeutic nature in which the patient feels free to disclose important (and often painful) past experiences. Such experiences often pertain to inadequate care or illness experience as a child (Craig *et al*, 1994). Two examples illustrate this:

> In the earlier example of the depressed man with an amputation (p. 41), it transpired that he had developed diabetes at the age

of 3; his parents had responded badly, blaming him for his diabetes and making him feel that he was 'damaged' and 'imperfect'. He never felt supported or loved by his parents and was frequently criticised and punished if he did not adhere strictly to his diet. His diabetes was very poorly controlled during his childhood, and it was not until he left home, and severed connections with his family that the control improved.

This patient compensated for his feelings of inadequacy by trying to be better than others; he became a high achiever at school. His early relationships, however, led to difficulty in trusting and feeling close to other people. He married and had two children, but the relationship did not last very long. Shortly after his marriage ended, diabetic complications arose with renal and vascular problems; the latter resulted in a below knee amputation. Post-operatively, anticoagulation for a DVT led to a haemorrhage and loss of sight in one eye, which meant that he could no longer work.

This man's way of coping with a serious, chronic illness was by becoming excessively hard-working and conscientious and succeeding at work. This avenue for bolstering his self-esteem, however, was thwarted when he lost the sight in one eye. Because of his mistrust and difficulties in getting close to people, he was unable to share with anyone the distress resulting from diabetic complications; he found that he had to face them alone, and had no friends he could turn to for support.

This extra insight into this man's inner psychological world, makes it clearer why he found it so difficult to accept that his leg had been amputated and why he subsequently 'acted out' by standing whilst travelling by bus resulting in further damage. The anger

---

Box 2.7 Dimensions of abnormal illness behaviour

An uncomfortable awareness of bodily events much of the time together with excessive fears and concerns about health and disease

Relentless search for causes and cures coupled with inability to accept reassurance from doctors even when this has been given clearly and on the basis of appropriate investigations

Adoption of life style around the sick role with repertoire of behaviours to sustain sick role

Inability to accept the suggestion that non-physical (i.e. psychosocial) factors may be relevant to one's condition

Disability out of proportion to detectable organic disease

Reinforcement of illness behaviours by the family, disability payments and health care providers

Inappropriate response to physical disorder – either excessive disability or denial of need for treatment/limitation of activities

and destructiveness he had felt for so long towards his parents, and towards his diabetes, was turned once again against himself.

Liaison case summaries

Some trainees find it difficult to marshall all the relevant facts of liaison cases and develop a coherent aetiological explanation of the patient's symptoms. To fully appreciate the complexities of a liaison case and to help formulate a management plan, it is useful to consider the following aspects which can be summarised at the end of the history and mental state examination:

(1) The reason for referral.
(2) Psychiatric diagnosis.
(3) Physical disease and the patient's reaction to it.
(4) Evidence of abnormal illness behaviour.
(5) The relationship between physical and psychological aspects of the case.
(6) The patient's personality and normal coping strategies.
(7) The patient's attitude towards psychiatric intervention.
(8) The staff's attitude towards the patient.

> A 48-year-old woman was referred to a psychiatrist from the gastroenterology department with a 29 year history of abdominal pain and no underlying organic pathology. In addition she described frequent belching, loose motions, flatulence, lethargy, lower backache, headaches, numbness in her feet, dizziness, blurred vision, neckache, discomfort on micturition, dry mouth, buzzing in her ears, sensitivity to noise, and paralysis of her right leg. Examination of her casenotes indicated that she had been seen in all departments of the hospital with various complaints – numerous investigations had not led to any satisfactory explanation of her symptoms in terms of organic disease. She had been confined to a wheel chair for the last 5 years because the abdominal discomfort made it difficult for her to walk. The paralysis in her right leg had recently begun following a suggestion from one of her physicians that she should give up her wheel chair and start a programme of rehabilitation. She believed the abdominal pain was the result of bowel cancer which now must have spread to her spine and caused the paralysis of her leg. She denied any psychological problems or difficulties and did not appear overtly depressed or anxious.

Although the above case appears quite complicated, a liaison case summary would be as follows:

(1) Reason for referral: multiple somatic complaints.

(2) Psychiatric diagnosis: somatisation disorder.

(3) No physical illness, although patient has a strong conviction that she has a physical illness and hypochondriacal beliefs that she has cancer.

(4) Abnormal illness behaviour: confined to wheel chair despite no physical reason why she cannot walk. Inability to use her hand when it was suggested she use her hands to propel herself in the wheel chair.

(5) Physical symptoms appear to be predominantly psychogenic in origin, although their presence reinforces the patient's belief in a physical aetiology. Thomas classification: 'somatic presentation of psychiatric disorder'.

(6) Personality and previous life experience has yet to be assessed but it will be important to check for any evidence of dependant traits, emotional deprivation during childhood, failure to separate from parents, physical illness when a child, and parental illness when patient was a child.

(7) The patient is wary and worried about psychiatric referral.

(8) The medical and nursing staff are exasperated with the patient and find her abnormal illness behaviour difficult to cope with.

This way of summarising a case is not meant to replace a psychiatric formulation, but it immediately identifies areas of the case which require further investigation, e.g. the patient's personality and life experiences. It clarifies the relationship between physical and psychiatric disorder and it highlights the need to address the concerns of the patient and the medical/nursing staff caring for the patient. It is just as useful for patients with physical illness. The liaison case summary for the man with diabetes (pp. 41 and 47) would be as follows:

(1) Reason for referral: refusal to consent to above knee amputation.

(2) Psychiatric diagnosis: depressive illness.

(3) Physical diagnosis: type I diabetes with peripheral vascular disease, renal disease and eye complications. Patient has longstanding anger and difficulty in accepting the diabetes.

(4) Abnormal illness behaviour: inconsistent adherence to diabetic diet and insulin regime over many years, inappropriate behaviour in relation to his artificial leg, refusal to accept further surgery despite possible life threatening consequences.

(5) Depressive illness: onset related to diabetes and negative aspects of relationships with parents, but depression now leading to refusal to accept further physical treatment. It has also released previously hidden feelings of anger about the diabetes; the physical status is deteriorating.

(6) Previous personality and life experiences: The patient has had difficulty in developing close, intimate and trusting relationships.

He was made to feel inadequate because of the diabetes and was never allowed to develop his own sense of control. He has compensated in the past by developing perfectionistic traits but this method of coping has broken down because of severe physical illness.

(7) He is accepting of a psychiatric referral and wants to talk about his problems.

(8) The medical and nursing staff have failed to recognise that he is depressed and feel angry and frustrated by his refusal to accept treatment.

Summary

The assessment of patients in liaison psychiatry takes time, skill and patience. The reason for the referral has to be understood, the patient has to be engaged in a detailed interview of psychological factors, new clinical signs and symptoms have to be elicited and the relationship between psychological and physical symptoms understood. In addition, the psychiatrist is unable to rely solely on the psychiatric diagnosis as usual; the psychiatric diagnosis is merely one piece of information in a complicated 'biopsychosocial' jigsaw.

The three most common errors junior psychiatrists make when conducting liaison assessments for the first time are: an over-emphasis on psychiatric diagnosis, a failure to link psychological and physical factors, and a failure to consult adequately with medical and nursing staff. The schema for conducting assessments outlined in this chapter are meant as helpful aids which, if employed, should produce more meaningful and useful psychiatric liaison assessments.

References

Bass, C. M. (1995) The role of liaison psychiatry. In *Psychiatric Aspects of Physical Disease* (eds A. House, K. Mayou & C. Mallinson), pp. 91–99. London: Royal College of Physicians & Royal College of Psychiatrists.

Beck, A. T., Ward, C. H., Mendelson, M., *et al* (1961) An inventory for measuring depression. *Archives of General Psychiatry*, **4**, 561–571.

Bridges, K. & Goldberg, D. P. (1985) Somatic presentation of DSM–III psychiatric disorders in primary care. *Journal of Psychosomatic Research*, **29**, 563–569.

Cavanagh, S. (1983) The prevalence of cognitive and emotional dysfunction in a general medical population using the MMSE, GHA and BDI. *General Hospital Psychiatry*, **5**, 15–21.

Cohen, S. I. (1982) The evaluation of patients with somatic symptoms – the 'difficult' diagnostic problem. In *Medicine and Psychiatry – A Practical Approach* (eds F. H. Creed & J. M. Pfeffer), pp. 105–118. London: Pitman.

Craig, T. K. J., Drake, H., Mills, K., *et al* (1994) The south London somatisation study. II: the influence of stressful life events and secondary gain. *British Journal of Psychiatry*, **165**, 248–258.

Creed, F. H. (1991) 'Life events'. In *The Scientific Basis of Psychiatry* (2nd edn) (eds M. P. I. Weller & M. W. Eysenck), pp. 491–508. London: W. B. Saunders.

—— (1992) Relationship of non-organic abdominal pain to psychiatric disorder and life stress. In *Medical Symptoms not Explained by Organic Disease* (eds F. Creed, R. Mayou & A. Hopkins), pp. 9–16. London: Royal College of Psychiatrists & Royal College of Physicians.

—— (1993) Stress and psychosomatic disorders. In *Handbook of Stress: Theoretical and Clinical Aspects* (eds L. Goldberger & S. Breznitz), pp. 496–510. New York: Macmillan.

—— & Guthrie, E. (1993) Techniques for interviewing the somatising patient. *British Journal of Psychiatry*, **162**, 467–471.

Endicott, J. (1984) Measurement of depression in out-patients with cancer. *Cancer*, **53**, 2243–2248.

Folstein, M. F., Folstein, S. E. & McHugh, P. R. (1975) "Mini-Mental State" a practical method for grading the cognitive state of patients for the clinician, *Journal of Psychiatric Research*, **12**, 189–198.

Hawton, K., Mayou, R. & Feldman, E. (1990) Significance of psychiatric symptoms in the general medical patient with mood disorder. *General Hospital Psychiatry*, **12**, 296–302.

Hopkins, A. (1992) The management of patients with chronic headache not due to obvious structural disease. In *Medical Symptoms not Explained by Organic Disease* (eds F. Creed, R. Mayou & A. Hopkins), pp. 34–46. London: Royal College of Physicians & Royal College of Psychiatrists.

House, A. (1988) Mood disorders is the physically ill – problems of definition and measurement. *Journal of Psychosomatic Research*, **32**, 345–353.

—— & Creed, F. (1993) Training in liaison psychiatry: recommendations from the Liaison Psychiatry Group Executive Committee. *Psychiatric Bulletin*, **17**, 95–96.

Jenkins, P. & Jamil, N. (1994) The need for professional services for mood disorders in the medically ill. In *Liaison Psychiatry. Defining Needs and Planning Services* (eds S. Benjamin, A. House & P. Jenkins), pp. 24–33. London: Gaskell.

Katon, W., Ries, R. & Kleinman, A. (1984) A prospective DSM–III study of consecutive somatisation patients. *Comprehensive Psychiatry*, **25**, 305–314.

Kroencke, K. & Mangelsdorff, A. D. (1989) Common symptoms in ambulatory care: incidence, evaluation, therapy and outcome. *American Journal of Medicine*, **86**, 262–266.

Lishman, W. A. (1987) *Organic Psychiatry* (2nd edn). London: Blackwell Scientific Publications.

Meakin, C. J. (1992) Screening for depression in the medically ill. *British Journal of Psychiatry*, **160**, 212–216.

Mechanic, D. (1961) The concept of illness behaviour. *Journal of Chronic Disorders*, **15**, 184–194.

Moffic, H. S. & Paykel, E. S. (1975) Depression in medical in-patients. *British Journal of Psychiatry*, **126**, 346–353.

Murphy, E. & Brown, G. W. (1980) Life events, psychiatric disturbance and physical illness. *British Journal of Psychiatry*, **136**, 326–338.

Pfeffer, J. M. (1982) The consultation process. In *Medicine and Psychiatry – A Practical Approach* (eds F. Creed & J. M. Pfeffer). London: Pitman.

Royal College of Physicians & Royal College of Psychiatrists (1995) *The Psychological Care of Medical Patients: Recognition and Service Care.* CR35. London: RCP/RCPsych.

Seltzer, A. (1989) Prevalence, detection and referral of psychiatric morbidity on a medical oncology ward. *Journal of the Royal Society of Medicine*, **82**, 410–412.

Zigmond, A. & Snaith, R. P. (1983) The Hospital Anxiety and Depression Scale. *Acta Psychiatrica Scandinavica*, **67**, 361–370.

3 The classification of psychiatric disorders and their relationship to physical disorders

Francis Creed & Elspeth Guthrie

Prevalence of psychiatric disorder • Detection of psychiatric disorder • Diagnosis and classification • Limitations of diagnostic systems in liasion psychiatry

---

This chapter briefly reviews the prevalence of psychiatric disorders in the general hospital, indicating difficulties with the measurement and detection of such disorders. This allows the trainee psychiatrist to realise the very selective nature of patients referred to the liaison psychiatry service. The chapter then discusses in detail the diagnostic classification of psychiatric disorders seen in the general hospital and the relationship between psychological and physical disorders seen in patients referred to the liaison psychiatrist.

Prevalence of psychiatric disorder

Psychiatric disorder is common in the general hospital setting and its prevalence is higher than in the general population. A variety of studies over the last 20 years have suggested that the prevalence ranges from 16–61% (Maguire *et al,* 1974; Moffic & Paykel, 1975; Knights & Folstein, 1977; Cavanaugh, 1983; Bridges & Goldberg, 1984). The wide variation in these figures results from the employment of different measures and the study of different hospital populations (Mayou & Hawton, 1986) (see Chapter 10).

Measurement of psychiatric disorder

The discrepancy in the prevalence of psychiatric disorders in the general hospital, relates in part, to the difficulties of measuring psychiatric disorder when many somatic symptoms are present (see House, 1988; Jenkins & Jamil, 1994). These somatic symptoms may result from the underlying physical disorder and do not relate to depression. Cavanaugh (1983) found the following symptoms were common in medically ill patients, but not particularly associated with depression: irritability, sadness, dissatisfaction, discouragement about the future and difficulty with decisions. These symptoms were considered to be manifestations of a normal psychological reaction to acute illness and hospitalisation, and unless persistent or severe, not indicative of depressive illness.

Spuriously high prevalence figures can be obtained when the psychological scale includes somatic items. For example, in rheumatoid arthritis, Pincus *et al* (1986) identified a number of 'disease related' items on the Minnesota Multidimensional Personality Inventory (MMPI; Graham, 1987). These items were: inability to work, not being in good physical health, not feeling well, fatigue, presence of pain. Exclusion of these items brought the MMPI scores of rheumatoid arthritis patients down to the same as the general population, dispelling the idea of a 'rheumatoid personality'. When Creed *et al* (1990) removed the somatic symptoms from the total Clinical Interview Schedule score (excessive concern about physical illness, fatigue, poor sleep and hypnotics) the prevalence of psychiatric disorder among rheumatoid arthritis patients fell from 36% to 19%.

In the study by Bukberg and colleagues (1984) the point prevalence of major depressive episodes in oncology patients dropped from 42% to 24% when all somatic symptoms were eliminated as diagnostic criteria for depression. Goldberg (1986) has recommended a revised General Health Questionnaire (GHQ) cut-off score for patients in general medical settings to increase the sensitivity and specificity of this instrument in this setting. The GHQ can provide a satisfactory screening instrument with such a raised threshold (Meakin, 1992).

Assessment of psychiatric disorder using clinical interviews

The following section will refer to prevalence surveys that have used standardised research interviews to make psychiatric diagnoses. This is not a comprehensive review but illustrates the method and the results which occur from using such an interview.

In-patients

Maguire *et al* (1974) used a two-stage screening process (GHQ (Goldberg, 1972) followed by a Clinical Interview Schedule (Goldberg *et al*, 1970)). After excluding those who were not medically well enough to participate in the study and those who had been admitted after a suicide attempt, 23% of the remaining patients had a psychiatric disorder. They noted that "while referral was related to severity of psychiatric disorder and previous psychiatric disorder, the degree to which the psychiatric illness intruded or created problems in management appeared more crucial in determining referral". Thus the liaison psychiatrist will not necessarily see patients with the most severe psychiatric disorder, rather, they will see those patients where management problems occur.

Table 3.1 Psychiatric disorder in medical in-patients (from Feldman *et al*, 1987)

Psychiatric disorder	All patients (%)		Affected patients only (%)	
	Male	Female	Recognised by house officer	Referred to psychiatrist
Anxiety/depression	12	16	44	7.6
Alcohol problems	18	4	40	4.5
Dementia and delirium (patients over 70)	23	38	not recorded	15

Feldman *et al* (1987) also used a two-stage assessment procedure; 453 general medical in-patients were screened for mood disorder, organic mental states and alcohol problems. Patients admitted following a suicide attempt were excluded. All patients scoring above threshold (4/5) on the General Health Questionnaire (GHQ; Goldberg, 1972) were interviewed using the Present State Examination (PSE; Wing *et al*, 1974), and in addition, assessments of cognitive function and alcohol abuse were carried out. Fifty-six patients (14.6%) had a diagnosable psychiatric disorder; 28 patients anxiety, 26 depression, one mania, and one obsessive–compulsive neurosis. The rates for psychiatric illness were similar for men (12.2%) and women (16%), although women between the ages of 17–54 were particularly at risk. The prevalence of affective disorder, cognitive disorder and alcohol problems for different gender and age groups are shown in Table 3.1. The authors found striking associations between the presence of psychiatric disorder and the following: a previous history of psychiatric disorder, current social difficulties and the use of psychotropic medication.

House officers detected just under half of all psychiatric disorders and underestimated the severity of them. Very few patients (3%) were referred to a psychiatrist; six because of dementia, two with alcohol problems, three with depression and one with an anxiety state. These findings indicate the highly selected nature of patients referred to a liaison psychiatrist.

In some units, the prevalence of psychiatric disorder is higher. Bridges & Goldberg (1984) studied the prevalence of psychiatric disorder in neurological in-patients, and found point prevalence rates of 53.2% for women and 27.4% for men.

Out-patients

One recent study will be used as an example (Table 3.2). It included 191 general medical out-patients attending the University Hospital in Amsterdam (Van Hemert *et al*, 1993) and used a similar design to that of

Table 3.2 Prevalence of anxiety/depression in medical out-patients according to final medical diagnosis (from Van Hemert *et al*, 1993)

	Definite organic diagnosis (*n*=91) %	Recognised syndrome (non-organic)[1] (*n*=42) %	No organic diagnosis (*n*=58) %
Anxiety/ depression	12	43	33
Somatisation/ hypochondriasis	5	21	18

1. For example irritable bowel syndrome or fibromyalgia

Feldman *et al* (1987). Affective disorders were defined as in the PSE (Wing *et al*, 1974) and somatoform disorders as defined in DSM–III–R (American Psychiatric Association, 1987). For the total group of patients the prevalence of psychiatric disorder amounted to 29%. Approximately 40% of the patients with psychiatric disorder fulfilled DSM–III–R diagnostic criteria for somatisation disorder or hypochondriasis.

This study showed that the prevalence of psychiatric disorder in medical out-patients with organic disease is approximately twice that of the general population. The prevalence of psychiatric disorder in patients with medically unexplained symptoms is approximately twice as great as those with organic disease (Van Hemert *et al*, 1993).

Detection of psychiatric disorder

Although the prevalence of psychiatric morbidity in the general medical setting is high, psychiatric disorder in many patients goes unrecognised by hospital doctors.

In-patients

Maguire *et al* (1974) found that 51% of the medical in-patients with a psychiatric illness had no evidence of such in their medical notes. In another study, Knights & Folstein (1977) informed the medical staff that they were assessing recognition of psychiatric disorder as reported in the notes; even so the physicians failed to identify 37% of patients with probable cognitive disturbance and 35% of patients with high scores on the GHQ (Goldberg, 1972).

In Bridges & Goldberg's (1984) study of neurological patients, 72% of the patients with psychiatric disorder were not recognised by the neurologists, when assessed by reference to the notes. This very high figure was partly accounted for by the fact that patients from the neurological unit do not see it as appropriate for neurologists to ask about the emotional aspects of their disorders.

In the Oxford study (Feldman *et al*, 1987) house officers judged half of the patients with psychiatric disorder as being psychologically well, and missed two of the four patients with the most severe disorders.

Out-patients

In their study on the effects of counselling on the psychiatric morbidity associated with mastectomy, Maguire *et al* (1980) assessed 152 consecutive patients using the PSE (Wing *et al*, 1974). They found that 53% of their control group developed psychiatric problems following the operation, and of these the majority (78%) were not recognised by the surgeons as having such disturbances. Brody (1980) reported that physicians failed to recognise 34% of patients who had high GHQ scores, even when the patients had seen the same physician on at least three different occasions during a six month period and the physicians knew the reason for the study.

Reasons for failure of recognition and referral

Many reasons have been put forward to attempt to explain why detection of psychiatric disorders in the general hospital is poor: the poor quality of psychiatric teaching at undergraduate level; the high turnover of acutely ill patients on some medical wards; the emphasis in medical training on obtaining facts rather than listening to patients, and the extreme fatigue and exhaustion common in junior doctors which may make them less receptive to emotional cues (RCP/RCPsych, 1995).

Seltzer (1989) discovered that nursing staff often recognised emotional problems in their patients but thought that referral to a psychiatrist was unnecessary because the psychological disorder was mild or the patient would be upset by the referral. In addition, Rosser & Maguire (1982) discovered that physicians thought that if they enquired into their patients' psychological state it would somehow be damaging to their patients. The medical and nursing staff were observed to actively avoid questioning patients with serious illnesses, which paradoxically was found to contribute to the patients' 'hidden' psychiatric problems. Maguire and colleagues have been studying this area for many years and have described characteristic barriers of communication between doctors and their patients. The different kinds of barriers and ways of preventing them from developing are described in Chapter 6.

Diagnosis and classification

Diagnosis and classification of psychiatric disorders seen in the general hospital is not always easy, partly because classification systems derived from patients in psychiatric departments have been regarded as inappropriate for patients in general medical settings (Mayou & Hawton, 1986). Many authors have called for new, multi-axial classification systems relevant to primary care and the general hospital (Goldberg & Bridges, 1988; Jenkins *et al,* 1988), however, such systems have yet to be routinely used in clinical practice.

There are two types of classification. First, the standard psychiatric schema which have been refined over the years, and both DSM–IV (APA, 1994) and ICD–10 (WHO, 1992) have more detailed sections than their predecessors concerning psychiatric disorders in the general hospital. The second form of classification, specifically devised for the general hospital setting, is one which encompasses the relationship between psychiatric and physical disorders (e.g. Thomas, 1983).

Diagnostic classification systems used in general hospital settings

These have been reviewed by Cooper (1990) who assessed the classifications in DSM–III–R (APA, 1987) and ICD–10, commonly employed in liaison psychiatry. In the next section, the DSM–III–R classifications described by Cooper have been upgraded to the terms used in DSM–IV.

Organic psychiatric disorders

These disorders, principally dementia and delirium, are essentially similar in the different diagnostic systems and general psychiatrists will be familiar with their use. Cooper points out the important section in ICD–10 concerning symptomatic mental disorders. Section F06 includes mental disorders, other than dementia and delirium, that are due to brain damage and dysfunction and to physical disease. This section is equivalent to the section on 'mental disorders due to a general medical condition' in DSM–IV (293.0), but DSM–IV includes delirium. Section F06 includes organic delusional disorder (293.81; DSM–IV), organic hallucinosis (293.82; DSM–IV), organic affective disorder (293.83; DSM–IV), organic anxiety disorder (293.89; DSM–IV) and organic dissociative disorder (293.9; DSM–IV). Section F07 includes organic personality disorder (310.10; DSM–IV), post-encephalitic syndrome and post-concussional syndrome.

The essence of these disorders is the presumption that interference of cerebral function underlies the disorder. This may be deduced from the following four criteria:

Table 3.3 Classification of somatoform and dissociative disorders under two diagnostic systems (ICD–10 and DSM–IV)

ICD–10	ICD–10	DSM–IV
F44	**Dissociative (conversion) disorder**	**Dissociative disorder**
F44.0	Dissociative amnesia disorder	Dissociative amnesia
F44.1	Dissociative fugue	Dissociative fugue
F44.2	Dissociative stupor	Dissociative identity
F44.3	Trance and possession states disorder	disorder
F44.4	Dissociative convulsions (or deperson-	Depersonalisation disorder
	alisation neurosis)	
F44.5	Dissociative convulsions	
F44.6	Dissociative anaesthesia and sensory loss	
F45	**Somatoform disorders**	**Somatoform disorder**
F45.0	Somatoform disorder	Body dysmorphic disorder
F45.1	Undifferentiated somatoform disorder	Somatisation disorder
F45.2	Hypochondriacal disorder	Hypochondriasis
F45.3	Somatoform autonomic dysfunction:	
	45.31 Oesophagus and stomach	**Conversion disorder**
	45.32 Lower GI disorder	
	45.33 Respiratory system	
	45.34 Urogenital system	
F45.4	Persistent pain disorder	**Pain disorder**
F45.8–9	Other, unspecified somatoform	Undifferentiated
	disorder	somatoform disorder
F48	**Other neurotic disorders**	
F48.0	Neurasthenia (fatigue syndrome)	
F48.1	Depersonalisation-derealisation	
	syndrome	
F48.8	Other neurotic disorders	
F48.9	Neurotic disorder, Unspecified	

(1) evidence of cerebral disease, damage or dysfunction
(2) a temporal relationship between the development of such disease and the onset of the mental syndrome
(3) recovery from the mental disorder following removal or improvement of the underlying presumed course
(4) absence of evidence to suggest an alternative cause of the mental syndrome (such as family history, previous episodes and precipitating stress).

An essential differentiating feature from delirium is the clear consciousness that should be apparent on cognitive testing as part of the clinical assessment. This is also evident if the patient is re-interviewed following the episode as they will be able to recall all its details, unlike the delirious patient who is generally amnesic for much or all of the episode.

> The metabolic state of a patient on renal dialysis deteriorated after delayed and omitted dialysis. The patient developed a typical manic state in which he spent excessively on his credit card (several thousand pounds over one weekend). He was convinced that he was superior to all the doctors treating him, he became irritable, slept poorly but showed relatively little increased activity. On mental state examination he showed no clouding of consciousness and his short- and long-term memory were good. Sedation and the reinstitution of consistent dialysis led to a marked improvement in his mental state. There had been no previous episodes of mania in the patient's personal history or in his family history.

This picture would be diagnosed as organic mood disorder (F06.3 in ICD–10) and as mood disorder due to a general medical condition (293.83 in DSM–IV).

A patient who presents a similar clinical picture in relation to drugs is classified as F1x.5 (292.84; DSM–IV), where mood and/or psychiatric symptoms occur during or immediately after psychoactive substance use but where there is little or no clouding of consciousness and the symptoms may continue for weeks or months. This state must be differentiated from delirium associated with intoxication (F1x.0) or withdrawal (F1x.4) where clouding of consciousness will occur.

Psychiatric disorders presenting with physical symptoms

There are two important categories under this heading. The first refers to the very common presentation of anxiety and depression with physical symptoms. The second, less common but more complex, presentations are those of the somatoform and associated disorders (see Table 3.3). The latter disorders are discussed in detail by Bass & Murphy in Chapter 5. They form a relative minority of patients referred to liaison psychiatrists. Creed *et al* (1993) recorded 40 patients with somatoform disorders among 279 referrals to a liaison service excluding suicide attempt patients. Their importance lies in the difficulty of diagnosis and the enormous cost to the general hospital.

It is important to note that the individual somatoform disorders are largely differentiated by behavioural aspects and the different emphases of the different disorders are shown in Table 3.4. It is also important that patients diagnosed as having a somatoform disorder may also warrant an additional diagnosis of depressive disorder.

Mixed anxiety and depression

Within the general medical setting there are many patients who have mixed anxiety and depressive symptomatology which does not reach diagnostic thresholds for either condition separately. These conditions, however, are important because they are associated with somatic presentation and considerable disability (Katon & Roy-Burne, 1991).

The relevant diagnostic category is F41.2 (mixed anxiety and depressive disorders). This should be used if neither the anxiety nor depressive symptoms reach threshold for one of the disorders and if autonomic symptoms (tremor, palpitations, dry mouth, stomach churning) are present. If the anxiety and depressive symptoms follow on from a severe life event the diagnosis of adjustment disorder (F43.2) should be used.

The term 'adjustment disorder' is used correctly for those patients who have difficulty adjusting to their illness and develop clear symptoms of distress within 3 months of the onset or diagnosis. It is important to separate two areas of adjustment disorder – adjustment to illness (evident prior to the current hospitalisation), and adjustment to hospital and staff.

Popkin *et al* (1990) proposed a distinction between those patients whose adjustment disorder is attributable to their medical illness and those who concurrently develop an adjustment disorder in relation to other social stresses (e.g. marital, financial problems, death of close relatives etc.). The latter have been found to be important, Creed *et al* (1993) found that 33% of patients who had a significant psychological reaction to their physical illness also had marked social stresses.

Psychiatric disorders associated with physiological dysfunction

Both ICD–10 and DSM–IV include a range of eating (F50), sleep (F51) and sexual (F52) disorders. These are similar to those seen in general psychiatry, and will not be discussed further here (see Chapter 4).

Psychological and behavioural factors associated with physical disorders

Section F.54 (ICD–10) refers to the presence of psychological or behavioural influences which are thought to have played a major part in the aetiology of physical disorders (classified in other chapters of ICD–10). Thus a patient with asthma would be categorised under the chapter for respiratory disorders but the presence of an important psychological precipitant, which may be the reason that the psychiatrist is asked to see the patient, would be categorised under Section F54. The psychological features (e.g. worry, emotional conflict, apprehension) may be mild in themselves and not justify use of any other psychiatric diagnostic term in ICD–10. They may sufficiently exacerbate the physical condition to warrant some specific management strategies. The equivalent section in

Table 3.4 European Consultation Liaison Workgroup guidelines for the differential diagnosis of ICD–10 somatoform somatisation disorder, hypochondriacal disorder and somatoform autonomic dysfunction (Huyse *et al*, 1996)

	Somatisation disorder (45.0)	Hypochondriacal disorder (45.2)	Somatoform autonomic dysfunction (45.3)
Multiple, recurrent and frequently changing physical symptoms	+	–	–
Chronic symptoms (2 yrs+)	+	±	–
Refusal to accept doctors reassurance	+	+	±
Social impairment due to symptoms	+	±	±
Attention to an underlying disease	–	+	±
Ask for treatment of symptoms	+	–	±
Ask for treatment of the disease	–	+	±
Delusional content	–	–	–
Symptoms of autonomic arousal	–	–	+

+, present; -, absent; ±, either present or absent.

DSM–IV is called 'psychological factors affecting medical condition' (Section 316).

Rare psychiatric disorders of special interest in general medical care

These are important categories. Section F68 (ICD–10) refers to the elaboration of physical symptoms for psychological reasons. Disability may be greatly out of proportion to underlying physical illness, severity of symptoms may be exaggerated; the patient often expresses dissatisfaction with the results of treatment and investigations and behaves in such a way to increase the amount of personal attention received in wards or clinics (abnormal illness behaviour). Such syndromes may be clearly motivated by the possibility of financial compensation, but this is by no means always the case. There may be intentional production or feigning of symptoms or disabilities – factitious disorders (F68.1) (300.16 or 300.19; DSM–IV) which are described in Chapter 5.

Although cumbersome, the term 'elaboration of physical symptoms for psychological reasons' is a preferable, and less perjurious, term than 'hysterical overlay' or 'functional overlay'; terms previously employed by physicians and surgeons for this type of disorder.

Psychiatric disorders frequently encountered in accident and emergency departments

Adjustment disorders are important in this setting. ICD–10 separates off the most acute of the adjustment disorders when these are the result of overwhelming stress, such as disasters, earthquakes and multiple bereavements (acute stress reaction F43.0). Post-traumatic stress disorder is now increasingly recognised and included in both ICD–10 and DSM–IV classifications.

It is striking that there are no categories in either ICD–10 or DSM–IV describing deliberate self-harm (parasuicide). This is on the premise that those patients with psychiatric illness who harm themselves will be classified elsewhere.

Relationship between physical and psychiatric disorders

The second type of classification used in the general hospital ignores the psychiatric diagnosis and classifies the disorder according to the relationship between physical and psychological disorders. Thomas (1983) evolved a typology for liaison referrals which he used to categorise consecutive referrals from physicians and surgeons to his service, excluding parasuicide.

Coincidental physical and psychiatric disorder

This category refers to patients whose physical and psychiatric conditions are unrelated. A patient admitted to an orthopaedic ward with a fracture sustained through a fall on ice, was found to have a history of schizophrenia and was referred to the psychiatrist. There was no link between the fracture and the schizophrenic illness.

Patients are sometimes referred to the psychiatrist simply because a past history of psychotic illness comes to light either through routine history taking or because the patient is on neuroleptic medication. This may prompt the staff on the medical or surgical unit to request a psychiatric opinion for fear that the patient might react badly to some aspect of the routine medical/surgical care.

In other cases, the medical or surgical staff may sensibly wish to review the current dose of neuroleptic medication and ensure that the

Table 3.5 Classification of patients according to system of Thomas (1983)

	Thomas (1983) (*n*=300) %	Creed *et al* (1993) Out-patients (*n*=159) %	In-patients (*n*=120) %
Coincidental psychiatric disorder	14	21	8
Cerebral complications of physical disease	14	1	12
Abnormal behaviour producing physical illness	5	3	11
Psychological reaction to physical illness	32	26	32
Somatic presentation of psychiatric disorder	30	45	28
Psychosomatic disorders	–	1	–
No psychiatric disorder	5	3	–

schizophrenia is well controlled with adequate support in the community. Such steps will be regarded as good clinical practice, though the reason for admission (e.g. poorly controlled diabetes) may be quite unrelated to the well controlled schizophrenia.

Cerebral complications of physical disease or treatment

Almost all physical illnesses may present with psychological symptoms – a way of classifying the physical illnesses which lead to psychological complications is shown in Table 3.6 (for further details see Lishman, 1987). It is important for the liaison psychiatrist to review all diagnostic possibilities – both physical and psychiatric – when faced with a difficult diagnosis problem. Psychiatrists should not assume that the physician or surgeon has been able to satisfactorily exclude all possible physical illness as the cause of the symptom. For example, cancer may present with depression and the latter may present before the cancer is evident (Whitlock & Siskind, 1979). The psychiatrist should be particularly alert to a middle-aged or elderly male presenting with depression for the first time in his life without family history or other predisposing factors and without a precipitating life event. Weight loss might be assumed to be a symptom of depression – in fact it may be a symptom of the underlying cancer. Cancer of the head or the pancreas has a particular reputation of presenting in this way but many cancers present with psychological symptoms before physical effects are noticed (Whitlock & Siskind, 1979). The suicide rate for patients with cancer is increased relative to the general population, and it includes some patients whose depression has not been diagnosed.

The combination of physical and psychiatric disorders may also present a management problem leading to psychiatric referral. For example, delirium is often well recognised and managed solely by the physician; referral to the psychiatrist may occur if there is a diagnostic or management problem, for example in the elderly, where perceptual difficulties may be prominent. Patients with temporal lobe epilepsy may also be referred if psychiatric symptoms occur.

It is common for the psychiatrist to be asked to advise about the management of depression following a stroke (Starkstein & Robinson, 1989). Robinson & Price (1982) reported that 30–50% of patients became depressed following stroke and suggested that the primary aetiological agent was the brain lesion. Others have found lower rates of depression following stroke and found depression to be associated with previous psychiatric history and the extent of the disability (for a review see Mulley & House, 1995). Assessment of depression after stroke is difficult and a trial of antidepressants may be required.

Abnormal behaviour producing physical illness

In this section, the primary disorder is seen as psychological and the physical disease is secondary to this. Examples are alcohol misuse in liver disease, injection of heroin leading to septicaemia or heart disease, anorexia nervosa leading to hormonal and metabolic abnormality and deliberate paracetamol ingestion leading to liver disease. Such disorders are dealt with in Chapter 4.

Psychological reaction to physical illness/treatment

This category refers to patients who develop depression or anxiety as a psychological response to their physical illness or its treatment. Diseases which commonly lead to such reactions include cardiovascular disease, chronic lung disease, neoplastic conditions, haematological problems, neurological disorders and arthritic conditions (Katon & Sullivan, 1990). The history should make it quite clear that the patient's anxiety/depression commenced concurrently with an exacerbation of the physical condition or a realisation of its serious and disabling nature.

The psychological reactions to physical illness have been reviewed by Lloyd (1977), who delineates factors in the patient (personality traits, age, previous experience of illness), the illness (severity of disability, extent of hospital treatment and potential fatality) and the social environment and support network. Sensky (1990) emphasises the importance of cognitive factors and the potential that cognitive therapy may have to offer in this respect. Two important points must be made in relation to this category:

(1) The psychological reaction to the physical disease may not be a simple one-to-one relationship. Several studies have failed to demonstrate a clear correlation between severity of physical illness and depression, indicating that additional factors may need to be considered. The commonest are predisposition to develop depression (evident from family history and previous personal history of depression, childhood deprivation) and precipitation by recent life events which may be independent of the physical illness (e.g. bereavement/marital separation) or related to it (e.g. loss of job) (Creed, 1990).

(2) Patients with a chronic painful condition, e.g. arthritis, who become depressed may present with increasingly painful joints. In the absence of increased disease activity or joint damage it may become apparent that a lowered pain threshold as a result of depression is responsible. Such increasing pain therefore represents a form of somatisation – presentation of somatic symptoms (increased pain) as a manifestation of the underlying depression. It is important to remember that the process of somatisation is very common in those with physical illness (Bridges & Goldberg, 1984).

Somatic presentation of psychological disorders

These are dealt with in detail in Chapter 5.

Psychosomatic disorders

This disease category developed in relation to the work of American analysts in the 1950s and concerns seven chronic diseases: peptic ulcer, ulcerative colitis, asthma, rheumatoid arthritis, essential hypertension, hyperthyroidism and eczema (Alexander, 1950). Selected patients with these conditions were referred for psychoanalysis and made substantial improvements as a result of improved self-confidence and reduced anxiety after successful analysis. As a result, several aetiological theories of psychosomatic disease were developed concerning specific personality factors or specific underlying conflicts. Subsequent systematic research showed, however, that many patients with these conditions, e.g. asthma, did not have the specific personality factors or increased anxiety (Zeally *et al*, 1970).

These theories are often portrayed in a simplistic way and it is frequently overlooked that Alexander believed in a multi-factorial model of disease and regarded the underlying dynamic conflict as only one element in the development of disease.

It is likely that a patient referred to the psychiatrist with a raised level of anxiety will be classified into the category 'psychological reaction to physical illness'; appropriate if the patient has life threatening asthma

Table 3.6 Examples of physical illness leading to psychological complications

	Acute	Chronic
Intracranial: generalised	Encephalitis	General paralysis of the insane (GPI) Normal pressure hydro-cephalus
Intracranial: focal	Temporal lobe epilepsy	Tumour Cerebral abscess
Extracranial	Any acute infection, Endocrine abnormality etc.	Thyroid disease Cancer e.g. pancreas

which provokes anxiety. The alternative is that high anxiety levels are leading to severe breathing difficulties. If this is the main aetiological factor, the patient could be classified as 'somatic presentation of psychiatric disorder'. It is this subgroup of patients who may respond well if given treatment for their anxiety. In some cases of asthma, anxiety is best understood as one of several multi-factorial aetiological agents (allergic and infective aetiological factors may also be present in the same patient). It would be appropriate to classify such a patient under the psychosomatic category but such patients are rarely referred to psychiatrists. Those who are referred usually have anxiety as the predominant, if not the only, aetiological factor.

Clinical use of this classification system

The use of this classification system in three studies is illustrated in Tables 3.5 and 3.7. The pattern of referrals in the series reported by Thomas (1983) is similar to that of in-patient referrals to a liaison psychiatry service in other reports (Senksy *et al*, 1985; Creed *et al*, 1993). The pattern of referrals of medical out-patients was different, however, with more patients referred with somatic presentation of psychiatric disorder and fewer with cerebral complications of physical disease (Table 3.5).

A similar pattern was found (Senksy *et al*, 1985) (Table 3.7) when the psychiatrist changed from a consultation style to a liaison style service, there was an increase in the proportion of patients referred because of psychological reaction to physical illness and somatic presentation of physical illness, and a reduction of patients referred with cerebral complications of physical illness. Any senior registrar in liaison psychiatry who works closely with a particular unit may experience this change in the pattern of referrals.

Table 3.7 Referral patterns in two different types of liaison
service (from Sensky *et al*, 1985)

	Consultation (*n*=83)	Liaison (*n*=59)
Coincidental psychiatric disorder	29	12
Psychiatric (cerebral) complications of physical illness or treatment	22	5
Physical complications of psychiatric disorder	23	19
Psychological reaction to physical illness or treatment	24	37
Somatic presentation of psychiatric disorder	17	39
Psychosomatic disorder	0	0
No psychiatric disorder	0	0

Limitations of diagnostic systems in liaison psychiatry

To illustrate the limitations of the different diagnostic systems in liaison
psychiatry, five cases of depressive disorder will be discussed in detail.
In each case the following will be considered: the reason for referral,
ICD–10 diagnosis, classification according to Thomas, physical diagnosis,
and degree of abnormal illness behaviour. These are the first five headings
of the scheme outlined in Chapter 2. Although all the patients are
depressed, there are important differences in each case which are
summarised in Table 3.8.

Case 1

The first case illustrates depression secondary to a physical illness
(rheumatoid arthritis).

> A 51-year-old woman with rheumatoid arthritis required repeated
> admissions to the medical ward because of painful and swollen
> joints. She appeared sad and despondent on admission and was
> noted by the nurses to be solitary and, at times, tearful. A
> psychiatric opinion for advice on the management of her
> depression was requested. It transpired that she had been feeling
> persistently depressed for several months, with sleep disturbance,
> lethargy and anhedonia, poor appetite and weight loss of two
> stone. She had occasional suicidal ideas, especially in the context
> of marital conflicts. After three months of antidepressant treatment
> and marital therapy her depressive symptoms responded, she
> reported less joint pain, reduced her dose of analgesia and did not
> require further hospital admissions.

This patient was markedly depressed (BDI score of 27) and her joint pains reflected her depression. The Thomas classification was 'psychological reaction to physical illness'. There was evidence of abnormal illness behaviour in her physical disability, which was disproportionate to a joint disease and she persistently sought medical treatment – both abnormal illness behaviours reversed when the depression was treated.

Case 2

The second case illustrates depression as a psychological reaction to physical illness, which then leads to denial.

> A 43-year-old woman with a history of breast cancer became more and more depressed in the months post-mastectomy. She felt tired and withdrew from her family and friends. She experienced numerous pains, lost one stone in weight, which she interpreted as evidence of recurrence of the cancer. She could not look at her mastectomy scar and failed to attend follow-up appointments at the hospital. It had been recommended that she have a course of radiotherapy, but she did not attend as she did "not want to think about it" and thought that "the treatment was pointless". This negative attitude and failure to attend for treatment led to psychiatric referral, which confirmed the depressive illness.

This woman's body image problem (see Chapter 6) was a result of her depressive illness. She had been unable to accept her illness or adapt to the loss of her breast following surgery. She has been acting in a way to deny her illness by not attending appointments or being able to look at her mastectomy scar. Her abnormal illness behaviour (denial) placed her at serious risk of further complications. This is also a psychological reaction to physical illness, but it takes a different form from case 1.

Case 3

This case also has depressive disorder which, in the absence of physical disease, led to psychiatric referral because of diagnostic difficulties.

> A 47-year-old woman was referred with an 18 month history of abdominal pain for which no organic cause could be found. In the few weeks prior to the onset of her symptoms, her father died and her husband suffered a brain haemorrhage. Although her husband recovered and there was no evidence of a residual neurocognitive deficit, their marriage was unhappy as he had always been demanding and argumentative. Her illness served as a clear function of reducing the extent to which she could respond to her husband's unreasonable requests for attention and care. Over the 18 month period her abdominal pain had, at times, been very disabling and she had given up her job. She had lost her appetite

and one and a half stone in weight, she had constipation with occasional episodes of diarrhoea. Each morning she woke early because of the pain and both she and her husband were convinced that she had developed cancer. Her doctors, in spite of numerous negative investigations and trials of treatment for irritable bowel syndrome, did not make a satisfactory diagnosis. She was referred to the psychiatrist with the question "could depression be causing this pain and weight loss and bowel dysfunction?"

Treatment of the depressive illness with antidepressants, marital therapy and help with her husband's own depression led to a complete remission of all of her symptoms and her return to work.

This case of depression would be classified as somatic presentation of psychiatric disorder presenting as abdominal pain and weight loss, where no physical disease is present. Like case 1, the abnormal illness behaviours disappeared with treatment of the depression.

Case 4

In this case it is presumed that the cerebral damage as part of the stroke was involved in the aetiology of the patient's depression.

A 68-year-old man was referred because of slow recovery from a stroke and a report from the physiotherapists that he showed poor motivation for mobilisation and rehabilitation. Nothing in the family or past previous psychiatric history indicated that this patient was likely to develop a depressive illness. During the weeks following his severe stroke, despite moderate improvement in his speech and mobility, his mood deteriorated; he lost interest in food and activity, slept poorly and lost weight. He developed pronounced depressive ideation and repeatedly said that life was not worth living. At times he would throw himself from a chair onto the floor and would fall over even when being helped to walk by a physiotherapist. Rapid improvement followed treatment with antidepressants.

This patient would be classified as having a cerebral complication of physical illness causing his depressive illness.

Case 5

In the final case, the patient presents with a depressive illness which is secondary to an underlying occult carcinoma.

A 63-year-old man was referred, like case 3, because of depression, weight loss and abdominal pain. The surgeons had not been able to find any obvious cause for his abdominal pain but were impressed by his despondency and tearfulness – they felt he

Table 3.8 Five cases of patients with depressive illness

	Case 1	Case 2	Case 3	Case 4	Case 5
Reason for referral	Tears in the ward	Failure to attend out-patient dept	Abdominal pain – cause?	Post-stroke depression, slow rehabilitation	Depression and weight loss
Psychiatric diagnosis	Depression	Depression	Depression	Depression	Depression
Physical diagnosis	Rheumatoid arthritis	Cancer	None	Cerebrovascular accident	Cancer
Abnormal illness behaviour	Excessive complaints of pain	Denial and refusal of treatment	Reduced activity, belief she had cancer	Falling and being unable to mobilise	None
Thomas Classification	Psychological reaction to physical illness	Psychological reaction to physical illness	Somatic presentation of psychiatric disorder	Cerebral complication of physical illness	Cerebral complication of physical illness

required psychiatric treatment. The psychiatrist agreed he had depressive disorder (Beck Score 29) but noted the absence of predisposing or precipitating factors for the depression and could find no explanation for the abdominal pain. Antidepressants were started but by the time of the second appointment the pain was worse and a report blood screen indicated a greatly raised erythrocyte sedimentation rate. Further investigations discovered a cancer of the pancreas which had not been visible on the previous scan.

This case was classified as cerebral complication of organic disease – the depression is assumed to be related to the cancer in this way.

These five cases of depression are all quite different, and the diagnosis of depressive disorder alone would not do justice to any of them. Standard psychiatric classification is inadequate in liaison psychiatry and other dimensions of behaviour and physical status are required before a case can be formulated and appropriate management outlined.

Summary

Diagnosis and classification is difficult in liaison psychiatry. The more detailed subclassifications included in ICD–10 are a significant improvement on the previous systems. Thomas' classification system (1983), however, remains a useful method of categorising patients in the general hospital as it contains a description of the relationship between physical diagnosis and psychiatric status. A multi-dimensional approach should be favoured which includes psychiatric diagnosis, physical diagnosis, classification according to Thomas, and a measure of abnormal illness behaviour.

References

Alexander, F. (1950) *Psychosomatic Medicine.* New York: Norton.

American Psychiatric Association (1987) *Diagnostic and Statistical Manual of Mental Disorders* (3rd edn, revised) (DSM–III–R). Washington, DC: APA.

—— (1994) *Diagnostic and Statistical Manual of Mental Disorders* (4th edn) (DSM–IV). Washington, DC: APA.

Bridges, K. W. & Goldberg, D. P. (1984) Psychiatric illness in in-patients with neurological disorders: patients' views on discussion of emotional problems with neurologists. *British Medical Journal,* **289,** 656–658.

Brody, D. S. (1980) Physician recognition of behavioural, psychological and social aspects of medical care. *Archives of Internal Medicine,* **140,** 1286–1289.

Bukberg, J., Penman, D. & Holland, J. C. (1984) Depression in hospitalized cancer patients. *Psychosomatic Medicine,* **46,** 199–212.

Cavanaugh, S. V. A. (1983) The prevalence of emotional and cognitive dysfunction in a general medical population: Using the MMSE, GHQ, and BDI. *General Hospital Psychiatry,* **5**, 15–24.

Cooper, J. E. (1990) The classification of mental disorders for use in general medical settings. In *Psychological Disorders in General Medical Settings* (eds N. Sartorius, D. Goldberg, G. de Girolamo, *et al*), pp. 49–59. Toronto: WHO and Hogrefe & Huber.

Creed, F. (1990) Psychological disorders in rheumatoid arthritis: A growing consensus? *Annals of the Rheumatic Disease,* **49**, 808–812.

——, Murphy, S. & Jayson, M. V. (1990) Measurement of psychiatric disorder in rheumatoid arthritis. *Journal of Psychosomatic Research,* **34**, 79–87.

——, Guthrie, E., Black, D., *et al* (1993) Psychiatric referrals within the general hospital: comparison with referrals to general practitioners. *British Journal of Psychiatry,* **162**, 204–211.

Feldman, E., Mayou, R., Hawton, K., *et al* (1987) Psychiatric disorder in medical in-patients. *Quarterly Journal of Medicine,* **63**, 405–412.

Goldberg, D. P. (1972) *The Detection of Psychiatric Illness by Questionnaire* (GHQ). Oxford: Oxford University Press.

—— (1986) Use of the General Health Questionnaire in clinical work. *British Medical Journal,* **293,** 1188–1189.

——, Eastwood, M. R., Kedwood, H. B., *et al* (1970) A Standardised Psychiatric Interview for use in community surveys. *British Journal of Preventative and Social Medicine,* **24**, 18–23.

—— & Bridges, K. W. (1988) Somatic presentations of psychiatric illness in primary care settings. *Journal of Psychosomatic Research,* **32**, 137–144.

Graham, J. R. (1987) *The MMPI. A Practical Guide* (2nd edn). New York: Oxford University Press.

House, A. (1988) Mood disorders in the physically ill – problems of definition and measurement. *Journal of Psychosomatic Research,* **32,** 345–353.

Jenkins, P. & Jamil, N. (1994) The need for specialist services for mood disorders in the medically ill. In *Liaison Psychiatry – Defining Needs and Planning Services* (eds S. Benjamin, A. House & P. Jenkins), pp. 24–33. London: Gaskell.

Jenkins, R., Smeeton, N. & Shepherd, M. (1988) Classification of mental disorder in primary care. *Psychological Medicine,* **12**, 1–59

Katon, W. & Sullivan, M. P. (1990) Depression and chronic medical illness. *Journal of Clinical Psychiatry,* **51**(Suppl. 6), 3–11.

—— & Roy-Burne, P. (1991) Mixed anxiety and depression. *Journal of Abnormal Psychology,* **100**, 337–345.

Knights, E. B. & Folstein, M. F. (1977) Unsuspected emotional and cognitive disturbance in medical patients. *Annals of Internal Medicine,* **87**, 723–724.

Lishman, W. A. (1987) *Organic Psychiatry* (2nd edn). Oxford: Blackwell Scientific Publications.

Lloyd, G. G. (1977) Psychological reactions to physical illness. *British Journal of Hospital Medicine,* **18**, 354–358.

Maguire, G. P., Julier, D. L., Hawton, K. E., *et al* (1974) Psychiatric morbidity and referral on two general medical wards. *British Medical Journal,* i, 268–270.

——, Tait, A., Brooks, M., *et al* (1980) Effect of counselling on the psychiatric morbidity associated with mastectomy. *British Medical Journal,* **182**, 1454–1456.

Mayou, R. & Hawton, K. (1986) Psychiatric disorder in the general hospital. *British Journal of Psychiatry*, **149**, 172–190.

Meakin, C. J. (1992) Screening for depression in the medically ill. *British Journal of Psychiatry*, **160**, 212–216.

Moffic, H. S. & Paykel, E. S. (1975) Depression in medical in-patients. *British Journal of Psychiatry*, **125**, 346–353.

Mulley, G. P. & House, A. (1995) Stroke. In *Psychiatric Aspects of Physical Disease* (eds A. House, R. Mayou & C. Mallinson), pp. 31–38. London: Royal College of Physicians/Royal College of Psychiatrists.

Pincus, T., Callahan, L. F., Bradley, L. A., *et al* (1986) Elevated MMPI scores for hypochondriasis, depression and hysteria in patients with rheumatoid arthritis reflects disease rather than psychological status. *Arthritis and Rheumatism*, **29**, 1456–1466.

Popkin, M. K., Callies, A. L., Coloh, E. A., *et al* (1990) Adjustment disorder in medically ill in-patients referred for consultation in a university hospital. *Psychosomatics*, **31**, 410–414.

Robinson, R. G. & Price, T. R. (1982) Post-stroke depressive disorders: A follow-up study of 103 patients. *Stroke*, **13**, 635–641.

Rosser, J. E. & Maguire, P. (1982) Dilemmas in general practice: the care of the cancer patient. *Social Science and Medicine*, **16**, 315–322.

Royal College of Physicians/Royal College of Psychiatrists (1995) *The Psychological Care of Medical Patients: Recognition of Need and Service Provision*. CR 35. London: RCP/RCPsych.

Seltzer, A. (1989) Prevalence, detection and referral of psychiatric morbidity in general medical patients. *Journal of the Royal Society of Medicine*, **82**, 410–412.

Sensky, T. (1990) Patients' reactions to illness. Cognitive factors determine responses and are amenable to treatment. *British Medical Journal*, **300**, 622–623.

——, Greer, S., Cundy, T., *et al* (1985) Referrals to psychiatrists in a general hospital – comparison of two methods of liaison psychiatry: preliminary communication. *Journal of Royal Society of Medicine*, **78**, 463–468.

Starkstein, S. E. & Robinson, R. G. (1989) Affective disorders and cerebral vascular disease. *British Journal of Psychiatry*, **154**, 170–182.

Thomas, C. J. (1983) Referrals to British liaison service. *Health Trends*, **15**, 61–64.

Van Hemert, A. M., Hengeveld, M. W., Bolk, J. H., *et al* (1993) Psychiatric disorders in relation to medical illness among patients of a general medical outpatient clinic. *Psychological Medicine*, **23**, 167–173.

Whitlock, F. A. & Siskind, M. (1979) Depression and cancer: a follow–up study. *Psychological Medicine*, **9**, 747–752.

Wing, J. K., Cooper, J. E. & Sartorius, N. (1974) *The Measurement and Classification of Psychiatric Symptoms*. London: Cambridge University Press.

World Health Organization (1992) *The Tenth Revision of the International Classification of Diseases and Related Health Problems* (ICD–10). Geneva: WHO.

Zeally, A. K., Aitken, R. C. B. & Rosenthal, S. V. (1970) Asthma: A psycho-physiological investigation. *Proceedings of the Royal Society of Medicine*, **64**, 825–829.

4 Deliberate self-harm, substance misuse and eating disorders

Michael Sharpe & Robert Peveler

Deliberate self-harm • Alcohol misuse • Drug misuse • Eating disorders

---

This chapter describes the presentation and management of deliberate self-harm, alcohol and drug misuse and eating disorders in the general hospital. The liaison psychiatrist may be asked to advise about the management of such patients. In some cases this will be an assessment before discharge, in others the management will require psychiatric in-patient or out-patient treatment, but in the most complicated cases the psychiatrist will have to be involved in the management of patients in the general hospital, advising the medical and nursing staff and being directly involved in the care of the patient over a period of time. Such management includes the suicidal patient who wishes to discharge themselves, alcohol or opiate withdrawal in the general hospital or eating disorders in conjunction with a serious physical illness, e.g. diabetes. These are complicated and difficult management problems; it is important that the trainee psychiatrist always involves the consultant psychiatrist and, if necessary, the regional expert for alcohol and substance misuse.

Deliberate self-harm

Deliberate self-harm (DSH) is a very common reason for attendance at casualty departments and for admission to general medical wards. There are over 100 000 admissions per annum in England and Wales; it is the most common reason for admission for women under 65 and the second most common reason for men (after ischaemic heart disease) (Hawton & Catalan, 1987). DSH therefore constitutes a major part of the workload of emergency medicine and is the 'bread and butter' of most liaison psychiatry services. The medical management of DSH is likely to require the involvement of the liaison psychiatrist because of the association with psychiatric disorder and the acknowledged risk of subsequent suicide.

Each hospital should have a stated policy regarding the management of DSH (DHSS, 1984; RCPsych, 1994). It has become accepted that patient assessment may be performed by non-psychiatrists, such as nurses and medical house-staff as long as they have received appropriate training and receive supervision from a psychiatrist. This policy derives from reports that assessments by medical staff (Gardner *et al*, 1982), social workers (Gibbons *et al*, 1978) and nurses (Hawton *et al*, 1981, 1987) are as satisfactory as those performed by psychiatrists and the repetition rate is no different. However, there is evidence that assessments by junior medical staff are not always accurate (Black & Creed, 1988) and there is particular concern about patients discharged from the A & E department without psychiatric assessment (Owens & Jones, 1988; Owens *et al*, 1991).

Presentation

For a patient presenting to A & E, the history of DSH is usually obvious and is the presenting complaint. In many cases either the patient or another person has called a doctor or ambulance soon after the act. The initial history may be inaccurate, however, with either a gross underestimate or exaggeration of the amount of drugs taken. Occasionally patients may present with the medical complications of DSH without giving a history of self-harm.

Methods

The most common method of deliberate self-harm is overdosing with easily available 'over the counter' tablets, particularly analgesics. The use of paracetamol (alone and in combination preparations) has become increasingly common in recent years, especially in young self-poisoners (Hawton & Fagg, 1992). It is important to detect its use because of the (treatable) risk of severe liver damage. Other drugs commonly taken in overdose include antidepressants and other psychotropic agents. Alcohol ingestion is commonly associated with the act. Deliberate self-harm may also result from self-laceration, jumping, hanging and attempted gassing with carbon monoxide from a car exhaust.

Box 4.1   Features in the history of DSH indicating high suicidal intent

Evidence of planning for suicide
Act performed when alone
Act unlikely to be discovered
Precautions to prevent discovery
All available drugs taken
Patient expected act to be fatal
Suicide note written
Patient made no effort to get help

Detection

Occasionally patients arriving unconscious or with unexplained severe illness may subsequently be discovered to have taken an overdose. The psychiatrist may also be asked to see patients in whom the physicians suspect an act of DSH which the patient denies. The best method of detection is a careful history of the sequence of events in the days prior to admission, together with an interview of an informant.

Management

The aims of management are to:

(1) minimise harm resulting from the act
(2) manage ongoing suicide risk
(3) detect and manage major psychiatric disorder
(4) offer help with associated psychosocial problems.

The first aim is principally the responsibility of the physician. The others are shared between physician and psychiatrist.

Psychiatric assessment may be delayed until the patient is alert. The interview should be conducted in private. A standard psychiatric history is suitable, but with an emphasis on the events leading up to the act of DSH, and on current problems. An interview with a relative or 'significant other' can yield useful information about the patient's personality, recent mental state, and the significance of the act of DSH.

Suicide risk

It is essential to assess the risk of suicide. While the majority of patients attending hospital following an episode of DSH do not repeat the act an important minority do. In the 12 months after initial presentation 15% will have re-presented with DSH, and approximately 1% will have committed suicide (Buglass & Horton, 1974). *The Health of the Nation* (Department of Health, 1992) specified reduction of suicide as one of the targets for mental health. If a large district general hospital sees approximately 800 DSH patients per annum from a catchment area of approximately half a million, and if 1.5% of these 800 patients commit suicide in the following year, this is 12 patients. The expected suicide rate for the half million population is approximately 40. This means that about one-quarter of all patients who eventually commit suicide in a 12 month period will have been seen at a general hospital following deliberate self-harm during the previous 12 months. This is why it is so important to detect suicide risk in this population.

The first step in assessing risk is to determine the degree of suicidal intent associated with the presenting act. Intent is best established by means of a detailed history of the events leading up to the DSH. Questions to include in the history are listed in Box 4.1. The interviewing psychiatrist may find it helpful to quantify the degree of intent by completing the Beck Suicidal Intent Scale (Beck, 1974). The next step in assessment is to estimate the risk of suicide based on the patient's personal characteristics and life situation. Increased risk is associated with the factors shown in Box 4.2 (Hawton & Catalan, 1987). Hopelessness is a particularly important predictor (Beck *et al*, 1985). The third step is to assess the patient's expressed current intent. Do they still feel the same? What would make them try again? Do they feel hopeless? Have circumstances changed since they made their attempt?

Finally, an overall clinical judgement concerning the short-term risk of suicide must be made on the basis of all these factors. An estimate may also be made of longer-term risk although this is more difficult to evaluate. The conclusion reached will be the major factor in determining immediate management.

It is important that a clear and detailed description of the patient's suicidal risk is recorded in the notes – this is not always done (Black & Creed, 1988) but it can contribute to the *Health of the Nation* target of reduction of suicide (RCP/RCPsych, 1995).

Psychiatric disorder

While symptoms of emotional distress are almost universal in patients admitted to hospital following DSH, symptoms amounting to a depressive illness occur in approximately 60% of patients (Newson-Smith & Hirsch, 1979; Urwin & Gibbons, 1979), but only 5–10% have psychiatric disorder of sufficient severity and persistence to require psychiatric in-patient treatment (Hawton & Catalan, 1987). The most common psychiatric diagnoses in this group are adjustment reaction, anxiety and depressive disorder. The majority of these disorders are transient and are resolved within 3 months (Newson-Smith & Hirsch, 1979). They are associated with acute stress, especially crises in relationships. A substantial proportion of patients also have personality disorders.

Box 4.2   Patient characteristics associated with increased risk of suicide

Older age
Male gender
Unemployed
Living alone
Poor physical and mental health
History of previous suicide attempts

A small but important minority will have more severe psychiatric disorders, most notably marked depressive disorder with pronounced hopelessness and suicidal ideation and psychotic disorders. These are usually readily apparent from the assessment interview. They may be less obvious, however, and should be suspected when the nature of the deliberate self-harm indicates marked suicidal intent and appears to be disproportionate to the patient's current social problems. Substance misuse is relatively common in this group and should be assessed as described later in this chapter.

Psychosocial problems

While the precipitating event is usually a crisis in an important relationship, other more chronic difficulties are frequently present (Bancroft *et al*, 1977; Farmer & Creed, 1986). Common areas of difficulty are listed in Box 4.3.

Treatment

A sympathetic and complete psychiatric assessment can itself be therapeutic by allowing the patient to show distress and helping them to clarify problems. After this initial assessment several treatment options are available. These include discharge to the general practitioner (GP), out-patient follow-up, and psychiatric admission. For an impulsive overdose of low suicidal intent the GP may be best placed to follow-up the patient. If the patient has serious psychiatric disorder or is considered at high risk of suicide more intensive intervention is indicated.

> A 21-year-old woman was admitted to a medical ward after taking 20 aspirin tablets in front of her boyfriend after seeing him with another woman. She was treated with gastric lavage. She subsequently regarded the overdose as 'stupid' and there was no evidence of continuing suicidal intent. It was clear that her action had been impulsive and there was no planned suicidal intent. Initial assessment did not reveal evidence of psychiatric disorder but, on further enquiry, she revealed a problem of severe debt as well as that of her boyfriend seeing another woman. Her boyfriend visited her while she was on the ward and there was a stated reconciliation. She was discharged from hospital after discussion with her GP, who agreed to see her after a few days. In addition, a referral to social services was made.

Out-patient treatment

Psychiatric out-patient follow-up may be required where the patient is considered to be at risk of suicide or has a psychiatric disorder but psychiatric admission is not considered appropriate. This practice varies widely between services (House *et al*, 1992). The principal difficulty with this form of management is the low compliance rate. However, attendance may be improved by giving an early appointment, usually within a week of discharge, preferably with the person who performed the initial assessment, and for the follow-up to occur in the general hospital rather than in a psychiatric unit.

Patients considered to be at risk of suicide should be seen frequently and the suicide risk regularly reviewed. Specific psychological or pharmacological treatment may also be given (see below).

Psychiatric admission

Psychiatric admission is required only for a small minority of patients. It is indicated by the presence of severe psychiatric disorder (particularly depression and schizophrenia), for patients who have become exhausted during a personal crisis, and for patients who present an immediate suicide risk. Admission for suicide risk should be considered when there is no other satisfactory form of management (such as the patient being looked after by a relative). The use of the Mental Health Act in such situations may occasionally be necessary.

> A 60-year-old man was admitted after trying to hang himself. At initial assessment he offered no clear explanation for his carefully planned attempt. Further psychiatric assessment revealed that he had been motivated by a desire to escape unidentified 'persecutors'. He was placed under Section 2 of the Mental Health Act and transferred to the psychiatric in-patient unit for further assessment of a possible paranoid psychosis.

Specific psychological interventions

The main approaches used are brief focused problem solving therapy and cognitive–behavioural psychotherapy (Hawton *et al*, 1989). There have been five UK trials of psychiatric intervention following DSH (Chowdhury *et al*, 1973; Gibbons *et al*, 1978; Hawton *et al*, 1981, 1987; Salkovskis *et al*, 1990). These have been reviewed by House *et al* (1992), who concluded that all the samples studied are too small to show a statistically significant reduction of repetition rate. In order to show a statistically significant reduction in repetition rate from 15% to 10%, for example, approximately 1000 patients in a randomised controlled trial are required. However, more recent studies of patients at high risk of repetition (having already taken at least two overdoses) suggest that this type of treatment can reduce the repetition rate (Salkovskis *et al*, 1990).

These forms of treatment do improve psychological and social well-being in a proportion of patients and four of the five studies mentioned above showed significant improvement in social problems. Psychological treatments may be conducted in the psychiatric clinic or patients may be referred to other agencies for counselling (e.g. Relate).

Use of medication

The prescription of psychotropic medication is not commonly indicated in the management of this group. Before prescribing, the psychiatrist should have evidence of persistent psychiatric disorder. The decision to prescribe should be based on a careful appraisal of the relative risks and benefits. If a drug is prescribed, relative safety in overdose is an important consideration. Alternatively, arrangements may be made for the patient to receive only small quantities of the drug at a time.

Other forms of follow-up

Depending on local facilities and the patient's particular problems, other forms of follow-up may be appropriate. The GP has an important role and should be informed of the patient's discharge, in advance if possible. A referral to social services may be appropriate where financial, housing and employment issues are prominent. Some liaison services offer open telephone access to patients seen after DSH. These may be used months or years after the initial contact.

Mental Health Act

Doctors have a duty to detain a person who they consider to be at immediate and grave risk of suicide. Doctors using reasonable physical force or medication to achieve this end will be protected by common law. In cases where more than brief restraint is required, or where transfer to a psychiatric ward for further assessment is required, Section 2 or 4 of the Mental Health Act should be used. Section 5 of the Act may be used to hold a person in a medical bed, pending transfer to a psychiatric unit.

Box 4.3   Common problem areas in patients presenting with deliberate self-harm

Relationship with partner or family
Employment or studies
Finances
Housing
Legal
Drugs and alcohol
Physical illness
Social isolation

Special problems

Self-cutting

A minority of DSH patients present with self-inflicted lacerations. The suicidal intent associated with the act should be assessed as described above. The motivations associated with this form of DSH are varied, however, and the act may function as 'tension relief', or expression of anger, rather than wish to die. Some patients may present repeatedly with superficial lacerations. This behaviour is difficult to modify and may be associated with severe personality problems. It is also associated with eating disorder, substance misuse, and childhood physical or sexual abuse.

If the patient wants help to gain control of the self-cutting, cognitive–behavioural techniques are probably the most useful and are described by Hawton (1990). More severe or disfiguring laceration is less common and is more likely to be associated with severe psychiatric disorder which may require management in its own right.

Use of violent methods

Violent methods are employed by a minority of patients and are more common in young males. These methods include hanging, shooting, jumping and attempted drowning. They are associated with a relatively high risk of subsequent suicide.

The chronic repeater

Patients who repeatedly present with DSH become a cause of concern, and frequently of exasperation, to those involved in their care. While such behaviours frequently represent a maladaptive response to stress in a person with severe personality disorder, it should be remembered that this type of patient has a relatively high risk of completed suicide. The liaison psychiatrist has an important role in such cases. Negative staff attitudes may become particularly pronounced and a mutually hostile relationship can develop between casualty staff and patient. Intervention should be directed at helping the staff to be neither over-attentive nor punitive. Supportive psychotherapy for the patient may be arranged on a regular basis, and not contingent on acts of DSH. It may also be useful to 'demedicalise' the distress by arranging for this supportive therapy to take place away from the general hospital.

Summary

Deliberate self-harm is a common reason for medical admission. Patients presenting with DSH are often disliked by medical and nursing staff. The assessment of persisting suicidal intent is essential, as is the detection of major psychiatric disorder which occurs in the minority of patients. Urgent psychiatric treatment may be required. Even when no urgent treatment is indicated the provision of help with the patient's psychological and social problems is desirable and may reduce the risk of repetition.

Alcohol misuse

Substance misuse is prevalent among general hospital patients, often goes undetected, and is an important contributory factor to physical ill-health. The substance most commonly misused is alcohol. The misuse of other drugs is an increasingly important cause of medical admission, however, especially when they are taken intravenously. The psychiatrist working in the general hospital therefore needs to have a high index of suspicion that alcohol or drug misuse may be contributing to a patient's illness, and to be aware of clues which may assist in the diagnosis of misuse. He also needs to be skilled in the management of chronic dependence on, and withdrawal from, addictive substances.

Substance dependence may be distinguished from substance misuse (Box 4.4). Persons who are not dependent on a substance may still suffer problems directly resulting from its misuse. These problems may be physical, psychological or social. Such persons may be regarded as problem users, or in the case of alcohol, problem drinkers.

The great majority of adults drink alcohol. The average alcohol consumption of men in the UK is estimated to be 20 units (a unit is a half-pint of beer, glass of wine or single measure of spirits) per week, and 10 units for women. The issue of whether or not there are safe upper limits for alcohol intake has been widely debated; the agreed acceptable limits were 21 units per week for men and 14 units for women until very recently when they were changed by the current government to 28 units per week for men and 21 units for women (Inter-Departmental Working Group, Department of Health, 1995). This change has been widely criticised in medical circles (Edwards, 1996). Alcohol intake is highest among young adult men, but is increasing among young women.

Prevalence of problem drinking in the general hospital

An informative account of alcohol problems in the general hospital is provided by Lloyd (1991). Approximately one-quarter of male medical admissions in the UK may be regarded as problem drinkers (Lloyd *et al*, 1982; Feldman *et al*, 1987). The group at highest risk is young male patients admitted to surgical, medical or orthopaedic wards (Barrison *et al*, 1982). The prevalence of problem drinking among female patients is lower, probably reflecting both lower consumption and greater unwillingness to admit to an alcohol problem.

Box 4.4 DSM–IV criteria for substance dependence and abuse

Substance dependence (key features)

A maladaptive pattern of substance use, leading to clinically significant impairment of distress, as manifested by three (or more) of the following:

(1) tolerance
(2) withdrawal
(3) the substance is often taken in larger amounts or over a longer period than was intended
(4) there is a persistent desire or unsuccessful effort to cut down or control substance use
(5) a great deal of time is spent in activities necessary to obtain the substance or recover from its effects
(6) important social, occupational, or recreational activities are given up or reduced because of substance use
(7) substance use is continued despite knowledge of having a persistent or recurrent physical or psychological problem that is likely to have been caused or exacerbated by the substance

Specify if with or without physiological dependence (i.e. either item (1) or (2) is present)

Substance abuse (key features)

A maladaptive pattern of substance use leading to clinically significant impairment or distress, as manifested by one (or more) of the following within a 12 month period:

(1) recurrent substance use resulting in failure to fulfil major role obligations at work, school or home
(2) recurrent substance abuse which is physically hazardous
(3) recurrent substance-related legal problems
(4) continued substance abuse despite persistent or recurrent social or interpersonal problems caused by the abuse

The symptoms have never met the criteria for substance dependence

---

There are several reasons why people admitted to hospital may be problem drinkers. Because problem drinking is prevalent in the population it is also common in persons admitted to hospital. In a number of patients, however, chronic heavy alcohol misuse has been an important cause of the physical disease that has led to admission. Patients may also be admitted to hospital because of the effects of acute intoxication with alcohol, or the effects of acute withdrawal.

**Box 4.5 Physical complications of excessive alcohol
consumption**

Gastrointestinal tract
    Gastritis and peptic ulceration; cirrhosis and carcinoma of
    the liver; oesophageal varices; pancreatitis; Mallory-Weiss
    syndrome
Nervous system
    Peripheral neuropathy; cerebellar degeneration; seizures;
    demyelination of the corpus callosum, optic tracts and
    cerebellar peduncles (rare); head injury; subdural haema-
    toma; dementia
Cardiovascular system
    Hypertension; stroke; cardiomyopathy
Reproductive system
    Impotence; infertility; foetal alcohol syndrome

Presentation

Alcohol has deleterious effects on many body systems, both by its toxic
effect and as a result of protein and vitamin deficiency (Box 4.5). The
most common associations are with gastrointestinal problems, cirrhosis
of the liver and injuries. Excessive drinking by pregnant women may
harm the unborn foetus, leading in severe cases to foetal alcohol
syndrome. Injuries to children may occur as a consequence of their
parents' heavy drinking.

Intoxication and overdose

The acute effects of alcohol intoxication are well known and may lead
to hospital attendance directly because of the physical consequences, or
indirectly because of its effect on behaviour (Lishman, 1990). Although
intoxication initially produces feelings of relaxation and mild euphoria,
at higher doses the sedative effects become more prominent. The patient
becomes uncoordinated and ataxic, and their speech becomes slurred.
Performance is impaired and seizure threshold lowered. Unconsciousness
occurs when the blood alcohol concentration rises to 300 mg per 100 ml
or more. Severely intoxicated patients smell strongly of alcohol, appear
ataxic and may be disinhibited or violent. Patients who have been involved
in road traffic accidents and fights are frequently intoxicated and alcohol
ingestion is frequently associated with acts of deliberate self-harm.

Withdrawal

It is not uncommon for alcohol withdrawal symptoms to occur in patients
admitted for elective surgery, typically in fit young men undergoing

orthopaedic procedures. Alcohol withdrawal is also an important differential diagnosis in cases of post-operative delirium, made more difficult because symptoms may initially be masked by anaesthetic drugs, and because an adequate pre-operative drinking history is rarely taken. An important clue lies in the time course between admission and onset of delirium – this is usually 2 days.

Delirium tremens occurs less often than uncomplicated alcohol withdrawal, but any patient consuming half a bottle of spirits or more per day is at risk. This delirium is characterised by disorientation, hallucinations and autonomic hyperactivity. Insomnia, tremor, sweaty palms, tachycardia and hypokalaemia are prodromal features which may serve to alert the clinician (Chick, 1989). Convulsions can occur in association with alcohol withdrawal.

Wernicke–Korsakoff syndrome

This is an acute encephalopathy which occurs in the chronically alcohol dependent, usually in the context of withdrawal. It is associated with thiamine deficiency. The encephalopathy presents with the signs of delirium with impairment of consciousness and disorientation, but in addition there is evidence of ataxia and opthalmoplegia. It can progress to Korsakoff's psychosis, a chronic organic brain syndrome characterised by severe and disabling memory impairment (Victor & Collins, 1971).

Detection

Detection of an alcohol problem is easy if the patient has presented acutely intoxicated, or with a physical illness that is clearly related to heavy drinking, such as alcoholic cirrhosis of the liver. In other instances the relevance of alcohol may be less obvious. The best way to detect alcohol related problems is to take a careful history. Studies have shown that junior medical staff record an adequate drinking history in only about half the patients they assess (Barrison *et al*, 1980).

It is also possible to screen medical populations for problem drinking using 'pencil and paper' instruments. The best known are the Cage Questionnaire (see Box 4.6), and the brief version of the Michigan Alcohol Screening Test (MAST; Pokorney *et al*, 1972).

Physical examination may reveal evidence of the stigmata of chronic alcohol misuse (liver disease, hepatic enlargement and cerebellar signs). Laboratory investigations which may aid the detection of excessive alcohol use include the mean red cell volume (MCV), gamma-glutamyl transpeptidase (γ-GT) and aspartate transaminase (AST) (Skinner *et al*, 1986). While blood alcohol concentration may be assessed directly or from analysis of urine, a breathalyser will give an estimate of the current blood alcohol level and is available in most casualty departments.

Management

If an alcohol problem is suspected a detailed drinking history and description of the current pattern of alcohol consumption should always be obtained (see Box 4.7) and followed up by a physical examination.

Problem drinking

It has been suggested that doctors fail to detect alcohol-related problems because they believe that there is little they can do to help patients cut down their intake. In fact there is evidence that early recognition of problem drinking, followed by simple advice and brief follow-up has a high success rate (Chick *et al*, 1985). More intensive follow-up may have impressive results, including significantly less time off work, less hospitalisation and reduced mortality (Kristensson *et al*, 1983).

Acute intoxication

The management of the acutely intoxicated patient is based on the principle of harm minimisation: there is no specific form of treatment which can accelerate the process of recovery. The patient should be provided with a suitable environment in which to recover from their intoxicated state. Violent behaviour should be managed with appropriate restraint, and every effort taken to minimise the risk to the patient of accidental injury. Maintenance of adequate fluid and food intake is important, and the small risk of other associated causes of delirium (hypoglycaemia, head injury) should be considered.

Acute withdrawal

The management of alcohol withdrawal in the dependent patient is a greater challenge. Withdrawal symptoms are most appropriately treated with a benzodiazepine such as chlordiazepoxide (initially at a dose of 10–20 mg, 6–8 hourly, increasing as required). The dose should be gradually tapered over the course of 4–5 days, or sooner, as symptoms abate. Maintenance of adequate food and fluid intake is essential, and parenteral fluid administration may occasionally be required. It is usual

---

Box 4.6　The 'CAGE' questionnaire

Have you tried to **C**ut down on your drinking?
Have you felt **A**nnoyed by someone criticising your drinking?
Have you felt **G**uilty about your drinking?
Do you take a drink first thing in the morning? (**E**ye-opener)

Subjects are 'CAGE-positive' if they answer yes to 2 or more items

---

Box 4.7 Assessment of alcohol misuse

Do you ever drink alcohol? If yes, how often?
What time of day do you have a drink?
What types of drinks do you have? (Beer, cider (need to know
brands to estimate strength), wine, sherry/port, spirits)
How much of each do you usually have?
What is the most that you drink in a day?
On how many days in the week do you not drink?
Has there been a time in the past when you have drunk more
    heavily than this?
Have you ever lost a job or suffered an injury through drinking?
Have you suffered any health problems from drinking?
What is your partner's view of your drinking? (needs
    independent confirmation)

---

to give oral multi-vitamin supplements, although these may not always be
well absorbed in patients with gastroenterological complications. The
use of a benzodiazepine lessens the risk of seizures, but if seizures do
occur then an anticonvulsant drug (e.g. phenytoin) should be given. If
sedation with chlordiazepoxide proves insufficient, haloperidol or
droperidol may be administered. Parenteral thiamine prevents the
development of Wernicke-Korsakoff syndrome.

> A 48-year-old academic was admitted after a fit. On assessment he
> was tremulous and disorientated. After a negative medical
> assessment the liaison psychiatrist was called. Review of the
> history using an informant revealed that the patient was drinking
> a bottle of whisky each day, but had stopped 2 days previously.
> Acute alcohol withdrawal was diagnosed and he was treated with
> intravenous fluid, thiamine and chlordiazepoxide. After counselling
> about his alcohol intake he agreed to attend an out-patient
> programme to help him remain abstinent.

Special problems

Chronic dependence

After the acute medical or psychiatric problem has been treated the
psychiatrist will be expected to help with management of the longer-term
problem. Clear educational advice about safe limits and the consequences
of exceeding these should be given, and backed up with information
about clinics and self-help organisations such as Alcoholics Anonymous.
If alerted by the hospital, the GP can play an important role in long-term
follow-up. If available, specialist alcohol treatment units may offer
admission or out-patient treatment.

Wernicke–Korsakoff syndrome

If this syndrome is suspected the management is similar to that of delirium tremens, with the important addition of large doses of intravenous thiamine. This should be given urgently. Failure to treat with thiamine may result in the development of Korsakoff's psychosis or even death.

Summary

Alcohol problems are the most common drug related problem in the medical setting. It is important that detection is improved as early advice and treatment can lead to substantial recovery in many cases.

Drug misuse

The term 'drug' is used to refer to a disparate group of psychoactive substances. Their use varies considerably according to fashion and availability. Drug misuse of all kinds has been increasing over the past 20 years (Royal College of Psychiatrists, 1987). The most widely used drug is cannabis, although the taking of amphetamines and LSD is also relatively common. Drugs that have enjoyed a recent increase in use include 'Ecstasy' (3, 4-methylenedioxymethylamphetamine, MDMA), ketamine and cocaine. While chronic opiate misuse is relatively uncommon, it has been estimated that 1% of young adult males use opiates at least occasionally (Department of Health, 1991).

Presentation

Most people who misuse illegal drugs understandably avoid contact with statutory agencies. They are unlikely therefore to attend hospitals and if they do will conceal their substance misuse. Some drug misusers will attend casualty departments in the hope of obtaining drugs, to seek attention for complications of drug misuse, or for treatment of unrelated illness. The complications of misuse include intoxication, withdrawal and associated diseases. Drug misusers are more likely to be encountered in inner city casualty departments. In one study 400 drug dependent patients were identified among casualty department attenders in London during a one month period (Ghodse, 1977). Out of 1000 attenders at an A & E department, 18.3% had drug related problems (Ghodse, 1981).

Intoxication and overdose

The user of any of the substances mentioned in this section may present to hospital in a state of acute intoxication because they are insensible, distressed, or unwell with physical disease.

Box 4.8   Opiate withdrawal syndrome

History of opiate use
Restlessness and insomnia
Myalgia
Sweating
Abdominal pain, vomiting and diarrhoea
Dilated pupils
Tachycardia
Pilo-erection and running nose and eyes

Both sedatives and opiates are dangerous in overdose and may be fatal. Some drugs (notably LSD, amphetamines, cocaine and cannabis) may produce an acute psychosis with delusions and hallucinations. This is usually, but not always, short-lived. There are special hazards associated with the use of Ecstasy (MDMA). Acute anxiety and paranoid psychotic reactions may occur, and death has been reported (Henry, 1992). Opiates and sedatives cause impaired consciousness and respiratory depression.

Withdrawal

Withdrawal syndromes are most marked in persons dependent on opiate and barbiturate drugs. The opiate withdrawal syndrome usually commences six to eight hours after the last dose, peaks at one to two days, and then wanes over a further seven to ten days. The symptoms and signs are listed in Box 4.8. The symptoms of barbiturate withdrawal are similar to those of withdrawal from alcohol. There is a significant risk of convulsions. Benzodiazepines are also known to cause a characteristic withdrawal syndrome, often presenting as severe anxiety with pronounced autonomic symptoms, impairment of cognitive function and sometimes perceptual disturbances.

Withdrawal syndromes may result from alterations to a long-standing drug regimen by medical staff who may not recognise the possibility of dependence.

Associated disease

Repeated intravenous injection of any substance (cocaine, opiates, amphetamine are commonly used by this route) may give rise to phlebitis, abscess formation and septicaemia. The major hazard of repeated intravenous administration of drugs, especially when adequate sterile techniques are not used, is the transmission of pathogenic viruses such as HIV (see below) and hepatitis B. Cocaine can also cause arrhythmias and sudden death, and its peripheral vasoconstricting effect can lead to gangrene of the nasal mucosa, resulting eventually in perforation of the nasal septum.

Solvent misuse is widespread among teenage children and may occasionally give rise to physical complications. The most serious of these are cardiac arrhythmias, myocardial infarction, cardiomyopathy, and death. Chronic central nervous system damage can also result (Sourindrihn, 1985).

Detection

Drug misuse should be suspected when a person presents to casualty with a specific request for drugs that are commonly misused, or with abnormal behaviour. Questions to include in the history are listed in Box 4.9. A urine drug screen may provide additional information. Dependence may also come to light during a hospital admission with evidence of withdrawal, or requests for drugs. Physical examination may reveal needle marks, phlebitis and facial marks from glue sniffing, constricted or dilated pupils, drowsiness or restlessness. The appropriate urine or blood sample will confirm intoxication. Drug misuse may also come to light when the patient presents with physical complications such as septicaemia, hepatitis or AIDS.

Management

In most instances the chief role of the psychiatrist is to assist in the correct diagnosis of a drug-related problem, to advise on immediate management, and to facilitate further referral to specialist agencies when appropriate. The Home Office and local registers will provide information about whether or not addicted patients seeking drugs (principally opiates) are also receiving them from other sources.

The aims of management are to:

(1) deal with intoxication and physical disease
(2) limit further harm from drug use ('harm minimisation')
(3) help the addict reduce or cease use where possible.

Intoxication

The management of severe intoxication is principally the task of the physician. The person who presents intoxicated with drugs may (as with the person intoxicated with alcohol) need a suitable place to recover. Some drugs may be reversed with specific antagonists (e.g. naloxone for opiates). The risk of respiratory depression and other physical complications should be considered. The liaison psychiatrist is likely to be called on once the person has recovered to provide further assessment and management of the substance misuse.

Planned withdrawal

It is sometimes difficult for physicians and surgeons to accept that little can be done to modify the behaviour of drug misusers who do not wish to relinquish their habit and the psychiatrist may need to help others to seek an outcome other than immediate abstinence. It may also be necessary to remind other doctors that they have a legal obligation to notify addicts using opiates and cocaine to the Home Office Drugs branch. In one study, only half of A & E attenders with opiate addiction were known to the Home Office (Ghodse, 1977). Details of the procedure are given in the British National Formulary.

The symptoms of opiate withdrawal can be managed most easily with oral methadone in gradually reducing doses, although diphenoxylate may be adequate when they are mild. Clonidine is also effective. The psychiatrist should be prepared to advise the physician and, if necessary, to supervise an in-patient withdrawal from opiates. This may be done in conjunction with the substance misuse consultant, who is well placed to arrange follow-up of the patient after detoxification, as well as provide help on the ward.

Harm minimisation

There is a strong case for considering objectives other than abstinence in the management of drug misusers who do not wish to cease use (Strang & Farrell, 1992). The aim of harm minimisation is to reduce the risk of physical harm to the user and the community. Specific aims include the encouragement of oral rather than intravenous administration, avoidance of needle sharing and the provision of information about the transmission

---

Box 4.9 Assessment of drug misuse

Do you ever use illicit/recreational/street drugs? If yes, how often?

What drugs do you use?

What routes do you use (ever intravenously)?

How much of each do you usually have?

What is the most that you use in a day?

On how many days in the week do you not use drugs?

Has there been a time in the past when you have used more heavily than this?

Have you ever lost a job or had problems with the law because of drug use?

Have you suffered any health problems from drug use (hepatitis B, HIV)?

What is your partner's view of your drug use? (needs independent confirmation)

of HIV and hepatitis B. In addition to education about these topics, where local policy permits, supplies of clean needles and syringes may be provided.

Special problems

Pain management in opiate dependent patients

Special difficulties arise when painful physical illness occurs in opiate misusing or dependent patients. The consulting psychiatrist may often be asked for an opinion about whether or not it is wise to give opiate analgesics to such patients. In general, a period of painful physical illness is not the best time to commence a withdrawal programme for such an individual. It is better to give adequate analgesia to relieve symptoms while the patient is in hospital, and return to the issue of habit change once this period is over. Opiate dependent patients may need considerably higher doses of opiate analgesics than are usually required to relieve pain.

> A 27-year-old woman was admitted to an orthopaedic ward after suffering a fractured pelvis in a road traffic accident. The liaison psychiatrist was called after she demanded large amounts of morphine for pain relief. On direct questioning she admitted to being addicted to heroin. The Home Office was informed. The psychiatrist negotiated with the staff for her to have larger than usual amounts of opiates for pain relief. She subsequently saw a drug counsellor and, although not wishing to give up her habit or to have a test for HIV, agreed to maintain contact with a drug misuse clinic, to transfer to oral methadone and to adopt safer sexual practices.

Acute drug related psychosis

This may respond to acute treatment with an antipsychotic drug such as chlorpromazine. Admission to a psychiatric ward for management and observation may sometimes be necessary.

HIV positive drug users

The diagnosis of HIV-infection depends on the detection of antibodies which appear 4–16 weeks after infection. Testing should only be done with the individual's consent and in the context of appropriate counselling. Individuals with antibodies are regarded as 'seropositive'. Several tests are needed to ensure the accuracy of the result, and a negative test cannot exclude recent infection. Education in the principles of harm minimisation is particularly important for seropositive persons and should include information, and if necessary ongoing counselling, concerning the hazards of needle sharing and sexual intercourse (Department of Health, 1989). Sexual promiscuity in such people should be taken very seriously, although the precise management of this problem will depend on the individual case.

Summary

Drug misuse is becoming more and more prevalent in the general population. The management of an acutely intoxicated patient is primarily a medical responsibility. The liaison psychiatrist should be able to offer advice about detoxification and to act as a link person for the patient to gain access to appropriate services when discharged from hospital

Eating disorders

Eating disorders (anorexia nervosa, bulimia nervosa and over-eating) are not usually the sole reason for admission to a general hospital, but they may complicate the management of other conditions, such as diabetes mellitus, and cause great concern among medical and nursing staff.

DSM–IV describes diagnostic criteria for these conditions (see Box 4.10). It is estimated that 1% of adolescent girls and young adult women may meet the criteria for anorexia nervosa, and 2–3% for bulimia nervosa. However, less severe disturbances of eating habits are much more common (Fairburn & Hope, 1988).

Presentation

An eating disorder may be an incidental finding in a patient presenting with another condition. It may, however, be the cause of physical abnormalities, or may underlie medically unexplained symptoms such as weight loss, vomiting, abdominal or menstrual complaints.

Detection

Patients are characteristically reluctant to admit to having an eating problem, and hence careful enquiry may be necessary. Questions to include are shown in Box 4.11. Young women are the highest risk group and may be found in several different medical specialities. The liaison psychiatrist should have a high index of suspicion when apparently healthy young women of normal or low weight present with medically unexplained symptoms. The most common presentations are to gynaecology for investigation of infertility, gastroenterology for investigation of abdominal pain, vomiting or diarrhoea, and orthopaedics with bone damage resulting from osteoporosis. Eating disorders may also

---

Box 4.10   DSM–IV diagnostic criteria for eating disorders

Anorexia nervosa (key features):
(1) Refusal to maintain body weight over a minimum normal weight for age and height, e.g. weight loss, leading to body weight 15% below that expected, or failure to make the expected weight gain during a period of growth leading to body weight 15% below that expected
(2) Intense fear of gaining weight or becoming fat even though underweight
(3) Disturbance in the way in which body weight, size or shape is experienced
(4) The absence of at least three consecutive menstrual cycles

Bulimia nervosa (key features):
(1) Recurrent episodes of binge eating
(2) Recurrent behaviour to prevent weight gain such as self-induced vomiting, use of laxatives or diuretics, strict dieting, fasting, or vigorous exercise
(3) A minimum average of two binge eating episodes a week for at least three months
(4) Self-evaluation is unduly influenced by body shape and weight
(5) The disturbance does not occur exclusively during episodes of anorexia nervosa

---

present as problems in the management of physical disease such as that of 'brittle diabetes'.

Anorexia nervosa

The most obvious pathological effect of anorexia nervosa is low weight. Other metabolic changes may occur as a consequence of restricted food intake. These include leucopenia, lymphocytosis, and hypoplasia of bone marrow. Hypokalaemic alkalosis is common among patients who vomit or misuse laxatives and may cause electro-cardiographic abnormalities, such as flattening or inversion of the T wave, ST segment depression and QT interval lengthening. Thyroxine (T4) levels are usually low in the underweight patient, and serum T3 levels also decrease. Amenorrhoea is accompanied by abnormal luteinizing hormone, follicle-stimulating hormone and oestrogen secretion. Reversible bone loss may result in pathological fractures in vulnerable bones such as the vertebrae.

Bulimia nervosa

Physical signs may also be seen among patients with bulimia nervosa, but are more variable in their occurrence. The bulimic patient is usually within the normal weight range. In a proportion of patients there is pronounced hypertrophy of the salivary glands, particularly the parotids, which is usually bilateral and painless. Patients who vomit repeatedly suffer erosion of dental enamel, and if they use their fingers to stimulate the gag reflex they may have a characteristic callus on the dorsum of the hand. Hypokalaemic alkalosis and raised serum amylase levels occur. Menstrual irregularities are common.

Management

The assessment of the patient with an eating disorder hinges upon a thorough history of eating habits, weight control behaviour, and attitudes to shape and weight (see Box 4.11). The diagnosis is usually made from the history but physical examination is required to assess the severity of physical complications. The patient should also be assessed for depressive disorder, suicide risk and substance misuse. The aims of management are to:

(1) reverse physical disturbance, including low weight
(2) normalise eating behaviour
(3) correct the attitudinal disturbance underlying the abnormal eating
(4) manage depressive disorder and suicide risk.

Physical disease and starvation

The management of physical disease is principally the responsibility of the physician. It has been suggested that anorexia nervosa may be mistakenly diagnosed in patients with wasting diseases (Jenkins *et al*, 1988). In practice this is unlikely if a careful history is taken, and it is ascertained that weight loss has been self-induced. If this feature is not elicited, then a thorough search for the physical causes of weight loss should be undertaken.

The treatment of eating disorders has been reviewed in detail by Garner & Garfinkel (1985). The initial aim for the treatment of anorexia nervosa is restoration of adequate nutrition. However, there are two main difficulties with this. The first is that resumption of an adequate diet runs counter to the patient's wishes and beliefs. The second is that the patient may initially be physically unable to consume normal amounts of food. Re-feeding can be accomplished in a general medical ward but this takes time (often 3 months or more), and it is important that at least some of the nursing staff are familiar with the problems which may be encountered. Patients may often use devious tactics to avoid an adequate food intake, such as hiding food or surreptitious vomiting. The liaison psychiatrist may play a useful role in supporting and advising nurses in such situations.

Treatment of abnormal beliefs and behaviour

The first psychotherapeutic task is to form a therapeutic relationship with the patient. Education about the nature and consequences of the eating disorder may then be given. Only after this should attempts be made to persuade the patient to normalise her eating behaviour. The prominent role of patient beliefs in the perpetuation of eating disorders makes psychotherapeutic intervention necessary. Cognitive–behavioural psychotherapy is well suited to this task and is usually conducted on an out-patient basis. There is good evidence for its efficacy in bulimia nervosa. The best form of psychological management of anorexia nervosa is less clear (see Garner & Garfinkel, 1985).

Drug treatments

Drugs do not have a major role to play in the management of eating disorders. In bulimia, antidepressant drugs reduce the frequency of overeating, but do not affect patients' disturbed attitudes to shape and weight or their extreme attempts to diet. There is no clear role for drug therapy in anorexia. Antidepressants may be considered when severe and persistent depression occurs in association with an eating disorder (see below).

Special problems

Coexisting physical disease

The presence of an eating disorder in a patient with diabetes mellitus provides a good example of the way in which problem behaviours may complicate the management of physical illness. The medical condition is worsened with impaired glycaemia control, and an increased risk of the physical complications of diabetes. The diabetes in turn provides the patient with a further potential method of weight control by reducing their intake of insulin. Furthermore, this particular combination of disorders is not rare, affecting up to 5% of young females with diabetes (Fairburn *et al*, 1991). An eating disorder should be considered, therefore, in any young female diabetic in whom difficulties with glycaemia control are encountered. Screening questions such as those listed in Box 4.11 may be helpful.

If the patient has anorexia nervosa, admission to hospital for weight restoration and glycaemia control may be indicated. If the weight loss is not too severe, out-patient management may be possible. It should be remembered that insulin is necessary for weight gain and that patients seeking to avoid weight gain may not only avoid eating, but may also deliberately omit doses of insulin. Treatment of the eating disorder is usually based on a cognitive–behavioural approach (Hawton *et al*, 1989).

Box 4.11   Assessment of eating habits and attitudes

Describe a typical day's food intake, beginning with breakfast
   and ending with the last food before bedtime
Do you have control over your eating?
Do you diet to control your body weight or shape?
Do you do anything else to control your body weight or shape
   (vomit, take laxatives or other drugs, exercise intensively)?
How do you feel about your current weight?
What weight would you like to be?
How would you feel if you gained 2lbs in weight?
How would you feel if you lost 2lbs in weight?
How important to you is your weight and shape?

This may be carried out by any adequately trained therapist, but it is desirable for the therapist to also have a good working knowledge of the medical management of diabetes.

The conflicting management imperatives of diabetes and eating disorder may necessitate modifications to the standard treatment of both (Peveler & Fairburn, 1989, 1992). Treatment of the eating disorder (which emphasises relinquishing strict dieting, and flexibility in eating habits) may require relaxation of 'tight' glycaemia control, and changes in eating habits and weight during the course of treatment will necessitate continual adjustments in diet and insulin dose. Hence, there is a need for effective liaison between psychiatrist and physician. Indeed if the psychiatrist is sufficiently well versed in the management of diabetes it may be advantageous for him to take over the management of the diabetes while treating the eating disorder.

> A 17-year-old girl of normal weight admitted with 'brittle' diabetes mellitus was found to be repeatedly inducing vomiting and omitting doses of insulin. The liaison psychiatrist found that she also engaged in binge eating of large quantities of food and had a strong desire to be thin. After stabilising her diabetes as an in-patient she was seen in the liaison psychiatry clinic where she received cognitive–behavioural psychotherapy from the psychiatrist who, with the advice of the diabetologist, also prescribed her insulin.

Severe weight loss

Low weight may occasionally lead to death by starvation or as a result of accident. The aim of management is to improve nutrition to reverse physiological and psychological changes. In most cases admission is to a psychiatric ward for intensive nursing and a behavioural programme of re-feeding. Occasionally starvation is so severe that admission to a medical ward is required for intravenous correction of electrolyte disturbance or intravenous feeding.

Depressive disorder

The effects of starvation may mimic the symptoms and signs of severe depressive disorder. However, if there is pervasive low mood and hopelessness the coexisting depressive disorder may require treatment. Care should be taken with the use of antidepressant drugs in the severely malnourished and lower doses may be required.

Suicide risk

There is a greatly increased risk of suicide in anorexia nervosa. While many patients with chronic anorexia suffer personality disturbances and may present a chronic risk of suicide, admission to a psychiatric unit may be required at times of increased intent. Intent should be assessed in the usual way (see below).

Use of the Mental Health Act

In cases of life threatening anorexia nervosa the use of compulsion may be considered. This may involve detention in hospital under the Mental Health Act, and the use of nasogastric or intravenous feeding. The Act is rarely used as it is counter to the longer-term aim of improving the patient's self-control over abnormal eating habits. However, its use should be seriously considered when there is a clear threat to life. This may occur as a consequence of severe weight loss or severe depression. Psychological treatment is not possible where starvation or depressive disorder, or both, cause cognitive impairment. Compulsion may also be needed to manage suicide risk.

Summary

To a greater or lesser extent many admissions to a general hospital can be said to be a consequence of a person's behaviour. Behaviour can lead to medical admission either by producing symptoms or by giving rise to actual physical disease. Behavioural problems will also occur in patients admitted with unrelated physical disease. Although not all such patients will meet criteria for psychiatric disorder, the liaison psychiatrist has an important role in the detecting and management of these problem behaviours.

References

American Psychiatric Association (1994) *Diagnostic and Statistical Manual* (4th edn) (DSM–IV). Washington, DC: APA.

Bancroft, J., Skrimshire, A., Casson, J., *et al* (1977) People who deliberately poison or injure themselves: their problems and their contacts with helping agencies. *Psychological Medicine*, **7**, 289–303.

Barrison, I. G., Viola, L. & Murray-Lyon, I. M. (1980) Do housemen take an adequate drinking history? *British Medical Journal*, **281**, 1040.

——, ——, Mumford, J., *et al* (1982) Detecting excessive drinking amongst admissions to a general hospital. *Health Trends*, **14**, 80–83.

Beck, A. T., Schuyler, D. & Herman, J. (1974) Development of Suicidal Intent Scales. In *The Prediction of Suicide* (eds A. T. Beck, H. L. P. Resnik & D. J. Lettiere). Maryland.

——, Steer, R. A., Kovacs, M., *et al* (1985) Hopelessness and eventual suicide: a 10 year prospective study of patients hospitalized with suicidal ideation. *American Journal of Psychiatry*, **145**, 559–563.

Black, D. & Creed, F. (1988) Assessment of self-poisoning by psychiatrists and junior medical staff. *Journal of the Royal Society of Medicine*, **88**, 97–99.

Buglass, D. & Horton, J. (1974) A scale for predicting subsequent suicidal behaviour. *British Journal of Psychiatry*, **124**, 573–578.

Chick, J. (1989) Delerium tremens. *British Medical Journal*, **298**, 3–4.

——, Lloyd, G. & Crombie, E. (1985) Counselling problem drinkers in medical wards: a controlled study. *British Medical Journal*, **290**, 965–967.

Chowdhury, N., Hicks, R. C. & Kreitman, N. (1973) Evaluation of an after-care service for parasuicide (attempted suicide) patients. *Social Psychiatry*, **8**, 67–81.

Department of Health (1989) *AIDS and Drug Misuse, Part 2*. London: HMSO.

—— (1992) *The Health of the Nation*. London: HMSO.

—— (1991) *Drug Misuse and Dependence*. London: HMSO.

Department of Health and Social Security (1984) *The Management of Deliberate Self-Harm*, (Hn [84] 25). London: DHSS.

Edwards, G. (1996) Sensible drinking. *British Medical Journal*, **312**, 1.

Fairburn, C. G. & Hope, R. A. (1988) Disorders of eating and weight. In *Companion to Psychiatric Studies* (eds R. A. Kendell & A. K. Zealley). Edinburgh: Churchill Livingstone.

——, Peveler, R. C., Davies, B., *et al* (1991) Eating disorders in young adults with insulin dependent diabetes mellitus; a controlled study. *British Medical Journal*, **303**, 17–20.

Farmer, R. & Creed, F. H. (1986) Hostility and deliberate self-poisoning. *British Journal of Medical Psychology*, **59**, 311–316.

Feldman, E., Mayou, R., Hawton, K., *et al* (1987) Psychiatric disorder in medical in-patients. *Quarterly Journal of Medicine*, **63**, 405–412.

Garner, D. M. & Garfinkel, P. E. (1985) *Handbook of Psychotherapy for Anorexia Nervosa and Bulimia*. New York: Guilford Press.

Gardner, R., Hanka, R., Roberts, S., *et al* (1982) Psychological and social evaluation in cases of deliberate self-poisoning seen in an accident department. *British Medical Journal*, **284**, 491–493.

Gibbons, J. S., Butler, J., Urwin, P., *et al* (1978) Evaluation of a social work service for self-poisoning patients. *British Journal of Psychiatry*, **133**, 111–118.

Ghodse, H. (1977) Casualty departments and the monitoring of drug dependence. *British Medical Journal*, *i*, 1381–1382.

—— (1981) Drug related problems in London accident and emergency departments: a 12 month survey. *Lancet*, *ii*, 859–862.

Hawton, K. E. (1990) Self-cutting: can it be prevented? In *Dilemmas and Difficulties in the Management of Psychiatric Patients* (eds K. E. Hawton & P. J. Cowan), pp. 91–103. Oxford: Oxford University Press.

——, Bancroft, J., Catalan, J., *et al* (1981) Domiciliary and out-patient treatment of self-poisoning patients by medical and non-medical staff. *Psychological Medicine*, **11**, 169–177.

—— & Catalan, J. (1987) *Attempted Suicide: A Practical Guide to its Nature and Management* (2nd edn). Oxford: Oxford University Press.

——, McKeown, S., Day, A., *et al* (1987) Evaluation of out-patient counselling compared with general practitioner care following overdoses. *Psychological Medicine*, **17**, 751–761.

——, Salkovskis, P. M., Kirk, J., *et al* (1989) *Cognitive–Behaviour Therapy for Psychiatric Problems: A Practical Guide*. Oxford: Oxford University Press.

—— & Fagg, J. (1992) Trends in deliberate self-poisoning and self-injury in Oxford, 1976–90. *British Medical Journal*, **304**, 1409–1411.

Henry, J. A. (1992) Ecstasy and the dance of death. *British Medical Journal*, **305**, 5–6.

House, A., Owens, D. & Storer, D. (1992) Psycho-social intervention following attempted suicide: is there a case for better services? *International Review of Psychiatry*, **4**, 15–22.

Inter-Departmental Working Group (1995) *Sensible Drinking*. London: Department of Health.

Jenkins, A. P., Treasure, J. & Thompson, R. P. H. (1988) Crohn's disease presenting as anorexia nervosa. *British Medical Journal*, **296**, 699–700.

Kristensson, H., Ohlin, H., Hulten-Nosslin, M. B., *et al* (1983) Identification and intervention of heavy drinking in middle aged men: results and follow-up of 24–60 months of long-term study with randomised controls. *Alcoholism*, **7**, 203–209.

Lishman, A. (1990) Alcohol and the brain. *British Journal of Psychiatry*, **156**, 635–644.

Lloyd, G. (ed) (1991) Alcohol and drug related problems. In *Textbook of General Hospital Psychiatry*. Edinburgh: Churchill Livingstone.

——, Chick, J. & Crombie, E. (1982) Screening for problem drinkers among medical in-patients. *Drug and Alcohol Dependence*, **10**, 355–359.

Newson-Smith, J. G. & Hirsch, S. R. (1979) Psychiatric symptoms in self-poisoning patients. *Psychological Medicine*, **9**, 501–507.

Owens, D. W. & Jones, S. J. (1988) The accident and emergency department management of deliberate self-poisoning. *British Journal of Psychiatry*, **152**, 830–833.

——, Dennis, M., Jones, S., *et al* (1991) Self-poisoning patients discharged from accident and emergency: risk factors and outcome. *Journal of the Royal College of Physicians of London*, **25**, 218–222.

Peveler, R. C. & Fairburn, C. G. (1989) Anorexia nervosa in association with diabetes melitus – A cognitive–behavioural approach to treatment. *Behaviour Research and Therapy*, **27**, 95–99.

—— & —— (1992) The treatment of bulimia nervosa in patients with diabetes mellitus. *International Journal of Eating Disorders*, **11**, 45–53.

Pokorney, A. D., Miller, B. A. & Kaplan, H. B. (1972) The brief MAST: a shortened version of the Michigan Alcoholism Screening Test. *American Journal of Psychiatry*, **129**, 342–345.

Royal College of Physicians & Royal College of Psychiatrists (1995) *The Psychological Care of Medical Patients: Recognition of Need and Service Provision*. London: RCP/RCPsych.

Royal College of Psychiatrists (1987) *Drug Scenes*. London: Gaskell.

—— (1994) *General Hospital Management of Adult Deliberate Self-Harm*. Council Report CR32. London: RCP.

Salkovskis, P. M., Atha, C. & Storer, D. (1990) Cognitive–behavioural problem solving in the treatment of patients who repeatedly attempt suicide: a controlled trial. *British Journal of Psychiatry*, **157**, 871–876.

Skinner, H. A., Holt, S., Sheu, W. J., *et al* (1986) Clinical versus laboratory detection of alcohol abuse: the alcohol clinical index. *British Medical Journal*, **292**, 1703–1708.

Sourindrihn, I. (1985) Solvent misuse. *British Medical Journal*, **290**, 94–95.

Strang, J. & Farrell, M. (1992) Harm minimization for drug misusers. *British Medical Journal*, **304**, 1127–1128.

Urwin, P. & Gibbons, J. G. (1979) Psychiatric diagnosis in self-poisoning patients. *Psychological Medicine*, **9**, 501–507.

Victor, M. & Collins, G. H. (1971) *The Wernicke–Korsakoff syndrome*. Oxford: Blackwell.

5 Somatisation, somatoform disorders and factitious illness

Christopher Bass & Michael Murphy

Operational definitions of somatisation • Prevalence of somatisation • Aetiology and pathogenesis • Somatoform disorders • Assessment of the somatising patient • Management • Factitious disorders

---

The term somatisation is used by clinicians and researchers to refer to a variety of phenomena and processes. Its meaning thus differs according to author and school of thought. In general, however, it refers to the presentation of bodily complaints assumed to arise from psychological disturbance but which are attributed by the patient to organic disease.

The development of bodily discomfort, such as pain and fatigue, appears to be a universal response to environmental stress and psychological trauma. Recently some researchers have contrasted somatisation with 'psychologisation', i.e. the attribution of distress to pathological mental processes. It has been suggested that psychologisation is a more recent phenomenon and occurs less frequently than somatisation (Goldberg & Bridges, 1988). Psychologisation may be more prevalent in developed countries with plentiful supplies of doctors, and in cultures where mental illness and emotional problems are less stigmatised. The popular dissemination of psychoanalytic ideas has undoubtedly contributed to this cultural trend.

Predictable differences between psychologisers and somatisers have been identified in primary care. Somatisers report less depression, lower levels of social dissatisfaction and are likely to have a less sympathetic attitude towards mental illness (Bridges *et al*, 1991). They are also more likely than psychologisers to have a history of in-patient medical care.

Somatisation is better understood as a process rather than an entity, and it should therefore not be regarded as a diagnosis. The term should not be confused with the somatoform disorders (including somatisation disorder), which are a group of psychiatric syndromes described in DSM–III and IV and ICD–10. Somatisation is common to these disorders, but most patients who somatise do not fulfil the criteria for these diagnoses. In this chapter we will discuss somatisation as well as the somatoform and related disorders, and reference to both DSM–IV (American Psychiatric Association, 1994) and ICD–10 (World Health Organization, 1992) will be made.

Operational definitions of somatisation

The term is sometimes used broadly to refer to the somatic symptoms that accompany diagnosable psychiatric disorders. It is common for anxiety disorders and mood disorders to present with physical complaints, particularly in general practice. In a study of patients in primary care Bridges & Goldberg (1985) defined somatisation in the following terms:

(1) consulting behaviour – the patient seeks medical help for somatic rather than psychosocial problems
(2) attribution – the patient attributes these symptoms to a physical cause
(3) psychiatric illness – the patient satisfies criteria for a DSM–III diagnosis of mental disorder
(4) response to intervention – treatment of the psychiatric disorder would cause the somatic manifestations either to disappear or revert to pre-illness levels.

These criteria are useful in research studies of acute and sub-acute somatisers in primary care settings, but criteria (3) and (4) do not always apply in practice, particularly in patients whose symptoms are chronic.

'True' and 'facultative' somatisation

In a study of all new inceptions of illness in primary care, Bridges & Goldberg (1985) found that the majority of patients with psychiatric illness (including adjustment reactions) presented with somatic rather than psychological complaints. Although they had somatised when consulting their GP, many of these patients readily changed their attributions when interviewed by the research psychiatrist. These patients may have complained of physical symptoms initially because they believed they were more likely to be taken seriously by their GP. However, they were able to acknowledge their psychosocial problems and recognise the link between these problems and their symptoms when interviewed by the psychiatrist. Bridges & Goldberg called these 'facultative somatisers' as opposed to 'true somatisers', who were unable to make such links.

Duration of somatisation

Although the course of a somatised illness may be acute, sub-acute or chronic, there are no generally agreed thresholds which separate acute or sub-acute from chronic forms. For the purposes of this chapter these periods are less than 4 weeks, 1–6 months and in excess of 6 months respectively. Pain researchers tend to use the arbitrary period of 6 months to define chronic pain, and similarly the diagnosis of chronic fatigue syndrome (CFS) requires a patient to have had fatigue for 6 months. It takes a great deal longer than 6 months to meet the criteria for somatisation disorder (DSM–IV) and a minimum period of 2 years is specified for the ICD–10 diagnosis of multiple somatisation disorder.

Chronic somatisation is usually more resistant to treatment and requires specialised psychological intervention (Bass & Benjamin, 1993). It is more likely to be associated with personality disorder and other significant psychopathology than acute somatisation (Kaminsky & Slavney, 1976; Stern *et al*, 1993). These chronically ill patients are more likely to be referred to psychiatrists.

The functions of somatisation

Using a disease model, symptoms and disability are simply the manifestations of disturbed bodily functions or structures. Until the 19th century this was how hysteria and hypochondriasis were perceived. Briquet, for example, thought hysteria was due to a disturbance of the 'affective' part of the brain. Freud later introduced the idea of secondary gain in hysteria, suggesting that symptoms could be maintained if they offered social advantages to the sufferer. This represents a change of perspective: the sick person is no longer simply a faulty organism, but a subject with intent (unconscious or conscious). Goldberg & Bridges (1988) argue that somatisation is a route through which people unsympathetic to psychological illness can enter the sick role while psychologically distressed. Medical anthropologists have also noted that the symptom complexes we call anxiety or depression are treated as physical illness in cultures where mental illness is stigmatised, for example neurasthenia in China (Kleinman & Kleinman, 1985).

A patient with physical disease is generally not held responsible for his condition. This is not always true of mental illness, which is more likely to be seen as of the patient's own making. Somatisation can thus avert blame. Instead of being held responsible for his 'personal problems', the patient enters the role of the passive victim. The avoidance of blame, including self-blame, may protect the patient from being as depressed as they might otherwise have been.

Powell *et al* (1990) have provided evidence to support this blame-avoidance function of somatisation. They compared depressive symptomatology and attributional style between a group of patients with CFS seen in a specialised medical setting with depressed controls seen in a specialised psychiatric setting. Although certain depressive symptoms were common to both groups, significant differences emerged between the CFS patients and the depressed controls with respect to self-esteem and guilt. The CFS patients tended to attribute their symptoms to external causes, for example viruses, whereas the depressed controls made inward attributions, i.e. they blamed themselves for their illness and experienced more guilt. Style of attribution is thought to influence the cognitive processes seen in depression; an 'inward' style is associated with greater psychological distress and lower self-esteem (Robson, 1988). External attribution also means the patient is less likely to be referred or accept referral to a psychiatrist. This avoids the stigma of being labelled psychiatrically ill.

However, there are also disadvantages of external attribution. Helplessness, lack of self-efficacy and diminished responsibility for one's own health and personal problems may become maintaining factors in a patient's illness. Furthermore, effective psychiatric or psychological intervention may be delayed. The following vignette illustrates some disadvantages of somatisation:

> A 31-year-old successful commodity broker presented with an 18 month history of loss of power in his voice, which was also husky and hoarse. Fifteen months previously his wife of two years had left him without warning and taken their one-year-old child with her. The ostensible reason for her leaving was his work addiction and refusal to spend time with his family. The patient felt devastated by these events but nevertheless carried on working until his physical symptoms led to referral to an ENT surgeon. All investigations, including indirect laryngoscopy and an MRI scan of the neck were normal, and the patient was reassured. Despite this he consulted three further ENT specialists before agreeing reluctantly to see a psychiatrist. This occurred ten months after the initial presentation of the symptoms and after £3000 in health insurance had been spent on normal investigations.
>
> At the time of his referral to a psychiatrist, his performance at work had deteriorated and his supervisor had suggested that all he needed to sort out his problems was a fortnight's vacation in the Caribbean. Significantly, the patient reported a number of depressive symptoms in addition to his throat problem. These included low mood and tearfulness, poor concentration, initial insomnia and fitful sleep, irritability, loss of interest in his work and extreme lassitude. He also accused his wife of being unreasonable and of having deserted him for no good reason. After three sessions with the psychiatrist the patient agreed to take antidepressant medication and could recognise the links between his marital problems and his bodily complaints. He also appreciated that his abusive work regime had contributed to the problems and that this would have to change in order for a reconciliation to occur with his wife. This eventually occurred three months after his psychiatric referral, but two years after the couple had separated.

This vignette illustrates a number of features typical of the histories of somatising patients:

(1) persistent or repeated medicalising of the problem, which leads to the neglect of the primary diagnosis and prolongation of the disorder

(2) the reluctance of the patient to accept psychiatric referral

(3) an important relationship between a major life event and the onset of somatic complaints (which were probably antedated by an affective disorder)

(4) the importance of enquiring about emotional as well as somatic complaints in patients with unexplained physical symptoms

(5) the cost of somatisation (£3000 before psychiatric referral).

Somatisation and psychiatric disorders

We have already emphasised that somatisation is not a diagnosis and should not be confused with the diagnostic group of somatoform disorders. A wide range of psychiatric diagnoses are associated with somatic presentations; it is useful to divide these into acute and chronic disorders (Table 5.1).

There have been several studies examining the psychiatric diagnoses of patients referred for psychiatric evaluation of unexplained somatic symptoms. Affective and somatoform disorders predominate (in contrast to patients in primary care where adjustment disorder is the commonest diagnosis). Katon *et al* (1984) found that 48% of patients had an affective disorder and 29% had somatoform disorders. In contrast, another American study (Slavney & Teitelbaum, 1985) found a reversed distribution with affective disorders being diagnosed in 9% and somatoform disorders in 34% of patients. In the only British study, Lloyd (1986) found that 33% had an anxiety disorder and 11% a somatoform disorder. It is important to note that in two of these three studies a substantial minority of patients received no diagnosis of any kind.

Why have psychiatrists been slow to recognise the importance of somatisation?

Until quite recently most psychiatrists received their training in mental hospitals and had little contact with somatising patients. Consequently, trainee psychiatrists were taught that somatic presentations of depression were rare or atypical. Given this segregation of psychiatrists from the rest of medicine, it has taken psychiatrists a long time to realise that somatic presentations are the rule rather than the exception in non-psychiatric settings, i.e. general practice and medical out-patient clinics. In some places psychiatrists continue to receive most of their training in psychiatric hospitals, and as a result never acquire the experience or confidence to manage this substantial group of patients. This problem could be addressed by making attachments in general hospitals obligatory for trainee psychiatrists. However, liaison psychiatry is yet to be recognised as an important component of psychiatric practice, with its own body of knowledge and skills.

Table 5.1 Psychiatric diagnoses in somatising patients (ICD–10 classification)

Acute	Chronic
Adjustment disorder	Somatisation disorder
Depressive episode	Undifferentiated somatoform disorder
Anxiety disorder	Hypochondriacal disorder (includes
Phobic disorder	dysmorphophobia)
Panic disorder	Persistent somatoform pain disorder
Dissociative (conversion) disorder	Factitious disorder

Prevalence of somatisation

In order to measure prevalence we need a precise operational definition of the disorder concerned and reliable and valid measures for ascertainment. We also need to define the population to be studied and decide the time period. We have already alluded to the problems with case definition. It is easier to specify operational criteria for syndromal diagnoses than it is to define the process of somatisation. Furthermore, as we have already hinted, criteria for research (e.g. Katon *et al*, 1984; Goldberg & Bridges, 1988) may not be the most clinically relevant. Definitions usually include the patient's concern with physical complaints and their organic disease attributions. They also have to take into account the possible relative contribution of any physical pathology.

In clinical practice there are likely to be considerable differences in the threshold for case identification used by different psychiatrists. Even those who have taken a special interest in somatisation disagree on some aspects. For example, it may not be possible to distinguish by conventional diagnostic methods between symptoms caused by peripheral organic pathology and psychophysiological disturbance; the syndrome of 'atypical facial pain' is an example (Murphy, 1990). Some psychiatrists will be reluctant to identify somatisation in the absence of a psychiatric diagnosis. The psychiatric diagnosis will also vary between psychiatrists: some will include only mood and anxiety disorders, others will include DSM–III–R diagnoses such as 'adjustment disorders with physical complaints' and 'psychological factors affecting physical conditions.' These two DSM–III–R diagnoses would not be accepted by some psychiatrists as 'cases' of mental disorder. When they have been included, over 90% of pain clinic patients have been diagnosed as having mental illness (Benjamin *et al*, 1988). The validity of the somatoform disorders as diagnoses has also been questioned (Murphy, 1990).

Community based studies of prevalence

The National Institute of Mental Health Epidemiological Catchment Area (ECA) study in the USA has provided extensive data on the mental health of community samples (Escobar *et al*, 1987*a*). Individuals selected from the adult population samples were interviewed using the Diagnostic Interview Schedule (DIS; Robins *et al*, 1981), which includes a section on the 37 somatic symptoms used to establish the DSM–III diagnosis of somatisation disorder (SD). The diagnosis of SD requires the presence of 13 somatic symptoms; a threshold that has been criticised for being too stringent. In an analysis of ECA data, Escobar *et al* (1987*a*) used the presence of four or more somatic symptoms in men (from the list of 37 in the DIS), and six or more in women, to arrive at an 'abbreviated somatisation construct'. In a sample of 3132 adults, 4.4% reached this abridged cut-off score for somatisation, whereas only 0.03% met criteria for the full DSM–III diagnosis of somatisation disorder. That is to say, 4.4% of the sample endorsed at least four somatic complaints in their lifetime (six in women) that were not explained by relevant organic disease (the authors called the number of positively endorsed symptoms the 'somatic symptom index' or SSI). As in patients with SD, patients fulfilling these modified criteria have been shown to make greater use of medical services and have high rates of functional disability (Escobar *et al*, 1987*b*).

Prevalence in primary care

Research in primary care may be more clinically relevant and shed more light on the process of somatisation. It has been estimated in one American study that up to 60% of patients visiting their family doctors were somatising (Katon *et al*, 1984). Bridges & Goldberg (1985) found that 26% of general practice attenders were somatisers with mental disorders, including those with adjustment reactions but excluding facultative somatisers. Bhatt *et al* (1989) found about 30% of GP attenders were somatising, with only minor differences between ethnic groups.

Kirmayer & Robbins (1991*a*) studied 685 patients attending two family practices. Three operational definitions of somatisation were used: (a) high levels of functional somatic distress, measured by a SSI of 4/6 (male/female) on the DIS; (b) hypochondriasis, measured by high scores on a measure of illness worry in the absence of evidence of serious illness, and (c) exclusively somatic presentations among patients with current major depression or anxiety. The authors found that 26% of patients met criteria for one or more form of somatisation, 16.6% met criteria for the abridged somatisation construct. Hypochondriacal worry was recorded in 7.7% and somatic presentations of depression or anxiety disorders accounted for 8% of all attendances. Although the majority of patients displayed only one type of somatisation, there was overlap.

Hospital studies of prevalence

Surveys of general hospital patients run into different problems. As many as 84% of long-term out-patient attenders have been reported as having physical complaints without a relevant physical diagnosis. This does not mean that they are all somatisers. Recent studies of general hospital patients referred to liaison psychiatry services report that about 40% are somatisers and 15% have somatoform disorders (Katon *et al*, 1984; de Leon *et al*, 1987). Somatoform disorders have been diagnosed in 12–53% of patients attending pain clinics (Benjamin *et al*, 1988), the wide range almost certainly reflecting different sampling methods.

Aetiology and pathogenesis

Genetic factors

Adoption studies have attempted to assess the contribution of genetic factors to adult somatisation. It has been reported that certain somatoform syndromes are associated with psychopathology in the biological parent, whereas others are associated with psychopathology in the adopted parent. For example, the biological fathers of female 'high frequency somatisers' (whose chief complaint was headache, backache, and abdominal distress on different occasions) had often committed violent crimes, whereas the adoptive fathers of female 'diversiform somatisers' (who had a greater diversity of complaints but less frequent disability) were more often alcohol misusers (Cloninger, 1986). Although these familial associations between somatisation, alcohol misuse and antisocial personality have been noted in a number of studies (Bohman *et al*, 1984), these data are complex and we are a long way from understanding the role of genetics in somatisation.

Pathophysiological mechanisms

It was part of the DSM–III–R definition of somatoform disorders that no pathophysiological mechanism accounted for the symptom (or symptoms): "although the symptoms of somatoform disorders are 'physical', the specific pathophysiological processes involved are not demonstrable or understandable by existing laboratory procedures and are conceptualised most clearly by means of psychological constructs". This criterion presumably meant that symptoms arising from increased autonomic activity (demonstrable by laboratory procedures and not a psychological construct) were not somatoform. This gave rise to difficulty with the diagnosis of somatisation disorder and hypochondriasis, conditions in which autonomic overactivity is often present. In routine clinical work, tests for these mechanisms are seldom performed. Other processes such as increased smooth muscle and striated muscle contraction, hyperventilation, vascular changes, sleep disorder and the effects of inactivity are difficult to ascertain, but may play a role in many patients with somatoform disorders. These processes, and their relationship to psychosocial factors, are described in more detail elsewhere (Sharpe & Bass, 1992). In DSM–IV the definition of somatoform disorders is less restrictive. Physical symptoms suggestive of a medical condition have to be present but the symptoms do not have to be entirely explained psychologically. They merely have to be not fully explained by a general medical condition.

Childhood experience

Several retrospective studies suggest that adults who somatise are more likely to have had childhood experiences of illness in significant others. This includes an excess of: (a) somatic complaints by parents; (b) illness or complaints of illness in the family generally; (c) family complaints of pain, and (d) a history of family members with physical handicap and deformity (Blumer & Heilbron, 1982). Particularly striking is the similarity between children's symptoms and those of their parents – especially for abdominal pain, headache, and backache (see Benjamin & Eminson (1992) for a more detailed review of this field). There is also some evidence to suggest that adults with chronic intractable pain are more likely to have been hospitalised as children (Pilowsky *et al*, 1982).

Childhood experience of illness appears to be a more important risk factor for adult somatisation when it is associated with lack of parental care. In a recent study, Craig *et al* (1993) found that important predictors of adult somatisation were parental lack of care followed by childhood illness. Craig and his colleagues have speculated that both lack of parental care and early childhood illness contribute to two separate pathways which come together in adulthood. In this hypothetical model, lack of care would raise the risk of emotional disorder in the face of later adversity, while the early childhood exposure to illness predisposes the individual to interpret innocuous sensations as indicative of physical illness. There is also research on the role of childhood sexual abuse in the aetiology of somatoform disorders (it is important to appreciate that sexual abuse is probably more likely to occur in settings where there is also a lack of care). Pelvic pain and abdominal functional symptoms are more common in women who have been sexually abused in childhood (Walker *et al*, 1988; Drossman *et al*, 1990).

Another form of child abuse is Munchausen's syndrome by proxy, in which a parent presents a child to doctors with symptoms or signs fabricated or induced by the parent (Bools *et al*, 1994). Often the symptoms claimed by the parent to afflict the child lead doctors to investigate and thereby further interfere physically with the child. Anecdotal evidence suggests that children who have had these experiences may later develop chronic somatoform syndromes (Meadow, 1982).

Gain and social reinforcement

Patients who receive sickness benefits, pensions or other disability payments may remain disabled longer than those who have no such insurance, even with diseases of similar severity (Better *et al*, 1979). Financial incentives may thus act as reinforcers of somatic symptoms. This seems particularly likely in distressed individuals with relatively few other resources. There is inconsistent evidence that litigation increases reported severity of pain. However, there is no good evidence that it induces or aggravates somatisation, prolongs the duration of symptoms, or that legal settlement leads to amelioration of symptoms in patients involved in compensation claims (Mendelson, 1991).

The behaviour of family members can reinforce somatic complaints, and the interest shown by family members or by a physician probably all contribute to the tendency to attend to bodily sensations or to seek help from physicians, or both.

Social support and confiding relationships

Pennebaker and his colleagues (1988) have suggested that failure to express emotion and the lack of a confiding relationship may cause physiological arousal, somatic symptoms and physical disease. They report, for example, that among individuals whose spouses died unexpectedly by suicide or car accident, the more the survivors had talked to others about the spouse's death, the healthier they felt (Pennebaker & O'Heeron, 1984).

Cognitive factors

The central tenet of the cognitive model is that symptoms are the results of a patient's interpretation (or attribution) of somatic sensations. These sensations may form part of their awareness of normal bodily processes as well as resulting from physical pathology. They may also be the somatic aspects of arousal, stress, anxiety, depression, anger, etc.

Most of the time we correctly interpret such bodily sensations as due to innocuous physical causes or stress, but sometimes we misattribute them to serious disease. There are many factors which make this more likely. Often there is an interaction between two types of factor: knowledge and previous experience of illness, and emotional arousal.

Knowledge of illness may come from previous personal experience of disease and illness, or from witnessing sick family members, friends and neighbours. These experiences may contribute to a patient's 'model' of illness and it is important to elicit this information in the history. Previous experience of doctors and medical care in general may also influence current illness behaviour.

Emotional arousal can be understood in terms of the interaction of personality and environmental stress. Once symptoms have occurred, they may be maintained by secondary factors such as anxiety, the reactions of friends and relatives, and the reactions and behaviour of doctors. Each of these factors may lead a patient who has suffered temporary physical discomfort in their back, abdomen or chest to experience prolonged over-concern.

This multi-causal interactive model of somatisation places importance on physical problems, illness beliefs, personality and life circumstances. It also points to ways in which medical intervention could reduce distress and disability by modifying the patient's interpretations of his symptoms. It is often insufficient to simply reassure the patient that there is no serious physical cause. It is important to provide the patient with a satisfactory alternative explanation for their symptoms and appropriate advice on how to cope with them. Sometimes misinterpretations are so long standing that there is need for specialist psychological treatment.

Consequences of somatisation

Failure to detect and adequately manage somatisation can have deleterious effects on both the patient and the health care system. Apart from failing to have his psychiatric illness treated, the somatising patient may undergo unnecessary tests and investigations with an attendant risk of iatrogenic illness. Addiction to prescribed drugs is not uncommon in chronic somatisers and may be to opiate analgesics, benzodiazepines, or both. If somatisation becomes chronic there is a risk of the patient becoming disabled, with adverse effects on family life and work capacity (Katon *et al*, 1991). As a consequence a patient's social network may

---

Box 5.1 The consequences of somatisation (Katon *et al*, 1984, 1991)

Unnecessary (and expensive) laboratory tests
Repeated hospitalisations
Iatrogenic illness e.g. polysurgery
Prescribed drug misuse
Poor doctor–patient relationship
Secondary impact on family and social network
Disability and loss of earnings
'Addiction' to health care system for social support

---

become restricted, with increasing reliance and/or dependence on the health care system, which becomes increasingly unlikely and unable to resolve the patient's difficulties (Box 5.1). Another invariable adverse consequence of inappropriate management of somatisation is deterioration of the doctor–patient relationship.

Counting the cost of somatisation

There are many reports showing that patients with somatoform disorders undergo frequently repeated expensive physical investigations – an obvious misuse of health service resources. There are also enormous cost implications for acute somatisation. Non-specific abdominal pain (NSAP), defined as abdominal pain lasting a maximum of 7 days for which no organic cause can be found, is the commonest presentation of abdominal pain to surgical wards (Gray & Collin, 1987). Many of these patients undergo laparotomies, which not only cost the health service a lot of money, but can also result in further morbidity. It has been estimated that 33 000 negative laparotomies are performed each year in the UK (Raheja *et al*, 1990), which at 1988 prices would cost £16.5 million (although not all these are for NSAP).

Shaw & Creed (1991) calculated the direct costs (to the hospital) of investigations, performed before referral to the psychiatrist, in consecutive patients presenting with somatic symptoms. In all patients the somatic symptoms were the presenting feature of a diagnosable psychiatric illness. The median cost per patient was £286 (range £8.40 – £2300). Out-patient visits accounted for the majority of the costs and there was some evidence that median costs for patients referred from gastroenterology were higher than those from other medical units. It is clearly important to understand those factors which lead to expensive in-patient investigation compared with those which lead to only a single out-patient visit.

Patients with SD can consume vast resources. Bass & Murphy (1991) estimated that the cost to the health service of a 10 year 'segment' of health care in a patient with SD was approximately £14 000. In the US it has been shown that psychiatric intervention with this group of patients can lead to substantial savings without any compromise in patients' satisfaction with their medical care (Smith *et al*, 1986).

Somatoform disorders

The term 'somatoform disorder' was introduced in DSM–III (1980) to describe a new diagnostic class of psychiatric syndromes whose essential features are:

> "Physical symptoms suggesting physical disorder for which there are no demonstrable organic findings or known physiological

mechanisms and for which there is positive evidence, or a strong presumption, that the symptoms are linked to psychological factors or conflicts".

In the 1992 version of *The International Classification of Diseases* (ICD–10), the World Health Organization has followed the American lead and includes a category of somatoform disorders. As in DSM–III (now DSM–IV) this innovation is related to an attempt to eliminate the concept of neurosis as a 'major organising principle'. There are, however, differences between the two concepts of somatoform disorder (see Table 3.3, Chapter 3). Firstly, ICD–10 has combined somatoform disorders with 'stress-related' and 'neurotic' disorders to form a single overall group that emphasises their historical association with earlier concepts of neurosis and their likely psychogenic aetiology. Secondly, conversion disorders are excluded from the ICD–10 group of somatoform disorders and grouped instead with dissociative disorders, thus retaining the traditional notion of hysteria which dates from the 19th century. Thirdly, ICD–10 includes somatoform autonomic dysfunction as a form of somatoform disorder.

There are six conditions classified as somatoform disorders in DSM–IV: body dysmorphic disorder, conversion disorder, hypochondriasis, somatisation disorder, pain disorder, and undifferentiated somatoform disorder. These diagnoses encompass what has previously been called hysteria or abnormal illness behaviour.

The ICD–10 does not include a specific category of body dysmorphic disorder (such cases are to be classified as a variant of hypochondriacal disorder). Another difference is that neurasthenia (fatigue syndrome) is included in ICD–10, not as a somatoform disorder, but as a separate category.

Both classificatory systems have many shortcomings (Murphy, 1990). The major criticisms are that the individual disorders are not distinct but rather merge into one another and overlap; the clinical descriptions are derived from hospital-based rather than community and primary care samples; and that the diagnostic criteria for some categories, e.g. somatisation disorder, are too restrictive for clinical use: as a consequence many chronic somatisers end up in a 'residual' category (undifferentiated somatoform disorder). In practice clinicians and researchers are reluctant to use a residual category to classify a common clinical problem.

Before the somatoform disorders are described in more detail, it is important to keep in mind the following point: the most common psychiatric syndromes associated with somatisation are not the somatoform disorders, but more common psychiatric syndromes such as depression, panic disorder and adjustment disorders.

Body dysmorphic disorder

DSM–III–R introduced the new category body dysmorphic disorder, which is retained in DSM–IV, and which broadly corresponds to the more familiar term dysmorphophobia (Birtchnell, 1988). Patients with this disorder present with excessive concern about trivial or non-existent physical abnormality, which they believe renders them misshapen or ugly. The concern may vary in intensity from mild sensitivity, through to preoccupation sufficient to motivate requests for corrective surgery. The body image disturbance of anorexia nervosa and the gender dysphoria of trans-sexualism are specifically excluded, as are beliefs about deformity of delusional intensity, which are classified with delusional disorder somatic type, and otherwise labelled delusional disorder (F22.0; ICD–10) or monosymptomatic hypochondriacal psychosis (Munro, 1988).

Mild sensitivity about one's appearance is a common attribute of normal people, and the DSM–III–R criteria do not guide the clinician on what is excessive. For this reason the reliability and validity of the diagnosis is doubtful, and it may be better to regard preoccupation with perceived abnormality as a symptom. Dysmorphophobia can occur in the course of psychiatric disorders, such as schizophrenia or major depression, and personality disorder is common. As such, the natural history and treatment of the symptom will depend on the associated disorder. Nonetheless there remain some individuals whose preoccupation, however intense, is not accompanied by features of other conditions, and who may go to great lengths in seeking surgery. They are unlikely to see any need for psychiatric consultation except as a preliminary to surgery.

The psychiatrist's role is liaison with GPs and surgeons in an attempt to avoid unnecessary surgery, which carries iatrogenic risks and serves merely to maintain the preoccupation. Serotonin re-uptake blockers, like fluoxetine or neuroleptics may be useful in some patients with body dysmorphic disorder (Phillips, 1991). In an uncontrolled study, Marks & Mishan (1988) reported that patients were helped by behaviour therapy: patients were systematically exposed to the situations that evoked dysmorphic discomfort, and persuaded to refrain from behaviours which reduced that discomfort. This treatment, exposure therapy, can also be used to treat illness phobias.

Conversion disorder (or hysterical conversion, HC)

The validity of hysteria is called into question more often than any other psychiatric disorder. Why should this be? The ever present possibility of underlying brain disease emphasises the need for diagnostic vigilance, but does not challenge the nosological validity of the syndrome. Toone (1990) has pointed out that the reason for this continuing state of dissatisfaction is that the diagnosis of conversion disorder is predicated on two sets of negatives: (a) signs and symptoms of physical ill-health which the physician refuses to accept, and (b) inferences by the physician of psychological disturbance which the patient usually rebuts. It is hardly surprising that many doctors find this state of affairs intolerable.

The uncertain distinction between hysteria and malingering is also a source of disquiet. Faced with a mismatch between the complaints of the patient and the objective evidence of organic disease, many doctors incline to extreme positions: to give the patient the benefit of the doubt and to assume that all is organically determined, or to reject the patient out of hand as a malingerer. The third course, to accept the possibility that the patient may have a self-perception of bodily dysfunction that is genuine but at the same time quite incompatible with anatomical and physiological mechanisms as they are presently understood, introduces a far more difficult concept (Toone,1990).

The essential difference between conversion disorder and other somatoform disorders is that "an alteration or loss of physical functioning" is required for the diagnosis, i.e. it is not diagnosed on the basis of symptom complaints alone. Pain is therefore not classified as a conversion symptom even if the examiner believes that conversion is the mechanism of symptom production. The diagnosis of somatoform pain disorder should be considered instead (see below).

In ICD–10 (1992) all forms of either dissociation and conversion are subsumed in one category, dissociative disorders (F44). This is further subdivided into (a) disorders of memory awareness and identity, and (b) disorders of movement and sensation. These disorders are delineated from somatoform disorders (F45).

The prevalence of HC is difficult to establish. One per cent of all diagnoses in postgraduate psychiatric and neurological centres, and 0.7% of all admissions to a group of neurosurgical units satisfy criteria for HC. The experience of developing countries is quite different: between 8 and 10% of all new out-patient referrals in Sudan, Libya, and India have HC (Toone, 1990).

In patients with hysterical symptoms it is important to establish an inconsistency between the patient's symptoms or observed disabilities and their state on physical examination. For example, a diagnosis of hysterical conversion can be confidently made in the patient who claims to be unable to move the left side of the body yet is persuaded to demonstrate unacknowledged strength in the antagonist muscles in the presence of normal muscle tone and reflex responses. Complaints of sensory loss or motor weakness are more amenable to this type of demonstration: periodic disorders such as epilepsy, or conditions that lack readily objectifiable physical signs, such as dystonia, are less so.

The psychiatrist's role in the management of hysterical conversion lies primarily in providing an explanation about the impact of stress on bodily function, and of advising occupational therapists and physiotherapists to minimise more persisting symptoms. This can be carried out using a combination of behavioural methods to reduce positive reinforcement or secondary gain, physiotherapy and graded exercise to encourage resumption of normal function, and a diversion of attention away from the symptom itself towards any possible causative or perpetuating psychosocial stressors (Toone, 1990). In some cases it is appropriate to use a sodium amytal or diazepam interview in an attempt to alleviate a symptom, especially if the complaints are of short duration. The following case illustrates this:

> A 43-year-old woman with multiple sclerosis had become increasingly disabled and wheelchair-bound one year before admission to hospital. During this time her husband had deserted her for another woman. She had a 22-year-old married daughter who lived 15 miles away. Two collapses at home had precipitated her admission, and in the A & E department she was noted to be falling to the ground in a histrionic manner. She soon became mute, stuporose and doubly incontinent and was admitted to the medical ward. Neurological examination and MRI scan on her brain failed to reveal any organic cause for her mutism, and she was referred for a psychiatric opinion three days after admission with a provisional diagnosis of 'hysterical mutism'.
>
> History revealed that on the day of admission the patient had been urged to move into warden-controlled accommodation, a move that she had vigorously opposed but which, given her disability, appeared increasingly likely. Neither had she accepted her husband's desertion, and her repeated attempts to retrieve her marriage had all failed.
>
> It was decided to carry out a diazepam interview and to encourage her to discuss some of these stressful topics. She was given 22mg of diazepam intravenously during the course of 50 minutes, but, apart from some semi-purposive movements of her upper arms there was little change in her state. However, five hours later she suddenly started talking and regained the capacity to move all four limbs. When interviewed the following morning she was alert, cheerful and talking in an animated fashion to the other patients. She thought that the date was 1962 and was convinced that she was in a cottage hospital 20 miles away (where her daughter was born). In most other respects her cognitive function was normal, and during the course of the interview she became appropriately tearful and distressed when discussing her husband's desertion and the attempts to evict her from her house. She was discharged home from hospital the following day and remained well three months after discharge.

Although it is not possible to be sure that the diazepam interview led to the resolution of her mute state, it is important to attempt to relieve hysterical symptoms as soon as they emerge. Intravenous sodium amytal or diazepam are the most commonly used drugs (Sargant & Slater, 1972). It is important to assign a key nurse to the patient and observe the patient closely for 24 hours after the interview. Whenever possible a videotaped recording of the interview should be made, and in some circumstances it may be appropriate to show this to the patient and to discuss the possible ways in which stress and life difficulties can lead to loss of function of a bodily part. This may allow the patient to reintegrate the experiences and to understand the nature of the link between life events and physical symptoms.

Somatisation disorder

Somatisation disorder (SD) was introduced in DSM–III in 1980 to denote a chronic condition characterised by numerous changing physical symptoms. This introduction followed three decades of empirical research on hysteria (Briquet's syndrome) supporting the reliability and validity of the diagnosis as operationally defined (Perley & Guze, 1962; Guze 1975). The diagnosis is based on "a history of many physical complaints or a belief that one is sickly, beginning before the age of 30, and persisting for several years" (APA, 1992). The diagnostic criteria require the patient to have had a minimum of eight stringently defined symptoms from a given list, restricting the diagnosis to a small minority of somatising patients (Box 5.2).

The diagnosis is rarely made in this country. In spite of the claims made for its validity, many British psychiatrists believe it is a spurious, peculiarly American invention. Most believe that these patients have affective disorders and anxiety disorders, often in combination with personality disorder (Stern *et al,* 1993*a*). However, our research suggests that conventional psychiatric treatment of these 'underlying' mood and anxiety disorders does not prevent the repeated episodes of physical symptoms, further consultations, investigations and inappropriate physical treatments (Bass & Murphy, 1991).

SD is classified on Axis I (mental illnesses) rather than Axis II (personality disorders) of DSM–IV. There have been several studies of the co-existence of Axis I diagnoses with somatisation disorder (comorbidity). These have shown a high lifetime prevalence of mood disorders and anxiety disorders in SD patients (Katon *et al,* 1984; Orenstein, 1989; Bass & Murphy, 1991). The term 'comorbidity' may be misleading: it is naive to assume that a patient with SD and a history of depression and anxiety disorders has three different illnesses, each with its own cause and pathogenesis.

The most typical SD patient is female, in her forties, has a complicated medical history, is often on invalidity benefit, has spurious physical diagnoses, is on numerous drugs and has had a hysterectomy. Concurrent and past symptoms of depression and anxiety are common. Most have been treated for these with antidepressants and benzodiazepines. Many patients are as disparaging about their psychiatric treatment as they are about their medical management. Over 70% of SD patients have a personality disorder as assessed by the Personality Assessment Schedule (PAS; Stern *et al*, 1993*b*). This is double the rate seen in patients with most other Axis I psychiatric disorders. Patients with SD are also more likely than other psychiatric patients to be rated as having severe rather than mild or moderate personality disorders. The social lives of SD patients are often impoverished. Current and past family life is often marked by discord, acrimony and bitterness. Patients may not be able to provide adequate parental care for their children who, more often than in other non-psychotic patient groups, end up in care (Zoccolillo & Cloninger, 1985).

Many patients with SD have grown up in families where one or both parents suffered physical disability. They are also more likely to have suffered a disability themselves in childhood, either chronically or recurrently, e.g. rheumatic fever or asthma. Another characteristic of patients with SD is that they find it difficult to describe their previous illness history in any coherent or systematic manner. Cloninger (1986) drew attention to this facet of SD patients as follows: these patients "recall their current situation and past history as a series of separate elements, mixed together or mingled without sorting, discrimination, or apprehension of functional relationship and temporal order". A typical case is described below (for more details see Bass & Murphy, 1991):

> A 36-year-old woman reported that her problems began *in utero* with maternal rubella. She thought she was blind and deaf as an infant, but recovered. Insulin-dependent diabetes was diagnosed at the age of 2, leading to numerous lengthy admissions before the age of 5. Both parents were physically fit, but her mother had always been anxious and received treatment for depression. Their marriage was unhappy and her father had affairs. He seldom talked to his family and caned the patient if she disobeyed him. The mother 'always whined' and was excessively dependent on the patient, who admitted to inducing hypoglycaemia as a child to 'punish' her parents.
>
> She attended an ordinary school until the age of 9, followed by a school for handicapped children. She reported 'fits' since age 2, but said that doctors never believed her mother's description of these (this scenario might be described as Munchausen's by proxy today). She has been in receipt of phenobarbitone since 9, despite attempts by doctors to stop it.
>
> She left school at 15 and worked in a handicraft shop until she retired on invalidity pension at 30. She married at 25, having previously been sterilised. The marriage ended after several years, during which her husband beat and raped her. She said "there was no love, only fear, in the marriage". She has never experienced any sexual desire and always had pain during intercourse.

At 18, following several admissions for keto-acidosis, she was referred to the diabetic clinic at our hospital where complaints 'neither typical of hypo- nor hyperglycaemia' were noted. Abdominal pains at 19 led to appendicectomy and loin pain was diagnosed as lumbar strain. Since age 23 she has complained of pain and paraesthesiae in her hands and feet. A bilateral carpal tunnel decompression at 26 failed to alleviate this and she was referred to a Raynaud's Unit. Several years later it was noted that she had 'a random response to two point discrimination' and that there was 'nothing the matter with her hands'.

At 27 she was investigated for 'visual deterioration' and diplopia but no cause could be found. From 27 to 30 she had intermittent aphonia which she later said was due to "the stress of my husband hitting me." At 29 she was investigated for abdominal pain. Tests suggested a gallstone and cholecystectomy was performed after 4 months of continuous pain. Findings were normal at operation and her pain persisted. This was then attributed to sacro-ileitis for which she received a variety of treatments including physiotherapy. After 10 months it was noted that 'every type of technique and grade of technique aggravated her condition'. She was then referred to a rheumatologist and investigated for low back pain. Tests were normal and she was treated with steroid injections, a corset and a raised shoe. A few months later, aged 31, she was referred to the pain clinic with neck and thoracic pain. Transcutaneous nerve stimulation, acupuncture, a soft collar and relaxation exercises had no effect. During the same period she was referred to an orthopaedic surgeon with numbness in her hands. Nerve conduction studies were normal and her symptoms were described as functional. The same year she saw a gynaecologist about pelvic pain and inter-menstrual bleeding. Dilatation and curettage were normal. At follow-up she reported haematuria and after a normal IVP was admitted for laparoscopy and cystoscopy, which were also normal. Her pelvic pain persisted and she had an abdominal hysterectomy at 33. Post-operative histology was normal. Following this she reported urinary incontinence and, despite normal urodynamic tests, requested surgery, which was refused. The gynaecologist then arranged for her to see a neurologist because of numb feet. Nerve conduction studies were normal but despite this 'a mild form of neuropathy' was diagnosed. This diagnosis was subsequently revised and she had myelography to rule out lumbar canal stenosis – which it did. Her gait then became abnormal and she was admitted. Nerve conduction studies were again normal and she was seen by an orthopaedic surgeon because she claimed her problem was scoliosis. The surgeon found no evidence of this and tried unsuccessfully to dissuade her from wearing a raised shoe. On discharge she was referred back to gynaecology with urinary incontinence and frequency.

At 34 she saw a chest physician for dyspnoea. Lung function tests and an echocardiogram were normal and a diagnosis of asthma was made on the history. She was put on anti-spasmodic and steroid inhalers and although the diagnosis was later changed to hyperventilation syndrome, she remained on these. A few months later she was referred from the chest clinic to a cardiologist with dyspnoea on exertion and palpitations. A treadmill test, thallium scan and 24 hour ECG tape were normal; a diagnosis of supraventricular tachycardia was made and she was put on verapamil.

At 35 she had more eye tests but they could not account for her visual symptoms. She was told that she might have a retinal disturbance and she has since worn dark glasses. A few months later she was referred again to a neurologist with tremor and numbness of her hands, diarrhoea and incontinence. She was concerned that she had multiple sclerosis and visual evoked responses were performed to reassure her. These were normal, but a history of MS was often recorded in subsequent notes. Other entries in her notes described her as a 'known diabetic neuropath' despite the lack of evidence for this.

The same year she was seen in the dermatology, oral medicine and the ENT departments because of pain in her throat which she said was associated with blood blisters. She also had persistent nausea that led to a negative barium meal. While attending the cardiology clinic she had further investigations for dizzy spells. A high serum phenobarbitone level led to the diagnosis of toxicity in 'a lady with cardiac disease'.

Her gait then deteriorated and she was admitted for a lumbar puncture. This and further electrophysiological studies were normal and a diagnosis of Briquet's syndrome was made (by an astute neurologist). Shortly after this, she was admitted to her local coronary care unit with chest pain, but tests were normal. A few months later she was admitted under the cardiologists at our hospital because of further chest pains. Coronary angiography was normal but she continued taking anti-anginal drugs. The pain was diagnosed as gastrointestinal in origin and ranitidine prescribed. Shortly after this she was referred to a psychiatrist by her dermatologist, who thought that psychological factors played a role her painful throat. The psychiatrist detected 'no formal mental illness', offered no advice about management and no follow-up.

This case illustrates the chaos, confusion and cost associated with SD. The potential for iatrogenic illness is often realised and, as in this patient, the notes allude repeatedly to a number of diagnoses and pseudo-diagnoses that have never been established. Physicians and GPs are often astonished, indignant or embarrassed when psychiatrists fail to establish a psychiatric diagnosis or advise on the management of patients who are manifestly disturbed or distressed and often disabled. They have every right to be.

Box 5.2 Diagnostic criteria for somatisation disorder (DSM–IV)

(1) History of many physical complaints, beginning before the age of 30, which occur over a period of years and result in treatment being sought or significant impairment in social, occupational or other important areas of functioning

(2) Each of the following criteria must have been met, with individual symptoms occuring at any time during the course of the disturbance:

    (i) four pain symptoms: related to at least four different sites or functions

    (ii) two gastrointestinal symptoms

    (iii) one sexual symptom

    (iv) one pseudoneurological symptom

(3) Either:

    (a) after appropriate investigation, each of the symptoms in criterion (b) cannot be fully explained by a known general medical condition or the direct effects of a substance (e.g. a drug of abuse or medication); or

    (b) when there is a related general medical condition, the physical complaints or resulting social or occupational impairment are in excess of what would be expected from the history, physcial examinination or laboratory findings

(4) The symptoms are not intentionally produced or feigned

Undifferentiated somatoform disorder

Many patients present with features of more than one somatoform disorder, and cannot readily be 'fitted' into one category. Some patients present with multiple unexplained symptoms, but not the requisite necessary for a diagnosis of somatisation disorder. A category – undifferentiated somatoform disorder – is intended in DSM–III–R for this latter group, but it is a testament to the failure of the classificatory system that this supposedly residual category is actually by far the most common somatoform diagnosis in community surveys, being much more prevalent than somatisation disorder (Escobar *et al,* 1987*b*).

Pain disorder

Pain is the most common complaint in medicine (Merskey & Spear, 1967); it is also a common way for psychiatric disorder to present, particularly depression. Among the somatoform disorders it is usually present in somatisation disorder and common in hypochondriasis. It is not, however, a sufficient symptom for the diagnosis of conversion disorder. In the 1980 edition of DSM–III, criteria for psychogenic pain disorder were identical to those for conversion disorder with the difference that the symptom was limited to pain. It was thus a requirement of the diagnosis for psychological factors to be "aetiologically involved in the symptom", as they were for conversion disorder. The separation of pain from conversion symptoms was not justified, as might have been expected, on the grounds of widespread dissatisfaction with the concept of hysterical pain, but rather on the basis that psychogenic pain tends to be chronic while other conversion symptoms are usually transient.

The term 'psychogenic pain disorder' was replaced by the term 'somatoform pain disorder' in response to the criticism that the former term was stigmatising (Williams & Spitzer, 1982). The description of the disorder and the criteria for its diagnosis were also modified. This was, in part, to take account of the findings from a study of patients with chronic pain published in 1982 (Blumer & Heilbronn). In DSM–IV the term is now 'pain disorder'. The revised criteria include:

(1) preoccupation with pain
(2) the pain causes significant distress or impairment
(3) psychological factors are judged to have an important role in the onset and maintenance
(4) it is not feigned
(5) it is better accounted for by a mood, anxiety or psychotic disorder.

These revised criteria no longer require any judgement about the aetiological role of psychological factors. The ICD–10 has also included a caveat in its description of somatoform pain that allows the diagnosis to be made without evidence of psychological aetiology.

Pain disorder is therefore a diagnosis of exclusion and is based on the presence of a single symptom. The term thus describes a diagnostic problem rather than a discrete syndrome. Indeed, it might be asked why a diagnosis based on these criteria should be regarded as a mental disorder at all.

Problems also arise with the classification of regional pain syndromes for which there are competing physical and psychological aetiological theories. Atypical facial pain is a good example. Claims have been made for temporo-mandibular joint disease and cervical spine disease, as well as vasomotor dysfunction, whereas others regard it as a conversion symptom, or as a "symptom of an underlying depressive state" (Lascelles, 1966). Other chronic regional pain syndromes, such as low back pain, headache, and chronic pain whose site is not specified, have also frequently been described as variants of depression (Roy *et al*, 1984). The evidence for these claims is, on the whole, unsatisfactory. Many studies have demonstrated that chronic pain sufferers frequently report depressive symptoms and depressed subjects frequently report pain. But failure to specify diagnostic criteria for depression, poor sampling methods, varying selection criteria, lack of suitable controls and the use of unreliable techniques for measuring pain and depression have all undermined this research effort (see Gupta, 1986, for a critical review).

The most recent and influential case for regarding chronic pain as a "variant of depressive disorder" has been argued by Blumer & Heilbronn (1982). They have described a syndrome called 'the pain prone disorder' which they claim is "a well defined psychobiological disorder with characteristic clinical, psychodynamic, biographic, and genetic features". They conceive this as "a form of masked depression, associated with a number of characteristic traits". To explain why this essentially depressive disorder is dominated by pain, they combine clinical observations with psychodynamic inference. They also present empirical data from a clinical study comparing 'pain patients' with rheumatoid arthritis sufferers to support their claims. However, the methodology (the choice of controls in particular) in this study and the authors' interpretation of their findings have been challenged (Turk & Salovey, 1984).

It is clear from Blumer & Heilbronn's own data that the clinical features they describe are neither sufficiently sensitive nor specific to be diagnostic criteria in the DSM–III sense. Rather than having delineated a syndrome by providing inclusion and exclusion criteria or specifying clear boundaries for the concept of pain-prone disorder, they have described a prototype based on their clinical experience. Neither do they make a convincing case for chronic pain as 'masked depression'. In Popperian terms this is a scientifically spurious hypothesis as it cannot be refuted by failing to demonstrate depression.

Hypochondriasis

The DSM–IV and the ICD–10 concepts of hypochondriasis differ little from Gillespie's 1928 definition of hypochondria. This emphasised the patient's preoccupation with having a physical disorder "far in excess of what is justified", as well as disease conviction that showed an "indifference to the opinion of the environment, including irresponsiveness to persuasion" (Gillespie, 1928). The DSM–IV (1994) diagnostic criteria for hypochondriasis are shown in Box 5.3.

The nosological status of hypochondriasis is unclear. Hypochondriacal symptoms occur in a variety of psychiatric disorders, and there is a substantial overlap with anxiety, depression and somatisation disorder. In distinguishing hypochondriasis from these conditions, much emphasis is placed upon its cognitive and behavioural elements which include, respectively, the misattribution of bodily sensations to the effects of illness, and the consequent repeated and unsuccessful reassurance-seeking.

The prevalence of hypochondriacal concerns in the general population is unknown. Since most measures are based on continuous scales, the distinction between cases of hypochondriasis and non-cases is often a matter of degree. Kellner (1985) estimated that hypochondriasis ranged from 3–13% in different communities and that illness worries, varying from rational concerns to constant, incapacitating fears, occurred in 10–20% of normal people. Barsky *et al* (1990) reported a 6 month prevalence of DSM–III–R hypochondriasis in a sample of general medical out-patients of between 4.2% and 6.3%.

Is hypochondriasis a discrete syndrome?

This question has attracted a lot of controversy. Much of this arose after a case note study by Kenyon (1964) of 521 patients with hypochondriacal complaints. Kenyon concluded that there was no evidence to support the view that hypochondriasis was a primary neurotic syndrome as described by Gillespie, but rather that, "on the available evidence, hypochondriasis is always part of another syndrome, most commonly an affective one". He recommended that the word hypochondriacal be retained only as an adjective to describe symptoms present in other disorders and personality traits.

While widely quoted and influential, Kenyon's study is methodologically flawed and does not justify his conclusion. Apart from the limitation of being a retrospective case note study, it was conducted in a psychiatric hospital population, introducing a selection bias towards the coexistence of other psychiatric disorder. No operational definitions of hypochondriasis or other disorders were used, and there is no statistical analysis of the data to support his interpretation of them. It has even been suggested that his data contradicts his conclusion (Appleby, 1987).

Subsequent studies have supported the notion of a primary hypochondriacal syndrome. Pilowsky (1967) devised a questionnaire

---

Box 5.3 Diagnostic criteria for hypochondriasis (DSM–IV)

(1) Preoccupation with the fear of having, or the belief that one has, a serious disease, based on the person's misinterpretation of bodily symptoms
(2) The preoccupation causes clinically significant distress or impairment
(3) The fear of having, or belief that one has, a disease persists despite medical reassurance
(4) Duration of the disturbance is at least six months
(5) The belief in (1) is not of delusional intensity, as in delusional disorder, somatic type
(6) The preoccupation is not better accounted for by other psychiatric conditions (e.g. generalised anxiety disorder)

called the Whiteley Index to investigate the concept of hypochondriasis. After establishing items which reliably distinguished hypochondriacal from non-hypochondriacal patients, the responses were used in a factor analysis. Principal component analysis identified three factors, each reflecting a different dimension of hypochondriasis. The factors were: bodily preoccupation, disease phobia and conviction of the presence of disease with non-response to reassurance (disease conviction). Subsequent similar work by Pilowsky and others has supported the validity of primary hypochondriasis (Pilowsky, 1970; Bianchi, 1973).

A study of 42 patients with hypochondriasis (DSM–III–R criteria) recruited from a general medical clinic, compared with a random sample of 76 out-patients from the same setting, was conducted to ascertain if hypochondriasis is a discrete syndrome. When primary hypochondriasis was defined as hypochondriasis without another major concurrent Axis I diagnosis, one-fifth of hypochondriacs had the primary condition and four-fifths had the secondary form (Barsky *et al*, 1992). However, there were no significant differences between the two groups, although disease fear was greater in the secondary hypochondriacs. Other interesting findings from this study included; hypochondriacs had three times the level of personality disorder as the comparison group, and one-fifth of the hypochondriacs also fulfilled criteria for somatisation disorder (see below).

Barsky *et al* (1986) examined hypochondriacal attitudes in a random sample of 92 consecutive medical out-patients. Their means of assessment were the Whiteley Index, a somatic symptom self-report scale (derived from the subscales of a number of different inventories), a structured interview and a review of medical records. They found that disease conviction, disease fear, bodily preoccupation, and somatic symptoms were significantly intercorrelated. In other words, they showed that these characteristics tend to occur together in the same individuals. They concluded that, in accord with previous work, there was considerable 'internal validity' and consistency in the syndrome.

They examined the distribution of hypochondriacal attitudes and somatic symptoms and found that there was no evidence of bimodality, or any discontinuity in measured variables between the most highly hypochondriacal individuals and the group as a whole. They therefore concluded that hypochondriasis was best viewed as a dimension of illness behaviour rather than as a discrete category.

In this study the strongest psychiatric correlate of hypochondriacal attitudes (Whiteley Index Score) was the Beck Depression Inventory Score (Salkind, 1969), which accounted for 33% of the variance. The degree of depression also emerged as a powerful predictor of somatic symptoms, accounting for 26% of the variance. Although these are strong correlations, it is also clear that a fairly high proportion of hypochondriasis could not be accounted for by depression. Thus the two conditions showed partial overlap. Overlap with anxiety disorders was not assessed in this study, the somatic symptoms commonly reported by most hypochondriacal patients were those of autonomic arousal.

The distinction between hypochondriasis and anxiety disorders

In DSM–IV hypochondriasis is only diagnosed when the individual's health concerns are not better accounted for by some other anxiety related or affective disorder. Hypochondriacal interpretations of panic attack symptoms are extremely common (Noyes *et al,* 1986) and cognitive models of panic give them a causal role in the pathogenesis of a panic attack (Clark, 1988). It has been suggested that an important difference in the development of panic attacks as opposed to hypochondriasis is the nature of the patient's illness beliefs (Warwick & Salkovskis, 1990). If a patient believes that they are vulnerable to an immediately catastrophic illness such as a heart attack, he will give selective attention to sensations consistent with this belief. For instance, this patient is more vigilant and more likely to detect an innocuous change in heart rate. Noting a 'missed beat' or an increased heart rate the patient becomes anxious that he is having a heart attack and his heart beats even faster. This in turn is interpreted as further evidence that something is wrong with the heart and further increases anxiety, thus setting up a vicious circle. Other somatic symptoms of anxiety may then develop with increasing autonomic arousal and receive further catastrophic interpretation. Hyperventilation, for example, may be interpreted as meaning that the patient is about to stop breathing and thus die. Similarly, giddiness may lead the patient to think that they are about to lose consciousness and then die. Such a patient might call on emergency medical services. If the panic attack is initially misdiagnosed as an acute medical emergency, which is often the case initially, the erroneous patient's beliefs gain further support.

This scenario can be contrasted with a patient who believes incorrectly, for whatever reason, that he has cancer. While also anxious, this patient does not anticipate any immediate medical catastrophe. He therefore does not develop the same level of arousal and is less likely to be caught in the vicious circle outlined above. If this patient's heart rate were to increase, he would be less likely to focus on the sensation, since it does not fit in with his beliefs about cancer.

The distinction between hypochondriasis and somatisation disorder

In ICD–10 it is suggested that the distinction between hypochondriasis and somatisation disorder (SD) is that in the former the patient is preoccupied by "the presence of the disorder itself and its future consequences" whereas in the latter the emphasis is on individual symptoms. It is also stated that in hypochondriasis there is "likely to be a preoccupation with only one or two possible physical disorders which will be named consistently, rather than the more numerous and often changing possibilities in somatisation disorder" (WHO, 1992).

There is little information on the co-occurrence of hypochondriasis and SD, although Oxman & Barrett (1985) found that hypochondriacal features were present in 38% of family practice out-patients with somatisation disorder. In our own (tertiary care) sample of patients satisfying DSM–III–R criteria for SD we found that while some patients with SD score highly on measures of hypochondriasis, like the Whitely index (see above), many do not. Comparing the scores of our SD patients with a comparable sample of medical out-patients studied by Barsky *et al* (1986), we found that fewer than half our cases had scores in the top quartile of the medical out-patients sample. Our SD patients also scored lower on this scale than did patients with panic attacks studied by Noyes *et al* (1986).

The distinction between hypochondriasis and somatisation disorder has been attacked as trivial (Vaillant, 1984). But while there is overlap, the accurate identification and analysis of hypochondriacal pre-occupations and behaviours may have important treatment implications. Cognitive–behavioural formulations of hypochondriasis, compatible with the DSM–III–R definition, have been proposed and are the rationale for cognitive–behavioural treatments (Warwick & Salkovskis, 1990). The outcome of this treatment still needs evaluation but early reports suggest that it may be effective. It is therefore important to identify different cognitive sets in patients with chronic somatisation. Many of our own cases of somatisation disorder, while showing disease conviction, have ideas and attitudes concerning illness that are distinct from hypochon-driasis. For example, patients with somatisation disorder are often not seeking reassurance that they are free of serious disease (as in hypochondriasis), but rather want their illness behaviour and sick role to be sanctioned by a diagnosis of physical disorder. Thus, a hypochondriacal patient may be anxious that he has multiple sclerosis and seek reassurance that he has not. By contrast, a patient with somatisation disorder may become angry at the suggestion that there is no serious physical disease to legitimise his invalid status.

Hypochondriasis as a personality disorder

It has been argued by Tyrer and colleagues (1990) that some hypochondriacal patients are more accurately classified as having a hypochondriacal personality disorder rather than a mental state disorder (in DSM–III terms they have an Axis II as opposed to an Axis I disorder). They cite cases in which hypochondriacal attitudes and behaviour are chronic maladaptive patterns which begin early and continue throughout life (see Box 5.4 for diagnostic description). Using the Personality Assessment Schedule (PAS), Tyrer *et al* found that 8.6% of patients with affective disorders had a hypochondriacal personality disorder. One would expect patients with SD to have a high rate of hypochondriacal personality disorder, or assume that they were different ways of labelling the same group of patients, but this is not so. We found a high rate of personality disorder in SD patients, but no cases of hypochondriacal personality disorder using the PAS (Stern *et al*, 1993).

In contrast to the association between antisocial and histrionic traits described in patients with SD (strictly speaking the association is with Briquet's syndrome), patients diagnosed with hypochondriacal personality disorder scored highly on scales measuring anxiousness and dependence. In their classification of personality disorders using the PAS, Tyrer & Alexander (1987) reported that hypochondriacal personality disorder most closely resembled anankastic personality disorder.

While some DSM–III–R cases of hypochondriasis match Tyrer's description of personality disorder, there are also some which begin later in life which do not. For example, some older patients develop prolonged hypochondriacal reactions following an acute physical illness, or after a life event.

Somatoform autonomic dysfunction

Unlike DSM–IV, the ICD–10 has a subcategory of disorder whose essential feature is symptoms arising from autonomic overactivity. This group is further subdivided according to the organ or system regarded by the patient as the origin of the symptoms (Table 5.2).

For a definite diagnosis the following four features should be present:

(1) persistent troublesome symptoms of autonomic arousal, e.g. palpitations, sweating, tremor
(2) additional symptoms referred to a specific organ or system, e.g. cardiovascular or gastrointestinal
(3) preoccupation and distress about the possibility of a serious disorder of the stated organ or system that does not respond to reassurance
(iv) no evidence of a significant disturbance of structure or function of that organ/system.

It is stated that somatoform autonomic dysfunction can be differentiated from generalised anxiety disorder by the predominance of "the psychological components of autonomic arousal such as fear and anxious foreboding in generalised anxiety disorder, and the lack of a consistent physical focus for the other symptoms". This sharp dichotomy between somatic and psychological components of anxiety is difficult to sustain in clinical practice. Many cases could be classified either way. Furthermore overlap with hypochondriasis is inevitable and many patients will fulfil

---

**Box 5.4 Criteria for diagnosing hypochondriacal
personality disorder (Tyrer *et al*, 1990)**

Excessive preoccupation with maintenance of health with
    associated behaviour (e.g. will only take a limited range of
    food and water, regular consumption of 'health-promoting'
    medicines in order to remain well)
The perception of minor ailments and physical symptoms is
    distorted and magnified into major and life-threatening
    disorder
Repeated recourse to consultation with medical and associated
    disciplines for reassurance, investigation and treatment
Rigidity of beliefs about health and life-style ensures their
    persistence

---

criteria for both diagnoses. This is because different variables are used to
define different categories and these are not mutually exclusive. For
example, cardiac neurosis is given as an example of somatoform
autonomic dysfunction in ICD–10 and as an example of hypochondriasis
in DSM–III–R. In the former case it is classified by origin of symptoms
while in the latter it is classified by psychological characteristics. It is not
a case of one or other being the correct classification.

Neurasthenia, 'ME' or chronic fatigue syndrome

There has been a recent explosive growth of media interest and medical
research in myalgic encephalomyelitis – ME, preferably called chronic
fatigue syndrome (CFS). Controversy centres mainly on whether the
syndrome has a viral or psychosocial aetiology, while some argue against
such dualistic thinking. It is doubtful whether the problem of chronic
fatigue is any more common now than previously. Wessely (1990) has
argued that ME is simply 'old wine in new bottles'. The old wine is
neurasthenia, which was first described in the early 19th century and
became one of the most common diagnoses in medicine in the latter part
of the 19th century. It later fell into disfavour, and although it was included
as a type of neurosis in ICD–9, it is rarely used in British psychiatric practice.
Although it had been present in DSM–II, it was omitted from DSM–III
(APA, 1980). With the recent resurgence of interest in chronic fatigue, it
has been retained in ICD–10, where it is classified with 'other neurotic
disorders', rather than as a somatoform disorder. According to ICD–10
there are two main forms of neurasthenia. The main feature of the first
type is mental fatiguability with difficulty concentrating and inefficient
thinking, while in the second it is "feelings of bodily or physical weakness
and exhaustion after only minimal effort accompanied by a feeling of

Table 5.2 ICD–10 subtypes of somatoform autonomic dysfunction

F45.3	Somatoform autonomic dysfunction (subtypes)
F45.30	The heart and cardiovascular system e.g. cardiac neurosis
F45.31	The upper gastro-intestinal tract e.g. dyspepsia and pylorospasm
F45.32	The lower gastro-intestinal tract e.g. irritable bowel syndrome
F45.33	The respiratory system e.g. hyperventilation
F45.34	The urogenital system e.g. psychogenic increase of frequency of micturition and dysuria
F45.38	Other

muscular aches and pains". A variety of other physical and mental symptoms are also described.

Fatigue is a common symptom for which no organic cause is found. Only a minority of patients presenting with fatigue to their GPs progress to CFS. Various operational criteria for the diagnosis of CFS have been suggested for research purposes (Sharpe *et al*, 1992). Such definitions describe a presenting syndrome rather than an aetiologically unitary condition. In CFS, fatigue is of at least 6 months duration; it is often accompanied by other symptoms such as pain; there is impaired functioning; and the symptoms are not explained by physical disease. Many psychiatrists would diagnose patients with CFS as having mood disorder.

In community surveys it has been found that chronic fatigue often coexists with other physical complaints such as non-cardiac chest pain, symptoms of the irritable bowel syndrome and breathlessness (Kirmayer & Robbins, 1991*b*). These symptoms occur together more often than they occur alone.

Assessment of the somatising patient

Preparatory work

This depends on where the patient is seen. In the case of a ward referral, it is always important to speak with the patient's key nurse, and to ask about the patient's behaviour on the ward, for example analgesic use, pain behaviours, interaction with other ward patients as well as medical and nursing staff. The behaviour of any relatives or other visitors should also be enquired after. An example of how this information can lead to the correct diagnosis is illustrated in the patient described on page 121. The medical notes should be scrutinised for information about previous illnesses, and whether organic pathology was found. Check whether medical diagnoses have been substantiated, or whether they are based on self-report alone; the case cited earlier (pp.121–123) was incorrectly described in her case notes as 'a known diabetic neuropath'. This demonstrates how diagnostic labels can go unchallenged, particularly by junior medical staff. Many patients with SD believe, and indeed may have been incorrectly told, that they have diseases which they do not have.

In out-patients referred for psychiatric assessment it is useful to send the patient a problem list to complete before the first visit. This asks the patient to list the major physical complaints, and report details about family, work and other difficulties. Questions about disabilities and handicaps can also be included. This exercise also encourages the patient to do some preparatory work and to think not only about their physical symptoms but also their social predicament. An example of a problem sheet is shown in Box 5.7.

As with in-patients, the medical and psychiatric notes should be reviewed before the assessment interview, together with the results of recent investigations. In some cases where patients have been seen at other hospitals it often helps to request these, or the GPs notes in advance. It takes a few minutes and can save hours of work.

The patient's attitude to the referral

An important initial task is to discover the patient's attitude to the referral. Most patients resent the implication of mental illness implicit in referral to a psychiatrist and may forcefully express this antipathy. Others may be more willing to accept that psychosocial factors may be contributing to their problems. A helpful way to gain the patient's cooperation is to explain:

> " Dr X has suggested that it might be worthwhile exploring whether emotional factors are contributing to your problems. We often find that stress can aggravate headaches, chest pain etc., and so a psychological assessment might help you and Dr X understand your complaints better. Then we could discuss whether any treatment might be helpful."

The illness history

The current illness episode

It is important to start with a detailed account of the patient's physical symptoms, their nature, onset and development. In particular, the interviewer should establish when and where the symptoms began, what the patient was doing at the time, what thoughts were associated with the symptoms, who called for the doctor or ambulance and why they did. Obtain the details of what the patient was told by the doctors (and relatives

---

**Box 5.7 Problem list mailed back by patients before out-
patient visit**

It would be very helpful if you could complete the following
problem list before the doctor sees you at Clinic. Do not
worry if you are unable to answer any of the questions.

What are the main problems at present?
1. Pain: Yes/No
   If YES, state site(s) of pain:
2. Other physical complaints: Yes/No
   If YES, state complaints:
3. Problems at work   Yes/No
4. Family problems   Yes/No
5. Problem with others, e.g. with
   colleagues, friends   Yes/No
6. Financial problems   Yes/No
7. Physical disabilities   Yes/No
   List one or two activities you can no longer
   carry out since the symptoms began
8. Other problems not included from 1–7   Yes/No
   If YES, please list here:

---

and friends), and what treatment was given. The following case illustrates
the importance of eliciting these details:

> A 56-year-old woman was referred with a 9 month history of chest
> pain and breathlessness. She had a normal exercise treadmill test
> and normal coronary angiogram. Her symptoms began at 2am one
> evening when she awoke gasping for breath with chest tightness
> and palpitations associated with extreme anxiety and panic. She
> thought she was going to die of a heart attack and her husband
> telephoned for an ambulance which took her to hospital. Earlier
> that evening she had suffered a puncture while driving her car on
> the motorway. Her car had to be towed to the local garage where
> her husband examined the tyres in the early evening. He
> discovered that all four tyres had been slashed, and that it was
> only by chance that the other three tyres had not developed any
> punctures. His wife became very distressed on hearing this news,
> and was too upset to eat her evening meal. She retired to bed
> early but had a restless night's sleep until she woke at 2am with
> her physical complaints.
>
> Over the next 9 months she had three admissions to hospital
> (two via the A & E Department) with the same symptoms. She was
> subjected to invasive tests, and spent six days in hospital. But the
> history of how the problem began, which obviously suggests a
> diagnosis of panic attacks, was not recorded in her medical notes,

and possibly had not been elicited. Yet it was elicited within the first 20 minutes of the psychiatrist meeting the patient. The patient's condition responded well to anxiety management, along with the techniques of reattribution and link-making described below.

Current occupational, social and physical disabilities should be established, with particular emphasis on behaviours avoided because of fear of harmful consequences or aggravation of symptoms. Patients sometimes avoid activities they erroneously think make their symptoms worse, thus unnecessarily increasing their disability. Questioning the patient about the effects of their illness provides a natural bridge to enquiries about other recent stresses, and about symptoms of anxiety and depression. This 'changing of the agenda' (Goldberg *et al*, 1989) must only be undertaken when the patient has had ample opportunity to describe their physical symptoms and disease concerns. Psychiatric assessment should include questions to establish whether the patient has a specific anxiety disorder (especially phobic anxiety), mood or somatoform disorder.

If cognitive–behavioural treatment is an option, then a more detailed assessment is necessary (for details see Sharpe *et al*, 1992). This establishes the patient's beliefs and associated behaviour, and obviously requires a good working knowledge of the cognitive–behavioural therapy model. The focus of this approach is on how a patient's symptoms, distress and disability are perpetuated by an interaction between psychological and physiological processes (see Chapter 9, Fig 9.1).

After obtaining a history of the symptoms the patient is asked what he believes or fears to be the cause and likely consequence of his symptoms. For example, a simple question such as "what is your worst fear about your symptoms?" can be revealing. The 14-item Whiteley Index (Pilowsky, 1967) is a useful adjunct to this part of the interview, and the patient's responses to individual questions, for example "would you believe the doctor if he told you he could find nothing wrong with you", provide useful topics for discussion. During this part of the interview the patient may disclose that one or more alternative practitioners is being consulted. This provides further opportunities to explore beliefs and assumptions about symptoms and health, some of which may contribute to the problem or be therapeutic obstacles. Patients may believe, for example that "doctors should be able to explain all my symptoms", or "too much anxiety may kill me". Such assumptions might explain seemingly irrational concerns the patient has about symptoms, and need to be considered in treatment.

The behaviour employed by the patient to cope with the symptoms may result in disability. It may also be perpetuating the symptoms and cognitions. Hence helping the patient to change their behavioural response to symptoms can reduce disability and symptoms, as well as facilitating cognitive change. Examples of behaviours that may need to be modified include dysfunctional responses to symptoms, such as lying down for 4 hours each day, over-breathing, taking symptom-relieving medication and repeatedly seeking reassurance (Salkovskis, 1989; Sharpe *et al*, 1992).

Previous illness experience

Assessment must take account of not only the current physical complaints, but also the patient's previous illness experience. It is useful to adopt a biographical approach, enquiring about childhood illnesses, experiences of physical and emotional symptoms at times of life transitions and stress, for example menarche, examinations, marriage, childbirth, divorce. Experiences of exposure to illness in the family and the impact these had on the patient should be obtained. This may be particularly important if parental illness resulted in lack of care, and where physical symptoms may have become a means of communication within the family.

In some patients with transient disorders this should be straightforward, but in others with many years of somatic complaints, e.g. patients with somatisation disorder, the history may take more than two hours and involve writing letters to different hospitals as well as a telephone call to the GP. If a chronic, persistent disorder is suspected, then it is advisable to ask the family doctor for either the patient's complete medical file or a precis of it. It is not uncommon, for example, for a patient to deny any medical problems beyond the earliest recorded entry in their hospital notes; subsequent discussion with the family doctor or scrutiny of the primary care file may reveal a history of multiple somatic complaints of 20 or 30 years duration. Information of this nature may be crucial to the management of the patient. A typical example of this is given below:

> A 63-year-old woman was referred in 1992 by her family doctor with a 4 year history of irritable bowel syndrome and other minor complaints. On detailed enquiry the patient denied any medical problems before 1984, and the medical notes contained no details before 1983. The GPs notes were requested, and they revealed an extensive history of multiple unexplained somatic complaints dating from the patient's early life. Indeed, a diagnosis of somatisation disorder was suggested (and subsequently confirmed on detailed chart review) by a glance at the computerised summary of the patient's medical records.

The past medical history may suggest unnecessary surgery, in particular hysterectomy in women. Some patients will be taking unnecessary drug treatment, for example antispasmodics for hyperventilation misdiagnosed as asthma, anti-anginal medication for non-cardiac chest pain.

Interviewing the somatising patient

General interview techniques that are required in liaison psychiatry have already been discussed in Chapter 2. Further skills for interviewing the somatising patient are now discussed. Interviewing patients with strongly held beliefs that their problems are somatic rather than psychosocial usually requires greater flexibility on the part of the interviewer than standard psychiatric assessment. Having the requisite interviewing skills is essential (Bird & Cohen-Cole, 1990). These include: empathic witnessing; being able to guide and control the interview if the patient becomes excessively circumstantial; regularly summarising and reflecting back when the patient discloses information about somatic complaints that might be linked to life events (see later), and recognising and reflecting the patient's feelings as soon as they appear. It is important not to adhere too rigidly to a conventional psychiatric history taking scheme in these patients, and efforts should be made to keep the interview fluid rather than compartmentalising information. Attention to patients' feelings is important in establishing a therapeutic alliance. More than one interview may be needed to make a full assessment.

Helping the patient to make links

It is always important to ask whether somatic complaints are accompanied by any symptoms of emotional distress. Whenever appropriate, an attempt should also be made to link the physical and psychological symptoms to relevant life events and contexts. This can be done using judiciously timed summarising statements inviting comment from the patient: "You told me that the chest tightness, tiredness and headaches began about 3 years ago soon after you lost your job, and at about that time you were also feeling very tense and tearful. Have I got that right?" This approach should help the patient to recognise that: (a) each physical complaint is being taken seriously; (b) that physical and emotional symptoms sometimes coexist, and (c) that both might be related temporally to a specific psychosocial stressor (in this case loss of job). This latter technique of making the link encourages the patient to establish links between his emotional state and somatic symptoms (Goldberg *et al,* 1989). An example of an interview with a somatising patient is given below:

> The patient, a 50-year-old woman, presented with a one year history of a variety of somatic complaints that had not responded to tranquillisers, reassurance from her GP, or the efforts of two alternative practitioners. She was referred from the chest unit after her second series of lung function tests had proved normal. Before the symptoms began she had been travelling weekly to Scotland to visit her sick but fiercely independent mother, who had strenuously resisted all the patient's attempts to help her.

After a series of arguments, which culminated in her mother informing the patient that a social worker or home-help would never be allowed through the front door, the patient became unwell. This argument proved to be an important precipitating factor. In the segment of interview that follows the specific interviewing skills are in parentheses.

Dr: When did you first notice things going wrong?

Patient: It was on my way home from my mother's. My stomach started churning and I noticed I was yawning a lot. I was still thinking about all that ranting and raving with my mother.

Dr: It seemed to upset you a lot.

Pt: Well, yes. It was the first time I had ever screamed at my mother. I was so furious that she declined all our help.

Dr: What happened next?

Pt: Soon after we arrived home I started to experience a churning in my stomach, tightness in the chest and difficulty with my breathing.

Dr: (eliciting ideas about aetiology) What thoughts would go through your mind when you had these symptoms?

Pt: I would try to keep calm, but I thought there was something seriously wrong with my chest. This made me feel very panicky. I had just had flu and I thought it was the after-effects of that, or even something like TB.

Dr: Why TB?

Pt: Because my brother and sister-in-law had TB many years ago.

Dr: What would bring these symptoms on?

Pt: Anything at all, nothing specific.

Dr: How long would they last for?

Pt: Up to one hour.

Dr: (summarising statement, reflecting back to patient) So these episodes came out of the blue, lasted for about an hour, made you worried about having TB and flu, and they were associated with extreme anxiety and panic? You also told me that they all began within hours of the distressing argument with your mother, is that correct?

Pt: Yes, that's right.

Dr: Did you make any connection between these two events?

Pt: Not at that time, no.

Dr: So what did you do next?

Pt: I saw my GP. I thought it was all medical and I wanted a chest X-ray, so she arranged this.

Dr: What were the results?

Pt: They were normal. I was very pleased but I was also very worried about what else could be causing my symptoms, because all I could think about was this "breathing thing".

Dr: How often was this happening?

Pt: Oh, two or three times a day, every day.

Dr: (asking about the effects of the symptoms) Did it affect your ability to go about your normal activities?

Pt: Not really, but when I had this feeling I also had a sensation that everything around me was unreal. Also noises seemed to be louder, it was quite odd.

Dr: (empathic statement) It sounds as if these experiences were quite unpleasant?

Pt: Yes, very uncomfortable.

Dr: So what did your GP do for your breathing problems and unreal feelings?

Pt: She gave me some tranquillisers called ativan, 1mg daily for 30 days.

Dr: Did they help?

Pt: Amazingly, yes. All my symptoms disappeared after a couple of weeks so I stopped taking them.

Dr: Really, so what happened after that?

Pt: Well, the symptoms came back even stronger.

Dr: Were they the same symptoms?

Pt: Yes, but this time they were more frequent and I also had difficulty with my speech.

Dr: (open question) Tell me a bit more about that.

Pt: Well, when I had an attack I felt I had a lump in my throat and that my voice was disappearing.

Dr: I see. Did the speech problem occur at the same time as the other symptoms of chest tightness, breathlessness and churning in the stomach?

Pt: Not really, no, they didn't appear to be related.

Dr: Were there any situations in which these symptoms were more likely to occur? For example, in shops, standing in queues, or in public transport? (enquiry into possible situational nature of panics).

Pt: Not really, no, but people said I looked terrible when I was out. For example, when I was in the supermarket last week someone came up to me and asked me if I was alright.

Dr: What do you think they were seeing that made you appear so conspicuous in the supermarket?

Pt: I think I looked distressed, upset. I was shaking and trembling (breaks down and cries).

Dr: (empathic statement) I can see how distressed you are talking about it now. It does seem as though you have been very upset, tearful, panicky and unable to cope in the last six months.

Pt: Yes, I suppose so, but I still can't get my breathing under control.

Dr: (summarising and checking) So let me see if I've got this right. Although the symptoms were helped briefly by the tranquillisers, it seems as if they got worse after you stopped them. Not only did the symptoms recur more frequently, but you had more of them. Is that correct?

Pt: Yes.

Dr: So what did you do next?

Pt: Well, my family decided that there must be something wrong. My son, who is married to a doctor, insisted that I went to the hospital for some lung function tests.

Dr: How did you feel about that?

Pt: I was very pleased, although at the same time, about three months ago, I was already seeing a herbalist. She had been recommended by my sister, and was treating me with some medicines, but quite frankly they were not helping at all.

Dr: Did you see any other alternative practitioners about your complaints?

Pt: Yes, an acupuncturist gave me 12 sessions of treatment last November. He charged me £20 per visit.

Dr: Did it help?

Pt: Not really, no. But since I have stopped going I have felt worse. My last appointment with the acupuncturist was 4 weeks ago.

Dr: So the last month has been pretty bad for you?

Pt: Yes, dreadful. The worst thing is these panicky feelings that I've been getting. I worry that my husband will die during these attacks and I will be left alone (tears).

Dr: I can see that these attacks are very distressing for you?

Pt: Yes, I don't know why I have these thoughts, because he is in such good health.

Dr: Let's talk a bit more about your emotional state at present, because it does sound as if you have been very upset. How have you been feeling in your mood in the last fortnight or so?

Mental state enquiry revealed a number of psychological symptoms including low mood on most days with suicidal thoughts; sleep disturbance with early morning wakening at 5 am; loss of appetite with weight loss of 6 pounds in the previous 2 months; loss of interest in her hobbies and pastimes; poor concentration and irritability; as well as feelings of anxiety and panic which were associated with depersonalisation. All these symptoms had to be elicited from the patient and were not mentioned in any of the previous correspondence. Her selective attention to the breathing difficulties, chest tightness, churning in the stomach, globus sensation and dysphagia had led the physicians to single-mindedly search for a somatic cause for her multiple complaints.

After this brief interview, which lasted half an hour, the main components were brought together in a summarising statement:

Now let me see if I have got this right. If I have left anything out then please let me know. It seems that in addition to all the physical symptoms that you have had over the last year or so you have also been feeling very sad, with poor sleep, inability to think clearly, irritability, and episodes of anxiety and panic during which you feel unreal. It seems as if most of these symptoms began within a few days of this serious argument with your mother, and that despite treatment with tranquillisers, alternative medicine and a number of investigations of your lungs, things have not improved. Have I got that right?

The patient appeared satisfied with this summary of her predicament and acknowledged that there were both physical and psychological components to the illness, although she still expressed understandable concern that she had no idea what was causing her breathing difficulties.

Providing patients with an explanation for their somatic symptoms is important. But this should only be attempted after each complaint has been listened to fully and the patient knows that they have been taken seriously, and when the patient has had an opportunity to explore the links between life events and the onset of somatic complaints. Pathophysiological mechanisms in somatisation are important, and it is often possible to provide patients with physiological explanations for their somatic complaints and explain how these are linked to psychological processes (Sharpe & Bass, 1992).

The psychiatric history

Because these patients are often reluctant to discuss psychosocial issues we prefer to leave a detailed assessment of the past psychiatric history to the end of the interview. This has already been suggested in Chapter 2.

The patient's family

There may be advantages in conducting the interview with the patient in the presence of one or more family members. This may be particularly apposite in those patients with chronic pain or recurrent unexplained complaints, when family members may have years of experience of the patient's complaints and behaviour. A family interview which takes account of the patient's role in the family may provide information less likely to emerge when the patient is interviewed alone. The attitude of each family member to the patient's condition can obviously influence its outcome. Evidence that they share or collude with the patient's hypochondriacal or morbid beliefs about the complaint is likely to have an adverse influence on the prognosis, and suggests that family therapy may be an appropriate treatment.

Self-monitoring

A period of self-monitoring may also be helpful, especially if cognitive–behavioural treatment is being undertaken. Following the initial assessment interview, the patient is asked to keep a diary of symptoms and activities. This can provide an accurate account of frequency and pattern of symptoms, the patient's activity level and its association with symptoms. It also introduces the patient to the active role they will be required to play in treatment. Medication use, especially for analgesics, should be included in self-monitoring. These written diaries provide a baseline from which change can be planned and improvement assessed. They can begin as simple activity records, and later be expanded to include recording of thoughts and coping behaviours as necessary.

Management

Engagement in treatment

By the time a comprehensive assessment has been carried out, the therapist should have developed a fairly clear idea of the patient's problems and should be able to present a summary of what the patient has disclosed, always inviting comment. Patient and therapist should come to some kind of agreement about this summary/formulation before treatment proceeds.

Next, the patient and therapist must agree on treatment goals. During this phase different expectations of treatment and how it should proceed should be reconciled, otherwise treatment will not be effective. Finally, the patient must agree to have no further tests or investigations, and appreciate that during the course of treatment further lengthy discussions of symptoms will be unproductive.

Preparing the patient for psychological treatment

Before treatment is commenced there are three important issues to address:

(1) all investigations should have been completed. The patient should be told that treatment is conditional on no further investigations being carried out

(2) the patient should be informed that a pain- or symptom-free existence may not be a realistic therapeutic goal. In some patients it may be more appropriate to help them cope better with their pain and disability, i.e. 'coping not curing'

(3) the nature of the treatment and its approximate duration should be carefully explained.

The aims and goals of treatment should be made explicit from the outset. There are a number of different treatment approaches and these will be discussed later. Some patients have chronic symptoms, marked invalidity and/or intractable psychosocial problems that are unlikely to respond to a brief, focused, psychological approach. It may be more difficult to negotiate treatment goals with these patients. Early attempts to negotiate treatment goals can lead to the impression that the patient's main goal is to reject psychological help. Some patients will insist that they want physical treatment to cure their somatic symptoms, or demand more tests to get to the bottom of what is wrong with them. The patient should be told that this is not the psychiatrist's role, and that there will be no more tests or physical treatments (unless antidepressants are indicated or new symptoms suggest intervening organic disease).

Which clinical features predict response to treatment?

Patient selection is clearly a critical factor. Diagnostic grouping is an unreliable guide because:

(1) there is considerable overlap in symptoms between the various somatoform syndromes
(2) the processes involved in producing the symptoms are diverse
(3) those factors maintaining the symptoms differ from patient to patient.

Any treatment will be unsuccessful if the patient is not satisfactorily engaged. Although there are no single predictive factors, some general rules serve as a guide. For example, psychological treatment is more likely to be successful if the patient:

(1) accepts that psychosocial factors are contributing to the clinical problem, and
(2) is able to negotiate mutually agreed treatment goals. Clearly, if the patient is engaging in treatment then this is an encouraging sign.

There is some evidence from research studies to suggest that certain clinical characteristics predict response to psychological treatment. These will be briefly described.

Sociodemographic factors

There is general agreement that younger age, continuing employment and absence of pain-contingent compensation payments are associated with a better response to treatment. Work satisfaction is an important predictor of the outcome of treatment (Mendelson, 1991).

Pain related factors

Certain pain characteristics predict poor response to treatment. These include constant, unremitting pain, and pain that is not aggravated by stress or anxiety (Guthrie *et al*, 1993). Patients with a long history of unsuccessful surgery for pain, and those who have not experienced a life event before pain onset have also been found to have a poor outcome (Feinmann *et al*, 1984).

Psychological factors

There is evidence that those patients with more dysfunctional illness beliefs and assumptions about aetiology have a worse outcome. Patients in this category continue to attribute their symptoms to a physical cause, despite evidence to the contrary (Butler *et al,* 1991). The relationship between outcome and the level of anxiety and depression has varied between studies. For example, Butler *et al* (1991) found that treatment-resistant depressive illness was associated with a poor outcome in CFS, whereas Guthrie *et al* (1991) found that IBS patients with low scores on scales measuring anxiety and depression, i.e. the absence of reported psychiatric distress, had a poor response to psychological treatment. One interesting finding that requires replication is that patients whose spouses had lower scores on the hypochondriasis scale of the MMPI reported greater improvement after treatment (Roberts & Rhinehardt, 1980).

Deyo *et al* (1988) demonstrated that patients recruited for treatment studies through lay publicity have a better outcome than pain clinic patients. Greater attention should be paid to the mode of referral and recruitment of subjects when reporting and interpreting the results of studies in this field.

Factitious disorders

In 1951 Asher introduced the term Munchausen's syndrome for patients who deliberately simulate symptoms of acute disease to gain admission to hospital with no obvious goal other than to be a patient. The patients he described gave dramatic but plausible histories, had numerous admissions to different hospitals, and had often undergone repeated laparotomies for simulated acute abdominal pain (Asher, 1951).

Numerous other reports of Munchausen's Syndrome have appeared since 1951, supporting and adding to Asher's original description. The prototypical case is an itinerant male, admitted via casualty – sometimes using an alias. Often the patient has a criminal record and is described as having psychopathic personality traits. Once in hospital the patient may develop new symptoms when investigation of the original symptom is negative.

The typical patient with Munchausen's establishes little rapport with staff, may appear restless, evasive or hostile. Medical and nursing staff may begin to feel that the patient is making excessive demands, is being manipulative or truculent. Regardless of whether the diagnosis is made, quarrels with staff may precipitate self-discharge and a repetition of the same events at another hospital.

Munchausen's syndrome is only one of several clinical scenarios in which the manifestations of disease are intentionally fabricated without obvious conscious motive. The term 'factitious disorders' encompasses this wider range of cases. Although Munchausen's syndrome is an example it is not the most common type. Indeed, it is clinically misleading to assume that it is a paradigm of factitious disorders. Recent reports of factitious disorders suggest that most cases are females who do not usually adopt a truculent or overtly hostile attitude to staff, and indeed may be model patients. They do not wander from hospital to hospital but rather wish to be cared for by the same doctor over many years, and they do not abscond when confronted. One should not therefore be misled by the Munchausen stereotype. It was noted in one series of cases that many of the patients were pleasant young women (Reich & Gottfried, 1983). Many were on friendly terms with nurses, knew their physicians on a first name basis, were familiar with their families and even worked in their offices or baby-sat for them. In such cases the physician sometimes found it difficult to accept that the patient's condition was self-induced – "because they had known the patients well for many years and had trusted them" – even when circumstantial evidence was overwhelming (Reich & Gottfried, 1983).

Factitious disorders with various presenting signs and symptoms have been described. These include factitious dermatoses (dermatitis artefacta) (Sneddon & Sneddon, 1975; Lyell, 1979), self-induced fevers and infections (Rumans & Vosti 1978; Aduan *et al*, 1979), haemorrhage and bleeding disorders (Daily *et al*, 1963; O'Reilly & Aggeler, 1979), factitious asthma (Downing *et al*, 1982), factitious diarrhoea, factitious hypoglycaemia (Tattersall, 1985), self-poisoning, e.g. with lead, feigned unconsciousness and factitious dystonia (Naish, 1979). An awareness of factitious disorders with a willingness to entertain the possibility are prerequisites to making the diagnosis. The following case illustrates this point.

> Mr JS, a 26-year-old single man, had been admitted to a medical ward two months prior to psychiatric referral. He was referred by his consultant physician who was concerned that he was becoming dependent on pethidine which he had been receiving for abdominal pain. The patient was originally admitted with dyspnoea and a diagnosis of asthma. The dyspnoea resolved shortly after admission, but new symptoms and signs emerged. These included fever, haematuria and abdominal pain. Numerous investigations, including repeated blood cultures, endoscopies, barium studies, ultrasounds, radio-isotope scans, cystoscopy and laparotomy had negative results. At the time of psychiatric referral a number of rare medical conditions, but not factitious disorder, were included in the differential diagnosis. The psychiatrist immediately suspected factitious disorder upon hearing the history and encountering the patient's hostility and evasiveness. Several pieces of information obtained from nursing staff added to the likelihood of this. First, the patient had received no visitors. Second, he had submitted himself to investigations and operations without question, concern or curiosity. Third, a night nurse had observed

that he spent long periods in the toilet. Since self-injection with pyogenic material and self-catheterisation of the bladder require instruments, the water cistern of the toilet was opened and an array of needles and cannulae were found. The patient discharged himself from hospital that day.

A distinction should be made between factitious disorder and malingering. In malingering the patient produces symptoms deliberately but has an obvious goal, for example, to avoid criminal conviction or conscription. In a factitious disorder the motivation to be a patient is obscure – even to the patient: there is no obvious environmental goal other than achieving patient status and being submitted to tests and operations.

In addition to the distinction from malingering, factitious disorders should be contrasted with somatoform disorders. With a somatoform disorder a patient has physical symptoms or signs without an organic explanation but, unlike a patient with a factitious disorder, is not deliberately producing them. Thus, patients with factitious disorders know they are producing symptoms even though they are unclear about their motives for doing so. In practice most cases of factitious disorder, somatoform disorder and malingering can be distinguished, but occasionally the distinction can be difficult to make and mixed pictures undoubtedly occur. It is worth noting that in all the reported series of factitious disorders, obvious or major mental disorder has been rare, although many of the patients have been described as immature, passive or as having personality disorders (Dadelson, 1979).

Eisendrath (1984) has suggested that factitious disorders be subclassified according to the level of enactment and divides cases into three types: (a) describing fictitious symptomatology only; (b) simulation of a disease, e.g. as when a patient places a few drops of blood in their urine to convince the physician of the presence of disease, and (c) the production of actual abnormalities of physical examination or laboratory tests, e.g. when a patient injects pyrogenic material into themselves or inflicts injury on themselves. It is not, however, clear that this classification is useful for deciding treatment or predicting outcome, although clearly patients in the third group are most at risk from self-harm. Factitious disorders can be fatal or life-threatening and are often severe and chronic (Spiro, 1968).

In a report of 41 cases from a Boston teaching hospital four subgroups of factitious disorder were identified: self-induced infections, simulated illnesses, chronic wounds and surreptitious self-medication (Reich & Gottfried, 1983). This series comprised 39 women and two men, and the average age was 33 years. Twenty-eight of the patients worked in medical settings. Among the patients who were surreptitiously interfering with the healing of chronic wounds (including stasis ulcers) most had frequent hospitalisation for skin grafts, debridement and wound care.

The term dermatitis artefacta is used to describe a wide variety of self-inflicted skin lesions including rashes, ulcers, bruises and blisters. It is an imprecise use of the term dermatitis, but it has widespread acceptance. Patients usually deny causing their lesions and the diagnosis can be difficult to confirm. Lesions may have bizarre unnatural shapes and edges, for example, with linear or geometric outline. They may occur in unlikely sites, but patients with medical knowledge can produce lesions in seemingly inaccessible sites and more closely mimic naturally occurring conditions (Sneddon, 1982). Patients have been known to use acids, alkalis, phenol, heated needles and scalpels to induce lesions and some have had amputations of fingers, hands, arms and legs. Almost all such patients are women and under 30 years (Sneddon & Sneddon, 1975). Some patients have been known to use rubber bands or tourniquets to produce chronic oedema of a hand or leg.

Patients with factitious illness who admit their simulation are usually unable to explain their behaviour in any depth. They may acknowledge that they feel more secure in hospital or describe their behaviour as an "escape from reality". Some patients simulating severe pain appear to be seeking opiates. Most patients with factitious disorders, however, evade discussion of their motives. It is occasionally possible to engage such patients in exploration of their family and personal backgrounds and reach some understanding of their behaviour, as in the following case history.

> DF is a 30-year-old secretary who has had insulin dependent diabetes since the age of 3. She has diabetic neuropathy and small vessel disease, further complicated by chronic ulceration of her feet and legs. She was under the care of a chiropodist specialising in the care of diabetic feet who suspected that she was interfering with the healing of her ulcers, and that some of her ulcers were self-inflicted. This suspicion was based on observations made over the previous 4 years. Self-induced lesions occurred at atypical sites and had bizarre anatomical features e.g. straight edges. Ulcers that failed to heal when treated openly, quickly healed under closed dressings and close supervision in hospital. The ulcers led to repeated admissions to hospital, and treatment included skin grafts which always failed to heal, probably because of interference. Eventually, infection and gangrene lead to an amputation of her lower left leg. The patient had been requesting an amputation for some time before her physicians thought it was indicated.
>
> The patient's mother, who also had insulin-dependent diabetes, had died four years previously with liver and kidney failure. She had been dependent on alcohol from before DF was born. As a child DF was told by her father that her mother's inebriated behaviour was due to diabetes. She recalls her mother frequently being carried home or to bed in what she later realised was a

drunken stupor. She also had frequent episodes of diabetic coma. DF was frightened by and ashamed of her mother's state; as a result she became too ashamed to bring friends home. She bitterly describes family outings and holidays that were ruined by her mother's drinking, and the chagrin on her 13th birthday when mother got too drunk to organise the party.

As the older of two children DF tried to control her mothers behaviour and took on the 'responsible role'. She would put her mother to bed and frequently shouted at her. Her father was away on business a lot of the time. DF now knows that he had affairs with women. He initially nagged his wife about her drinking, but in later years ignored her. They never talked, and by the age of 7 DF was preparing meals while mother was in bed. She would also go shopping with her father on Saturdays and as she got older accompanied him on social occasions when other men were with their wives.

DF's father is a 66-year-old architect. In describing their relationship DF was inconsistent and ambivalent. She idealised him, but also said that he patronised her and did not give her emotional support when she needed it. She feels they have a close relationship even though they have never talked about her mother. DF had appealed to him to help her with her mother, but he ignored her. She knew that he was unhappy about her mother's drinking from about the age of 6. DF has one younger brother who 'patronises' her rather than showing real care. He checks up on how DF is eating and has often commented "if you were a good diabetic you wouldn't have got like this".

DF has had frequent hospital admissions and visits throughout her life because of poor control of her diabetes. She describes a recurring dream she has had since childhood in which she attends the diabetic clinic which is held on the 1st floor overlooking a stairwell. In the dream the 'good diabetics' stay up at the top with the doctors and nurses, while the 'bad ones', i.e. poorly controlled such as DF, are thrown over the side into the stairwell.

At school DF was quiet and compliant. Few people ever came to their house when she was a child and she had few friends. She first left home at 21, but returned after a few months to look after her mother despite 'hating' her. DF spoke disparagingly of her mother's psychiatrist who she had appealed to for help at the time.

DF left home again at 28 to live alone 40 miles away. Her mother was on her own and died 6 months later. DF visited her during these 6 months and helplessly watched her health deteriorate, often wishing that "the stupid cow" would die. After her mother's death she did not cry and simply went to work as usual not telling anyone what had happened. She said it took a few years for her to realise that she was dead and she never experienced grief, only the persistence of her contempt. The diagnosis of factitious disease was first considered around the time of her mother's death. None of the professionals involved in her care were told of the death at the time. She spent a high proportion of the next 3 years in different hospitals because of her ulcers and the amputation.

DF talked of having only one friend, one of the nurses who had looked after her. She had never had any sexual relationships or boyfriends and commented: "I am a loner because of what happened when I was younger. I have to find ways of looking after myself. I am a coper". She expressed resentment about the fact that people always saw her as coping so well – "If I ask for help people change the subject". On the other hand DF described her own role in creating this impression – "I am automatically cheerful – something in me takes over". Medical and nursing staff who knew her well described DF as "difficult, prickly, oversensitive, manipulative and a professional patient".

The staff were concerned that challenging DF about the cause of her ulceration would lead to her discharging herself from specialist care. During her first interview with the psychiatrist, however, DF said that her brother believed she produced her own ulcers to get attention. She did not admit that she did, but nor did she deny it. When asked why she might injure her feet and legs which were already diseased, her reply suggested complex motives. She was disgusted by her ulcerated feet and legs; they were a continual reminder of her diabetes and she would rather be 'an amputee'. She resented the doctors who had the power to decide matters like amputation and renal transplant for diabetic patients, and yet were 'useless' when it came to helping her mother. Her manner became grandiose and competitive as she talked about how she knew more about diabetes than many professionals.

Adopting a biographical perspective enables one to establish meaningful connections and reach some understanding of a patient's behaviour. Factitious disorders can be viewed as abnormal illness behaviour or abnormal care-eliciting behaviour. DF's self-destructive behaviour appears to give her a sense of control over her disease and at the same time occupy the sick role. There is a temporal association between her factitious disorder and the death of her mother suggesting a difficulty with the bereavement. This in turn is not surprising given the complicated ambivalence in their relationship. Her mother's inability to care for DF and her frightening out of control behaviour were presumably, in DF's mind, linked from an early age with diabetes. But DF is, like her mother, diabetic. Her self-injury appears to be partly motivated by a wish to rid herself of the external signs of her diabetes, her 'diabetic feet', and can be understood as an attack on part of herself that she identifies with her mother and her diabetes. DF's self-destructive behaviour may thus be an irrational attempt to deal with severe emotional trauma.

Once factitious illness is diagnosed the patient may evoke strong feelings in staff. There is often anger at the patient for being deceptive, embarrassment, fear of exposing or shaming the patient, and bewilderment. The doctor may fear precipitating an angry outburst after which the patient storms off. There is occasional worry that exposure of the deception may lead to suicide. On the other hand if the doctor does not confront the patient with the deception they may feel they are colluding with or even encouraging the patient's behaviour.

Although angry self-discharge is typical for Munchausen's syndrome, the literature suggests that it is far less likely to occur with other forms of factitious disorder, and there are no reports of patients committing suicide after confrontation. In the Boston series (Reich & Gottfried, 1983), 33 patients were confronted with evidence that their disorders were self-induced and none discharged themselves or became suicidal. Only 13 acknowledged causing their symptoms, yet even among those who did not some improvement occurred after confrontation, with four of the most chronic cases becoming asymptomatic.

Management

Confrontation of the patient with factitious illness should be carefully planned, and a joint approach involving both the physician and psychiatrist is advised. It is always easier to confront these patients when there is tangible evidence of fabrication e.g. a supply of syringes or illicit medication in the patient's locker. The doctor should sympathetically acknowledge the seriousness of the patient's problems, and how he has felt compelled to aggravate these. This is followed by a 'hand-over' to the psychiatrist, at the bedside if necessary, emphasising that this is routine practice. A typical interview with the patient might be as follows:

> Physician: "We have found this syringe/ medication in your locker and we believe that you have been injecting/medicating yourself with pus/blood/lead sulphate tablets. In our experience patients who do this sort of thing usually have stresses in their lives that they have had difficulty adjusting to or coming to terms with. My colleague Dr Murphy (the psychiatrist) has had a lot of experience of helping patients with this kind of problem and may be able to help you".

It is important to inform the patient that emotional support is available and that he will not be abandoned or rejected. There are no systematic evaluations of this kind of intervention strategy and it is obvious that it has to be adapted to the particular circumstances of each patient. Even when the offer of psychiatric help is taken up, some patients will continue to inflict harm on themselves, continue their deceptions and some may even develop factitious psychiatric disorder.

Summary

Somatisation is the most frequent form of presentation of psychiatric illness in the general hospital and primary care setting. Few psychiatrists gain enough experience of patients who somatise to be able to adequately diagnose and treat them. The management of chronic cases of somatisation can be extremely difficult and the psychiatrist needs to develop additional skills to be able to engage and hold patients in treatment.

Somatisation is a relatively new area in terms of modern research. The prevalence of the disorder has been clearly established in a number of different settings and new ways of treating somatisation are being developed and tested. There is little empirically based research on patients with factitious disorder because of its relative rarity. When the condition is suspected, it usually causes great concern among medical and surgical staff who find it difficult to understand or empathise with such patients. The liaison psychiatrist is ideally placed to provide support and guidance to both patient and members of staff.

References

Aduan, R. P., Fauci, A. S., Bale, D. C., *et al* (1979) Factitious fever and self-induced infection. A report of 32 cases and review of the literature. *Annals of International Medicine*, **90**, 230–242.

American Psychiatric Association (1980) *Diagnostic and Statistical Manual of Mental Disorders* (3rd edn) (DSM–III). Washington, DC: APA.

—— (1987) *Diagnostic and Statistical Manual of Mental Disorders* (3rd edn, revised) (DSM–III–R). Washington, DC: APA.

—— (1994) *Diagnostic and Statistical Manual of Mental Disorders* (4th edn) (DSM–IV). Washington, DC: APA.

Appleby, L. (1987) Hypochondriasis: acceptable diagnosis? *British Medical Journal*, **294**, 857.

Asher, R. (1951) Munchausen's syndrome. *Lancet*, i, 339–341.

Barsky, A., Wyshak, G. & Klerman, G. (1986) Hypochondriasis: An evaluation of the DSM–III criteria in medical out-patients. *Archives of General Psychiatry*, **43**, 493–500.

——, ——, —— *et al* (1990)The prevalence of hypochondriasis in medical out-patients. *Social Psychiatry and Psychiatric Epidemiology*, **25**, 89–94.

——, —— & —— (1992) Psychiatric comorbidity in DSM–III–R hypochondriasis. *Archives of General Psychiatry*, **49**, 101–108.

Bass, C. & Murphy, M. (1991) Somatisation disorder in a British teaching hospital: the unnatural history of a non–disease. *British Journal of Clinical Practice*, **45**, 237–244.

—— & Benjamin, S. (1993) Management of chronic somatization. *British Journal of Psychiatry*, **162**, 472–480.

Benjamin, S., Barnes, D., Berer, S., *et al* (1988) The relationship of chronic pain, mental illness and organic disorders. *Pain*, **32**, 185–195.

—— & Eminson, P. M. (1992) Abnormal illness behaviour: childhood experiences and long-term consequences. *International Review of Psychiatry*, **4**, 55–70.

Bhatt, A., Tomenson, B. & Benjamin, S. (1989) Transcultural patterns of somatization in primary care: a preliminary report. *Journal of Psychosomatic Research*, **33**, 671–680.

Bianchi, G. (1973) Patterns of hypochondriasis: a principal component analysis. *British Journal of Psychiatry*, **122**, 541–548.

Bird, J. & Cohen-Cole, S. A. (1990) The three-function model of the medical interview. An educational device. *In Methods in Teaching Consultation–Liaison Psychiatry* (ed M.S. Hale), pp. 64–88. Basel: Karger.

Birtchnell, S. A. (1988) Dysmorphobia – a centenary discussion. *British Journal of Psychiatry*, **153** (suppl. 2), 41–43.

Blumer, D. & Heilbron, M. (1982) Chronic pain as a variant of depressive disease: the pain-prone disorder. *Journal of Nervous and Mental Disease*, **170**, 381–409.

Bohman, M., Cloninger, C., von Knorring, A., *et al* (1984) An adoption study of somatoform disorders: III Cross-fostering analysis and genetic relationship to alcoholism and criminality. *Archives of General Psychiatry*, **41**, 872–878.

Bools, C., Neale, B. & Meadow, R. (1994) Munchausen's syndrome by proxy: a study of psychopathology. *Child Abuse and Neglect*, **18**, 773–788.

Bridges, K. & Goldberg, D. P. (1985) Somatic presentation of DSM–III psychiatric disorders in primary care. *Journal of Psychosomatic Research*, **29**, 563–569.

——, ——, Evans, G. B., *et al* (1991) Determinants of somatization in primary care. *Psychological Medicine*, **21**, 473–483.

Butler, S., Chalder, T., Ron, M., *et al* (1991) Cognitive behavioral therapy in the chronic fatigue syndrome. *Journal of Neurology, Neurosurgery and Psychiatry*, **54**, 153–158.

Clark, D. (1988) A cognitive model of panic attacks. In *Panic: Psychological Perspectives* (eds S. J. Rachman & J. Mayer). New Jersey: Lawrence Erlbaum Associates.

Cloninger, C. R. (1986) Diagnosis and classification of the somatoform disorders. In *Diagnosis and Classification in Psychiatry* (ed. G. Tischler), pp. 243–259. New York: Cambridge University Press.

Craig, T. K., Boardman, A. P., Mills, K., *et al* (1993) The south London somatisation study: I. Longitudinal course and the influence of early life experiences. *British Journal of Psychiatry*, **163**, 579–588.

Dadelson, T.(1979) The Munchausen's spectrum: borderline character features. *General Hospital Psychiatry*, **1**, 11–17.

Daily, W. J. R., Coles, J. M. & Creger, W. P. (1963) Factitious anaemia. *Annals of Internal Medicine*, **58**, 533–538.

de Leon, J., Saiz-Ruiz, J., Chincilla, A., *et al* (1987) Why do some psychiatric patients somatize? *Acta Psychiatrica Scandinavica*, **76**, 203–209.

Deyo, R. A., Bass, J. E., Walsh, N. E., *et al* (1988) Prognostic variability among chronic pain patients: implications for study design, interpretation and reporting. *Archives of Physical Medicine and Rehabilitation*, **69**, 174–178.

Downing, E. T., Braman, S. S., Fox, M. J., *et al* (1982) Factitious asthma: physiological approach to diagnosis. *Journal of the American Medical Association*, **248**, 2878–2881.

Drossman, D. A. Sexual and physical abuse in women with functional or organic gastrointestinal disorders. *Annals of Internal Medicine*, **113** , 828–833.

Eisendrath, S. J. (1984) Factitous illness: a clarification. *Psychosomatics*, **25**, 110–117

Escobar, J. I., Burnam, M., Karno, M., *et al* (1987*a*) Somatization in the community. *Archives of General Psychiatry*, **44**, 713–718.

——, Golding, J. M., Hough, R. L., *et al* (1987*b*) Somatization in the community. Relationship to disability and use of services. *American Journal of Public Health*, **77**, 837–840.

Feinmann, C., Harris, M. & Cawley, R. (1984) Psychogenic facial pain programme in out-patients with chronic pain. *Journal of Psychosomatic Research*, **34**, 13–19.

Gillespie, R. (1928) Hypochondria: its definition, nosology and psychopathology. *Guy's Hospital Report* **78**, 408–460.

Goldberg, D. & Bridges, K. (1988) Somatic presentations of psychiatric illness in primary care setting. *Journal of Psychosomatic Research*, **32**, 137–144.

——, Gask, L. & O'Dowd, T. (1989) Treatment of somatisation: teaching techniques of reattribution. *Journal of Psychosomatic Research*, **33**, 689–695.

Gray, D. W. & Collin, J. (1987) Non-specific abdominal pain as a cause of acute admission to hospital. *British Journal of Surgery*, **74**, 239–242.

Gupta, M. (1986) Is chronic pain a variant of depressive illness? A critical review. *Canadian Journal of Psychiatry*, **31**, 241–248.

Guthrie, E., Creed, F., Dawson, D., *et al* (1991) A controlled trial of psychological treatment for the irritable bowel syndrome. *Gastroenterology,* **100**, 450–457.

(1993) A randomized controlled trial of psychotherapy in patients with refractory irritable bowel syndrome. *British Journal of Psychotherapy*, **163**, 315–322.

Guze, S. (1975) The validity and significance of hysteria (Briquet's Syndrome). *American Journal of Psychiatry*, **132**, 138–141.

Kaminsky, M. J. & Slavney, P. R. (1976) Methodology and personality in Briquet's Syndrome: a reappraisal. *American Journal of Psychiatry*, **133**, 85–88.

Katon, W., Ries, R. K. & Kleinman, A. (1984) Part II: a prospective DSM–III study of 100 consecutive somatisation patients. *Comprehensive Psychiatry*, **25**, 305–314.

——, Lin, E., Von Korff, M., *et al* (1991) Somatisation: a spectrum of severity. *American Journal of Psychiatry,* **148**, 34–40.

Kenyon, F. (1964) Hypochondriasis: a clinical study. *British Journal of Psychiatry*, **100**, 478–488.

Kellner, R. (1985) Functional somatic symptoms and hypochondriasis. *Archives of General Psychiatry*, **42**, 821–833.

Kirmayer, L. J. & Robbins, J. M. (1991*a*) Three forms of somatization in primary care: prevalence, co-occurrence and socio demographic characteristics. *Journal of Nervous and Mental Diseases*, **179**, 647–655.

—— & —— (1991*b*) Functional Somatic Syndromes. *In Current Concepts of Somatization* (eds L. Kirmayer & J. Robbins), pp 79–106. Washington, DC: Academic Psychiatric Press.

Kleinman, A. & Kleinman, J. (1985) Somatisation: the interconnections in Chinese society among culture, depressive experiences and the meaning of pain. In *Culture and Depression* (eds A. Kleinman & B. Good). Berkeley: University of California Press,

Lascelles, R. (1966) Atypical facial pain and depression. *British Journal of Psychiatry*, **112**, 651–659.

Lloyd, G. G. (1986) Psychiatric syndromes with a somatic presentation. *Journal of Psychosomatic Research*, **30**, 113–120.

Lyell, A. (1979) Cutaneous artefactual disease: a review, amplified by personal experience. *Journal of the American Academy of Dermatology*, **1**, 391–407.

Marks, I. & Mishan, J. (1988) Dysmorphophobic avoidance with disturbed bodily perception: a pilot study of exposure therapy. *British Journal of Psychiatry*, **152**, 674–678.

Meadow, R. (1982) Munchausen's syndrome by proxy. *Archives of Disease in Childhood*, **57**, 92–98.

Mendelson, G. (1991) Psychological and social factors predicting responses to pain treatment. In *Proceedings of the 6th World Congress of Pain* (eds M. R. Bond, J. E. Charlton & C. J. Woolf), pp. 193–206. Elsevier Science Publishers.

Merskey, H. & Spear, F. (1967) *Pain: Psychological and Psychiatric Aspects*. London: Balliere, Tindall & Cassell.

Munro, A. (1988) Monosymptomatic hypochondriacal psychosis. *British Journal of Psychiatry*, **153** (suppl. 2), 37–40.

Murphy, M. R. (1990) Classification of the somatoform disorders. In *Somatization: physical symptoms and psychological illness* (ed. C. Bass). Oxford: Blackwell.

Naish, J. M. (1979) Problems of deception in medical practice. *Lancet*, **ii**, 139–142.

Noyes, R., Reich, J., Clancey, J., *et al* (1986) Reduction in hypochondriasis with treatment of panic disorder. *British Journal of Psychiatry*, **149**, 631–635.

O'Reilly, R. A. & Aggeler, P. M. (1979) Covert anticoagulant ingestion: a study of 25 patients and review of world literature. *Medicine*, **55**, 389–399.

Orenstein, H. (1989) Briquet's syndrome in association with depression and panic: a reconceptualisation of Briquet's syndrome. *American Journal of Psychiatry*, **146**, 334–338.

Oxman, T. E. & Barrett, J. (1985) Depression and hypochondriasis in family practice patients with somatization disorder. *General Hospital Psychiatry*, **7**, 321–329.

Pennebaker, J. W. & O'Heeron, R. C. (1984) Confiding in others and illness rate in spouses of suicide and accidental death victims. *Journal of Abnormal Psychology*, **93**, 473–476.

—— & Susman, J. R. (1988) Disclosure of traumas and psychosomatic processes. *Social Science and Medicine*, **26**, 327–332.

Perley, M. G. & Guze, S. B. (1962) Hysteria: the stability and usefulness of clinical criteria. *New England Journal of Medicine*, **266**, 421–426.

Phillips, K. A. (1991) Body dysmorphic disorder – the distress of imagined ugliness. *American Journal of Psychiatry*, **148**, 1138–1149.

Pilowsky, I. (1967) Dimensions of hypochondriasis. *British Journal of Psychiatry*, **131**, 89–93.

——— (1970) Primary and secondary hypochondriasis. *Acta Psychiatrica Scandinavica*, **46**, 273–285.

——, Bassett, D. L., Begg, M. W., *et al* (1982) Childhood hospitalisation and chronic pain in adults: a controlled retrospective study. *International Journal of Psychiatry in Medicine*, **12**, 75–84.

Powell, R. Dolan, R. & Wessely, S. (1990) Attributions and self esteem in depression and the chronic fatigue syndrome. *Journal of Psychosomatic Research*, **34**, 665–673.

Raheja, S. K., Mcdonald, P. J. & Taylor, I. (1990) Non-specific abdominal pain – an expensive mystery. *Journal of the Royal Society of Medicine*, **83**, 10–11.

Reich, P. & Gottfried, L. A. (1983) Factitious disorders in a teaching hospital. *Ann Intern Med*, **99**, 240–247.

Roberts, A. H. & Rhinehardt (1980) The behavioural management of chronic pain: long-term follow-up with comparison groups. *Pain*, **8**, 151–162.

Robins, L. N., Helzer, J. E., Groughan, J., *et al* (1981) National Institute of Mental Health Diagnostic Interview Schedule. *Archives of General Psychiatry*, **38**, 381–389.

Robson, P. (1988) Development of a new self-report questionnaire to measure self-esteem. *Psychological Medicine*, **19**, 513–518.

Roy, R., Thomas, M. & Mattas, M. (1984) Chronic pain and depression: a review. *Comprehensive Psychiatry*, **25**, 96–105.

Rumans, L. W. & Vosti, K. L. (1978) Factitious and fraudulent fever. *American Journal of Medicine*, **65**, 745–755.

Salkind, M. R. (1969) Beck Depression Inventory in general practice. *Journal of the Royal College of General Practitioners*, **18**, 267–271.

Salkovskis, P. M. (1989) Somatic problems. In *Cognitive Behaviour Therapy for Psychiatric Problems* (eds K. Hawton, P. Salkovskis, J. Kirk, *et al*). Oxford Medical Publications.

Sargant, W. & Slater, E. (1972) *An Introduction to Physical Methods of Treatment in Psychiatry* (2nd edn). Edinburgh: Livingstone.

Sharpe, M. & Bass, C. (1992) Pathophysiological mechanisms in somatization. *International Review of Psychiatry*, **4**, 81–97.

——, Peveler, R. & Mayou, R. (1992) The psychological treatment of patients with functional somatic symptoms: a practical guide. *Journal of Psychosomatic Research*, **36**, 515–529.

Shaw, J. & Creed, F. (1991) The cost of somatisation. *Journal of Psychosomatic Research*, **35**, 307–312.

Slavney, P. R. & Teitelbaum, M. L. (1985) Patients with medically unexplained symptoms. *General Hospital Psychiatry*, **7**, 21–25.

Smith, G. R., Monson, R. A. & Ray, D. C. (1986) Patients with multiple unexplained symptoms. Their characteristics, functional health, and health care utilisation. *Archives of Internal Medicine*, **146**, 69–72.

Sneddon, I. B. (1982) Simulated disease: problems in diagnosis and management. The Parkes Webber Lecture. *Journal of Royal College of Physicians*, **17**, 199–205.

Sneddon, I. & Sneddon, J. (1975) Self-inflicted injury: a follow-up study of 43 patients. *British Medical Journal*, **3**, 527–530.

Spiro, H. (1968) Chronic factitious illness. *Archives of General Psychiatry*, **18**, 569–580.

Stern, J., Murphy, M. R. & Bass, C. (1993a) Attitudes to the diagnosis of somatisation disorder among British psychiatrists. *British Journal of Psychiatry*, **162**, 463–466.

——, —— & —— (1993b) Personality disorders in patients with somatisation disorder. A controlled study. *British Journal of Psychiatry*, **163**, 785–789.

Tattersall, R. (1985) Brittle diabetes. *British Medical Journal*, **291**, 555–557.

Toone, B. K. (1990) Disorders of hysterical conversion. In *Somatization: Physical Symptoms and Psychological illness* (ed C. Bass). Blackwell Scientific Publications.

Turk, D. & Salovey, P. (1984) Chronic pain as a variant of depressive disease: a critical reappraisal. *Journal of Nervous and Mental Disease*, **172**, 398–404.

Tyrer, P. & Alexander, M. (1987) Personality Assessment Schedule. In *Personality Disorders: Diagnosis, Management and Course* (ed. P. Tyrer). Bristol: Wright.

——, Fowler-Dixon, R. & Ferguson, B. (1990) The justification for the diagnosis of hypochondriacal personality disorder. *Journal of Psychosomatic Research*, **34**, 637–642.

Vaillant, G. (1984) The disadvantages of the DSM–III outweigh its advantages. *American Journal of Psychiatry*, **141**, 542–545.

Walker, E., Katon, W., Harrop-Griffiths, J., et al (1988) Relationship of chronic pelvic pain to psychiatric diagnosis and childhood sexual abuse. *American Journal of Psychiatry*, 145, 75–80.

Warwick, H. & Salkovskis, P. M. (1990) Hypochondriasis. *Behaviour Research and Therapy*, **28**, 105–117.

Wessley, S. (1990) Old wine in new bottles: Neurasthenia and ME. *Psychological Medicine*, **20**, 35–53.

Williams, J. B. & Spitzer, R. L. (1982) Idiopathic pain disorder: A critique to pain-prone disorder and a proposal for a revision of the DSM–III category of psychogenic pain disorder. *Journal of Nervous and Mental Diseases*, **170**, 410–419.

World Health Organization (1992) *The Tenth Revision of the International Classification of Diseases and Related Health Problems* (ICD–10). Geneva: WHO.

Zoccolillo, M. & Cloninger, C. R. (1985) Parental breakdown associated with somatisation disorder (hysteria). *British Journal of Psychiatry*, **147**, 443–446.

6 Psychological reactions to physical illness

Peter Maguire and Peter Haddad

Psychological adjustment • Organic factors in the development of psychological disorders • Psychiatric disorders: diagnosis and treatment • Managing difficult situations • Hidden psychological morbidity • Reducing key concerns • Summary

---

Psychological adjustment

The prevalence of psychiatric disorder in the general hospital is very high with many patients suffering from either anxiety states or depression (see Chapter 3). The development of physical illness confronts patients and their families with several psychological hurdles. If these are not resolved they can cause persisting psychological distress and precipitate psychiatric disorder. These issues are discussed below and summarised in Box 6.1.

Uncertainty about the future

A diagnosis of a serious physical illness is associated with uncertainty as clinicians are often unable to provide exact information about prognosis. Key questions such as, "Will my treatment be curative?", "How long will I live?", "What will go wrong next?", are difficult to answer. In some patients, even when apparently cured, there is still a possibility of recurrence and premature death.

Clinical practise may exacerbate these uncertainties. Patients often see different doctors on each hospital visit. Each doctor may assume that the previous doctor discussed the illness, prognosis and treatment with the patient. So important points may never be explained properly or patients may be given conflicting information. Sometimes, clinicians withhold information from patients in a misguided attempt to protect them, which may also heighten their uncertainty.

Some degree of worry is normal. Some patients, however, become plagued by worries about the future. They cannot control these thoughts or distract themselves. Any reminder that they have a physical disease, like a magazine article or television programme, further intensifies their fears. Regular follow up visits can also reactivate worries that complications, or evidence of relapse or progression will be found. Worries are likely to be especially intense if they have had adverse

157

experiences of physical illness in close friends or relatives, particularly if the friend or relative was reassured that all would be well, but still died.

Search for meaning

People faced with a serious illness usually try to find an explanation for it. They will ask, "Why me?", "Why now?" and "What did I do to bring this on myself?". Psychological adaptation is more likely if an adequate explanation can be found. With certain diseases this is relatively easy, for example, in coronary heart disease risk factors have been identified including a strong family history, a diet high in saturated fats, lack of exercise and heavy smoking. In other conditions, such as multiple sclerosis, no strong risk factors are available. This leaves a vacuum into which patients and relatives project non-scientific theories. Popular lay theories include the role of diet or a virus. Patients who accept these theories either blame themselves for their predicament, or pursue alternative methods of treatment with a desperate urgency.

Patients with cancer often blame themselves, and self-blame lowers self-esteem which leads to demoralisation. These changes are likely to persist if patients see no way of changing their personality, life style, or of avoiding the main stressors. In some instances patients may project their blame onto key relatives or employers which engenders great bitterness. This hinders patients' ability to adapt and may cause a serious breakdown in personal relationships.

Loss of control

Patients cope better with life threatening illnesses if they believe that they can contribute towards their recovery. In coronary heart disease they can seek to lose weight, adopt a healthier diet, give up smoking or increase their exercise. In cancer there are no strong risk factors apart from smoking and patients may feel helpless. Helplessness is also likely to occur if patients feel that they have already done their best to preserve their health. Thus a woman who presents for help as soon as she finds a breast lump but is found to have metastatic cancer will feel let down and resourceless.

Other patients seek to fight their illness. They change one or more aspects of their lifestyle, such as diet, utilise psychological techniques (i.e. relaxation, visualisation, yoga or meditation), or become involved in volunteer organisations and self-help groups. They usually cope well unless their way of dealing with the illness becomes an over-riding preoccupation.

Loss of control is felt by many patients with physical illness as they are encouraged to adopt the role of passive recipients. This can be

---

Box 6.1 Psychological hurdles confronting patients with physical illness

Uncertainty about the future
Searching for meaning
Loss of control
Sense of failure
Stigma
Being secretive
Sense of isolation

---

exacerbated by the specialised nature of some treatments, such as radiotherapy, chemotherapy and bone marrow transplantation for cancer or the involvement of special wards, for example for patients with AIDS.

Side-effects of treatment, for example, lethargy and nausea, can exacerbate feelings of loss of control as patients may no longer be able to perform activities of daily living. This process also occurs in the terminal stages of illness when patients may need help with the simplest of tasks such as sitting up or turning over in bed. Accepting this loss of independence can be especially difficult for people who dislike placing their trust in others.

One of the attractions of unorthodox treatment is that patients feel they can contribute to their recovery. The more effort the patient puts into the treatment, for example eating a specially prepared and elaborate diet, the greater the sense of control.

Sense of failure

Patients often feel their bodies have let them down. Since death in childhood is particularly uncommon the parents of children with physical illness often feel this sense of failure acutely. They failed to ensure that the child reached healthy adulthood. Marked feelings of personal failure increase the likelihood of depressive illness.

Stigma

Physical illness and handicap is associated with stigma. Patients often convey this by using words such as 'dirty', 'unclean', and 'contagious'. Similarly, serious illnesses such as AIDS can evoke feelings of revulsion and fear in others. Parents are often reluctant to allow their children to play with a child who has cancer or AIDS. When one mother described the attitude of other children towards her daughter who had leukaemia she said "It's as though she's got leprosy". The whole family of the cancer patient may feel stigmatised.

The attitude of others need not be so unkind. Fallowfield (1990) quoted a 36-year-old lady with lung cancer describing the impact on others:

> "I felt immediately that you had entered a special place, a place I came to call 'The land of the sick people'. The most disconcerting thing, however, was not that I found that place terrifying and unfamiliar, but that I found it so ordinary, so banal. I didn't feel different, didn't feel that my life had radically changed at the moment that the word cancer became attached to it. The same rules held. What had changed, however, was other peoples' perceptions of me. Unconsciously, even with a certain amount of kindness, everyone – with the single rather extraordinary exception of my husband – regarded me as someone who had been altered irrevocably."

Verres (1986) reported that when healthy individuals were asked about their attitudes to cancer patients, fear of contagion was rarely expressed directly. However, precise questioning about the degrees of intimacy that people would engage in with a known cancer patient showed that over a third would not share utensils used by patients, many would not eat anything cooked by someone with cancer, and even more would avoid any physical contact. In a second study, 61% of health individuals admitted that they would avoid contact with a friend who had cancer. In the same study more than 50% of cancer patients felt that other people avoided them.

Stigma is more likely when the general public associates a particular illness with socially undesirable behaviour. For example, cervical cancer is associated with sexual promiscuity, AIDS is associated with homosexuality. Misconceptions by the public about the role of viruses and oncogenes in causing cancer may also fuel fears that cancer is infectious.

Being secretive

When patients worry about the acceptability of their diagnosis to close friends, relatives or employers they may decide to keep their diagnosis secret. They may also do this to protect loved ones from anguish. Secretiveness is associated with a poor psychological adaptation because it precludes patients receiving emotional support.

Sense of isolation

In addition to a sense of being stigmatised three other factors contribute. First, friends and relatives find it embarrassing to meet the patient or his close family as if they ask how the patient is doing they might hear bad news. Second, contact may remind them of their own mortality – something most individuals choose to deny until they have a serious illness or accident. Third, it is deeply distressing to watch someone you know, respect, or love deteriorate physically or mentally, especially if they suffer unpleasant symptoms such as pain, weight loss or vomiting. Thus, relatives and friends find it easier to avoid or reduce contact with the patient and his family.

> A young man with testicular cancer reported: "The effect of my illness on my friends hit me suddenly several months ago. I was walking down the road and I saw one of my friends approaching. He suddenly turned down a side street – I know it was to avoid me".

Psychological consequences of treatment

Certain treatments for physical illness may involve radical surgery, radiotherapy or powerful drug treatments with severe side-effects.

Surgery – loss of a body part

Surgical treatment may involve the removal of a body part like a breast or limb. The patient then has to come to terms with a change in body image. This will be difficult if the body part was important to their sense of psychological well-being. Up to 25% of women fail to adapt to the loss of a breast despite being given an adequate external breast prosthesis (Maguire *et al*, 1983). Three types of problem may develop in relation to loss of a body part. First, a patient may be unable to accept that he is no longer physically whole. This loss of physical integrity causes the patient to feel vulnerable psychologically, which makes it harder to adapt to other stressful life events. Second, a patient may feel a heightened sense of self-consciousness and worry that people have only to look at her to realise that she has lost a body part (e.g. breast or limb), even when the loss is concealed by baggy clothes or artificial aids. Finally, some individuals feel less sexually attractive and are unable to be reassured by their partners' claims that they love them as much as before surgery.

Continued inability to adapt to the loss of a body part whether it is due, for example, to breast loss or amputation of a limb, is highly correlated with subsequent psychiatric morbidity including affective disorders and sexual difficulties (Maguire *et al*, 1978).

Surgery – loss of a body function

Examples of surgery resulting in the loss of a body function include the loss of control over defecation following the formation of a stoma after surgical resection of the large bowel in ulcerative colitis, loss of the voice after laryngectomy in the treatment of cancer of the larynx and loss of fertility following hysterectomy for severe menorrhagia.

Up to one-third of patients who have a stoma formed after resection of a cancer of the large bowel become morbidly anxious and/or depressed (Williams & Johnson 1983; Thomas *et al*, 1987*a*,*b*). They cannot accept the stoma because it represents an 'obscene part of themselves' or they cannot adapt to the bag. They fear the bag will bulge, leak, smell, burst or make a noise. They worry that it could have a serious effect on personal relationships and employment. Sometimes individuals are frightened to leave the security of their own homes because they may have 'an accident'. Others only venture outside when they have carefully mapped out the position of public toilets. Some patients avoid going on holidays abroad because changes in diet may affect stoma function adversely or because there is no escape or privacy if there is a problem with the bag. Those who have yet to form a close relationship face a difficult dilemma. Should they mention their stoma to a potential partner and at what point? Fears associated with the bag and of rejection contribute to sexual difficulties.

Loss of fertility is a concern to many women following gynaecological surgery. Those who have not completed their families or have no children have to accept that they will have no more children. Loss of fertility may also exacerbate feelings of loss of control; fertility is a personal issue, an integral body function which every adult expects to be able to regulate for themselves.

Radiotherapy

Radiotherapy is often given after surgery or chemotherapy in patients with cancer. It is usually explained to patients on the basis that it will destroy any residual cancer cells. This can have a paradoxical effect when patients were led to believe they had a good prognosis.

> Pt: They said that all they needed to do was to remove the lump. I thought I was clear. Then they said I needed radiotherapy as an insurance. How can I square the two? I am getting more and more worried that the cancer is still there.

General side-effects of radiotherapy include fatigue and sore skin. Others depend on the area that is irradiated; for example, diarrhoea may follow radiotherapy to the abdomen, while treatment to the upper chest may result in hoarseness and a cough. There is a strong relationship between adverse effects caused by radiotherapy and subsequent psychiatric morbidity (Devlen *et al*, 1987).

Chemotherapy

Chemotherapy increases psychological morbidity especially when given in combination. Psychiatric morbidity is linked to the degree of toxicity especially gastro-intestinal effects like nausea, vomiting and diarrhoea (Devlen *et al*, 1987), and the length of treatment (Hughson *et al*, 1986).

Conditioned nausea and vomiting occur in up to 25% of patients receiving chemotherapy (Morrow, 1982). This also contributes to the development of anxiety and depression. Characteristically a patient experiences nausea and vomiting during the first one or two courses of treatment. Then the patient finds that any sound, sight or smell which reminds him of treatment provokes the same adverse effects. This can lead to phobic avoidance of treatment.

In men and women chemotherapy can cause infertility by destroying germ cells in the gonads (Whitehead *et al*, 1982). In women, infertility may be accompanied by a premature menopause. Men can now bank sperm prior to chemotherapy so that there is the possibility of fathering children later if their partners have artificial insemination. However, there is no current technology to store womens' eggs prior to chemotherapy. Women may be able to have hormone replacement treatment (HRT) after chemotherapy to prevent menopausal symptoms, though this is usually contraindicated in breast cancer.

Other treatments

Early studies of the effects of bone marrow transplantation have suggested that fears about treatment related mortality, concerns about the donor, and the experience of prolonged isolation, increase psychiatric morbidity in the short and long term. Larger scale and longer-term studies are needed to clarify the nature of these problems and their aetiology.

Organic factors in the development of psychological disorder

Organic factors in the aetiology of psychiatric disorder can be divided into treatment and disease related factors.

Organic factors related to treatment

Surgery can contribute to sexual problems by causing anatomical damage to the genitalia. This may occur with surgery for vulval, vaginal, cervical and penile carcinomas. For example , a vulval malignancy may be treated by a radical vulvectomy in which the labia, clitoris, mons pubis and surrounding skin are all removed leaving extensive scarring. As well as the psychological impact of such an operation, sexual intercourse will be affected by the apparent shortening of the vagina, the increased prominence of the pubic bone, vaginal stenosis which can accompany the scarring, and the loss of the clitoris which affects orgasmic potential.

Any kind of abdominal surgery may also cause damage to the nerve supply to the genitals, resulting in impotence and ejaculatory difficulties in men and failure of arousal and inability to experience orgasm in women. The psychiatrist should try to differentiate psychological and organic aetiologies so that correct management can be given.

Radiotherapy can cause sexual problems through direct physical damage. For example, in women with cancer of the cervix delivering radiotherapy through internal sources causes anatomical damage to the vagina, including stenosis, fibrosis and fistulae (Bos Branolte *et al*, 1988). It is possible that radiotherapy may cause depressive illness by a direct effect on the brain. This may explain why women undergoing breast conservation followed by radiotherapy experience as much psychiatric morbidity as those undergoing mastectomy (Fallowfield *et al*, 1986; Maunsell *et al*, 1989). Children who receive cranial irradiation suffer mild cognitive impairment. Whether adults are also at risk of such impairment is uncertain.

Chemotherapy may act directly on the brain to cause an affective disorder. This is more likely to occur when chemotherapies are used in combination. There is also evidence that chemotherapy can cause impairment of short-term memory (Devlen *et al*, 1987).

Steroids cause psychiatric disturbances including delirium, schizophreniform psychoses, elation and depression. The clinical picture often defies simple classification and consists of a complex mixture of affective, schizophreniform and organic elements. Furthermore, the picture may fluctuate rapidly. Psychiatric syndromes may also be precipitated by the sudden cessation of steroids.

Organic factors related to disease

Physical illness can cause a wide range of psychiatric disturbances through direct effects on the brain. This effect can be mediated in two ways. Firstly, via the direct destruction of brain tissue either by a tumour, brain metastases or infection. Secondly, via non-direct effects resulting from systemic illness. This effect may be mediated by a metabolic or an infectious mechanism.

Primary brain tumours account for about 3% of cancer deaths. They are the second most common tumour in children under the age of 15 years, accounting for 20% of all childhood tumours. The symptoms of a primary brain tumour depend on the site of involvement. In addition, any tumour may cause the non-specific symptoms of raised intracranial pressure including morning headaches and vomiting. Diagnosis is usually made by CT scan. The course of most brain tumours is one of progressive, gradual worsening of symptoms.

The tumours which most commonly metastasise to the brain include those of the lung, breast, alimentary tract, prostate and pancreas. Of these lung tumours are the commonest. Cerebral metastases are usually multiple and rapidly growing. Sometimes they can produce clinical signs before the primary lesion, particularly when this is on the lung. The signs depend on the areas involved. Two other forms of metastatic CNS involvement deserve mention. Firstly, an encephalitic form of metastatic carcinoma occasionally occurs where there is no discrete metastatic deposit but diffuse infiltration of carcinomatous-cells throughout the brain parenchyma. The second form of involvement is carcinomatosis of the meninges.

A vast number of conditions can produce organic psychosyndromes. These include encephalopathies, myelopathies, neuropathies, muscular disorders, metabolic disorders, etc. Only the encephalopathies, however, are likely to present to the liaison psychiatrist. The clinical picture may include confusion, errors in thinking, behavioural abnormalities, disorders of consciousness and abnormal motor signs. Often the resulting syndrome is a delirium, although the clinical picture can be more subtle.

Metabolic encephalopathies may follow the destruction of a vital organ. For example, hepatic metastases may lead to hepatic encephalopathy, bone metastases may cause hypercalcaemia, kidney metastases may cause uraemia, while lung metastases may cause pulmonary encephalopathy. The failure of these peripheral organs may follow intercurrent infections or dehydration.

Encephalopathies may also result from opportunistic CNS infection. The brain, meninges, and subarachnoid space may be invaded by microbes via the bloodstream (during septicaemia), by metastasis (from a focal infection elsewhere in the body), or through direct extension from nearby structures (e.g. sinuses). Although the usual signs of meningitis are pyrexia, stiff neck, diffuse headache and mental state changes, only the latter may be present in immunosupressed patients. A brain abscess may present with signs of a mass lesion or diffuse encephalopathy.

Depressive illness may be a prodromal feature of patients who develop cancer, and in some of these cases the depression may represent a non-metastatic complication of the cancer.

Box 6.2 Non-organic, psychiatric conditions that occur in association with physical disease

Adjustment disorder
Anxiety states
Affective disorders
Body image problems
Conditioned responses
Sexual problems
Eating disorders
Alcohol misuse
Opiate dependence
Post-traumatic stress disorder
Abnormal illness behaviour

Psychiatric disorders: diagnosis and treatment

The main non-organic, psychiatric conditions associated with physical illness are summarised in Box 6.2. These are a mixture of psychiatric diagnoses and behavioural responses to illness.

Adjustment disorders

These states are commonly encountered following the sudden development of an acute illness or the sudden deterioration of a chronic illness. The symptoms consist of an exaggeration, in terms of either duration and/or intensity, of the emotions seen in the normal stress response. Depressive symptoms are the most common, for example low mood, guilt and hopelessness. They are often accompanied by anxiety.

Psychological intervention must be brief and aimed to facilitate the individual's natural adjustment to his new physical status. Treatment is focused on helping patients to express their feelings about the illness, come to terms with it, and find suitable coping strategies to deal with it. Box 6.3 lists the steps which should be addressed when managing a patient with an adjustment disorder in the context of physical illness.

The liaison psychiatrist may need to see the patient on a regular basis to facilitate the expression of distress and provide support. It may, however, suffice to advise nursing and medical staff on how to help the patient through support, explanation and correction of any misconception that the patient may have. Specific behavioural and cognitive strategies may also be employed, for example, deep muscular relaxation to control anxiety symptoms. On rare occasions there is a place for the short-term use of medication to relieve distressing symptoms. A one week prescription of temazepam 10–20mg nocte prn may enable a patient to sleep better. Similarly, a one week prescription of a short acting benzodiazepine may combat daytime anxiety. Small doses of neuroleptics can also be prescribed to help with anxiety, but their use may be contraindicated if the patient has certain physical complications (see Chapter 10). If depressive symptoms are marked it is often worth commencing an antidepressant.

The systematic investigation of brief psychological interventions in the acute stage of illness has been limited. One area to receive attention, however, has been in patients with myocardial infarction (MI). There are now several controlled intervention studies that have employed brief, mainly behavioural, treatments in post-MI patients (Gruen, 1975; Langosch *et al*, 1982; Oldenburg *et al*, 1985). Their findings suggest that psychological intervention during the acute phase of the illness is beneficial, although the results must be viewed with caution, as most studies have quite serious methodological flaws including for example, small numbers, lack of random assignment and failure to define the treatment intervention.

A more recent study by Thompson & Meddis (1990) investigated the preventative effect of psychological intervention given at an early stage following illness. They prospectively evaluated an in-hospital programme of counselling provided to first time MI patients by coronary care (CCU) nurses. In this study, the psychological intervention was carried out by staff already working on the unit, rather than by psychologists or counsellors brought in from outside. Patients were randomised in cohorts of 10 either to the counselling intervention, or to an 'as usual' control group. Patients who received the counselling reported significantly lower levels of anxiety than controls, both immediately following the MI and when re-assessed six months later. They also reported less anxiety about returning to work and their spouses, who were also evaluated, reported significantly lower levels of anxiety than the spouses of controls. The key point about this study is that it demonstrates that a relatively simple psychological intervention, conducted by staff already involved in the care of the patient, can have a significant long-term impact on patients' well being.

A study of women awaiting mastectomy for breast cancer has also demonstrated the powerful effect of a simple intervention (Burton *et al*, 1991). In this study 200 women were randomly allocated to one of four groups; preoperative psychological assessment interview plus a 30 minute psychotherapeutic intervention; preoperative assessment plus a 30 minute 'chat' to control for the effects of attention; preoperative assessment only; or routine hospital care. The psychotherapeutic intervention was client-centered and conducted by a consultant surgeon, as was the 30 minute chat. The psychological assessment (45 minutes) was carried out by an experienced clinical psychologist, and included a detailed exploration of the woman's emotional status and her fears regarding surgery.

Preoperative assessment with or without additional 30-minute intervention from the surgeon was found to have lasting protective effects against body image distress (Burton *et al*, 1991) and HADS anxiety scores at 3 months and 1 year post-surgery. Patients in the three groups that received a psychological assessment were significantly less likely to be cases for both anxiety and depression on Present State Examination (Wing *et al*, 1974) criteria at 1 year than patients in the routine hospital care group. Little benefit was found in outcome for the psychotherapeutic intervention over the chat except that significantly fewer women were depressed at 1 year follow-up.

The striking finding from this excellent study is the powerful, long-term, protective effect of a simple psychological intervention, targeted at a specific group of patients during the acute stage of an illness. It suggests, as with the study of Thompson & Meddis (1990) that in patients with MI, self-disclosure and exploration of emotional issues during the acute illness, are the key factors in conveying protection against later emotional distress.

Anxiety states

Anxious mood should be diagnosed when a patient complains of persistent inability to relax or stop worrying; this represents a significant quantitative and qualitative change and the patient cannot distract him or herself or be distracted by others. An anxiety state should be diagnosed if there are four or more other symptoms including initial insomnia; irritability; sweating; tremor or nausea; impaired concentration; indecisiveness and spontaneous panic attacks. Patients with such generalised anxiety may also have irrational fears of specific situations, such as meeting groups of people (social phobia) or leaving the house alone (agoraphobia).

Specific treatment may be required for specific phobias (e.g. needles or chemotherapy) or with more generalised anxiety concerning coping with a serious illness such as multiple sclerosis, cancer or diabetes. In each case, psychological treatment is preferable to anxiolytic drugs.

Many medical rehabilitation programmes run by physiotherapists or general nurses include relaxation training and advice about reduction of stress and anxiety. When more specialised treatment is required, this is best administered by a clinical psychologist, who will employ relaxation (for generalised anxiety/tension), systematic desensitisation (for phobias), biofeedback, cognitive–behavioural or dynamic psychotherapy according to the nature of the complaint, the patient's personality and the psychologist's own training.

In patients with severe anxiety, certain drugs may be helpful when used for short periods, to help the patient settle so that he can learn anxiety management techniques. Brief treatment with benzodiazepines or low doses of a major tranquilliser, e.g. thioridazine, are helpful for in-patients but it is essential that these are reduced and stopped before discharge. Certain somatic symptoms, for example, palpitations and tremor respond well to beta-blockers.

If the patient has strong anticipatory anxiety prior to admissions for particular treatments or investigations, such as for chemotherapy in patients with cancer, the psychiatrist should recommend that the patient takes anxiolytics in small doses for two or three days beforehand to cover the treatment. If this approach is insufficient a major tranquilliser or an antidepressant should be tried. When somatic symptoms predominate a beta-blocker will be helpful.

If the anxiety is triggered by realistic uncertainty about prognosis the psychiatrist should advise the clinician to check whether the patient wishes to be told those signs and symptoms that might herald a recurrence of physical illness or further deterioration. Patients who wish to have such markers should then be asked how often they would like to be monitored. They usually nominate sensible intervals of time.

Depressive illness

Management of depressive disorders must always include careful consideration of predisposing, precipitating and maintaining factors. Where the depression appears closely bound up with a life threatening, disabling or near terminal illness, the patient should be encouraged to air any worries and helped to adjust to his new physical status. Where depression persists at the level of depressive disorder an antidepressant is indicated, irrespective of the original cause.

The difficulties of accurately assessing depression in the medically ill have already been discussed in Chapters 2 and 3. Key symptoms include: persistent low mood for 2–4 weeks which is significantly greater quantitatively and qualitatively compared with periods when the patient has been unhappy; sleep disturbance; irritability; impairment of attention and concentration; restlessness or retardation; loss of energy; social withdrawal; negative ideation; suicidal ideation; diurnal variation of mood; loss of appetite or weight, and constipation.

The liaison psychiatrist should advise that any depressive illness is treated promptly with antidepressants, which are effective but tolerable to people suffering adverse effects of physical illness. The use of antidepressants in liaison psychiatry is addressed in Chapter 10. It is important to advise the prescribing physician on several points about the prescription of antidepressants. First, that they do not cause physical or psychological dependence. Second, they are necessary because the depression is due to a change in the body's chemistry caused by the stress of the illness or its treatment. Third, the drug will need to be taken for at least 4–6 months to prevent any relapse of depression and the prescribing of such drugs is only the first step in helping a patient who has additional complaints like body image problems. Fourth, the antidepressant medication must be taken regularly as prescribed and not just when the patient is feeling low. Fifth, the patient must be warned of common side-effects of the particular antidepressant being prescribed. Finally, the clinician should inform the patient that any improvement may take 2–4 weeks.

Most patients with depression will respond to antidepressant medication. However, the clinician should be advised to refer the patient for reassessment if he fails to do so. When there are maintaining factors, such as inappropriately negative views of prognosis or body image it may be necessary to employ cognitive strategies, or alternatively suggest referral to a clinical psychologist. In other patients there may be interpersonal difficulties and a more dynamic approach may be helpful. Only a very small number of patients suffering from depression associated with physical illness will need admission to a psychiatric unit because the suicidal risk is usually low. However, chronic physical illness and pain, especially in the elderly, correlates with an increased risk of suicide.

Body image problems

The core feature in all body image disorders is that the patient becomes inappropriately preoccupied with the idea that their body is abnormal, incomplete or is in some way damaged. It is essential to check whether the patient can look at the affected part and the resultant emotional reaction. The degree to which the patient avoids looking and prevents others doing so should be established.

Behavioural treatments are useful in treating these disorders and specific treatments include graded exposure, desensitisation and cognitive therapy. Patients may also be referred when the surgeon wishes a psychiatric opinion about the appropriateness of reconstructive surgery. Suitable patients include those who have behavioural avoidance of looking at the affected part, want the surgery for themselves rather than because of pressures from somebody else and have a realistic view of the likely outcome and possible complications.

Conditioned responses

Conditioning can become so severe in patients undergoing certain kinds of chemotherapy or radiotherapy that the patient is left in a terrible dilemma; if they continue with the treatment it will become intolerable, if on the other hand they stop treatment they may die or become seriously ill.

Box 6.3 Steps to follow in the management of patients with an adjustment disorder

Reduce patient's fear and uncertainty by clear explanation of nature of illness and its treatment and prognosis. This should be repeated on several occasions by medical and nursing staff

Give an optimistic but realistic outlook regarding recovery

Facilitate patient's reactions to and feelings towards illness

Encourage expression of both positive and negative feelings

Allow patient to reflect on loss and explore possible coping mechanisms to deal with it

Involve patient in the decision making process regarding his/ her care

Involve patient's family and plan patient's rehabilitation before discharge

Inform patient's GP of the adjustment disorder so the mental state can be monitored following discharge

---

It is important that physicians try to prevent conditioned responses occurring in the first place by the use of effective anti-emetic regimes, and the recent development of the selective 5–HT$_3$ receptor-antagonist anti-emetics has contributed considerably to this. Conditioned responses are more likely to develop with long courses of chemotherapy that involve highly emetic agents, for example cisplatin.

If conditioned vomiting has become established, several approaches can be used. Reducing anxiety by behavioural methods can help, as in addition to feeling less anxious patients often experience less nausea and vomiting. One possible explanation for this is that somatic anxiety symptoms (e.g. abdominal churning, feeling hot, a lump in the throat) which result from anticipation of chemotherapy are interpreted as signs of incipient nausea and vomiting. Patients become more anxious so exacerbating their somatic anxiety symptoms. When vomiting occurs it reinforces the link between the somatic anxiety symptoms and vomiting. Removing the anxiety breaks this cognitive loop. A short-acting anxiolytic, like oxazepam, can be taken for 1–2 days prior to the infusion to reduce anxiety. In addition, the patient may be given intravenous sedation (e.g. midazolam) prior to starting chemotherapy. The amnesic effect of midazolam will also mean that the patient will have less memory of the treatment. An alternative approach is to use systematic desensitisation to break the conditioned link between cues associated with chemotherapy (e.g. the sight of a drip, the smell of the hospital) and nausea and vomiting.

Sexual problems

Sexual problems are common in the general population but are particularly widespread in general medical and surgical patients. The true prevalence is difficult to measure because of the social restrictions governing the disclosure of information about sexual behaviour. In addition, doctors do not routinely enquire about sexual activity even when prescribing drugs that are well recognised as having a deleterious effect upon sexual performance.

Certain conditions such as renal disease and diabetes have very high rates of sexual dysfunction. In renal disease 90% of males have erectile failure and 80% of women are anorgasmic. In diabetes between 35–60% of men report sexual problems, with the highest rates seen in older men with more severe diabetic disease. For example, all men over 50 with diabetic retinopathy are impotent. Men report more sexual difficulties in relation to physical illness than women. For example, in diabetes, the prevalence of sexual problems in women is approximately 35%.

A model for understanding sexual dysfunction in physical illness has been described by Bancroft (1989) and should include three important factors:

(1) recognition of the direct physical effects of the condition
(2) the psychological effects of the condition
(3) the effects of drugs and other physical treatments on sexuality.

It is interesting to note that sexual problems are more prevalent in patients with hypertension who have received treatment than in untreated patients. This is a result of the side-effects of antihypertensive agents. Table 6.1 lists some of the common drugs used in the general hospital setting which can interfere with sexual functioning. It is important to note that many of the antidepressants have a marked effect on sexual function, yet psychiatrists rarely ask routinely about sexual function.

The sensate focus method of sex therapy pioneered by Masters & Johnson (1970) is effective in treating sexual dysfunction which is psychological in aetiology. Before embarking on this it is important to exclude any underlying depressive illness, particularly when the complaint is of decreased libido or impotence. Some problems may require referral to an appropriate sex therapist. However, simple advice may be all that is needed. For example, vaginal dryness secondary to radiation damage may be relieved by the use of a lubricant gel. A woman whose vagina is shortened as a result of a total hysterectomy for endometrial or cervical cancer may find the missionary position too painful for intercourse. Advising her that the female-superior position will give her more control over the depth of penetration may relieve this. Patients often have difficulty discussing sexual problems with their partners. Facilitating openness and giving permission to try different forms of love-making can help. This is

Table 6.1 Drug effects on sexual function

Drug type	Examples
Anticholinergics	Procyclidine, benzhexol
Anticonvulsants	carbamazepine
Antidepressants	
Tricyclics	Dothiepin, imipramine
SSRI	Paroxetine, sertraline
MAOI	Phenelzine, tranylcypromine
Antihypertensives	
Beta-blockers	Propranolol, atenolol
Noradrenergic blocking agents	Guanethidine, bethanidine
ACE inhibitors	Captopril, enalopril
Centrally acting drugs	Methyldopa, clonidine
Benzodiazepines	Temazepam, diazepam
Diuretics	Indapamide, spironolactone
Neuroleptics	Thioridazine, chlorpromazine
Sex hormones	Medroxy-progesterone acetate, combined oral contraceptives

In addition to these prescribed drugs, excessive alcohol consumption is a common cause of impaired sexual function.

particularly important with older people who are more inhibited about discussing sex. It is important to remember that increasing age is no bar to sexual activity; many people in their seventies and older have active and enjoyable sex lives.

Eating disorders

Eating disorders in association with physical illness have already been discussed in Chapter 4. It is important to emphasise that relatively mild eating problems from a psychiatric point of view can result in complex clinical problems in patients with underlying physical disorder.

Alcohol misuse

There are several reasons why alcohol misuse is associated with physical illness, these are discussed in Chapter 4. Alcohol abuse can occur, however, as a direct response to developing severe illness, the patient turning to drink to gain relief. The patient may drink as a result of depression which has arisen in relation to the illness.

Opiate dependence

Occasionally a patient with physical illness whose disease is static or who has been cured, complains of dependence on the opiate analgesics required in greater quantities earlier on in the illness. This situation is rarely encountered, but is easily treated by gradual opiate withdrawal. It is often helpful to convert all opiate analgesics to the equivalent amount of methadone mixture. As this is a liquid it can be gradually reduced. In addition it is less habit forming as it has a relatively long half-life.

Post-traumatic stress disorder (PTSD)

Many patients admitted to the general hospital or seen in the Accident and Emergency department have experienced severe physical trauma or have been involved in some kind of accident or assault. PTSD has become a well recognised psychiatric complication of such experiences (Schottenfeld & Cullen, 1986; Mayou, 1992). Patients report frequent and distressing re-experiences of the traumatic event. Avoidance and numbing is common, with associated disturbances in attention and arousal. In addition, many patients experience a variety of physical complaints that may be mistaken for organic pathology and are often the focus of the patients' distress and the cause for consultation with professionals (McFarlane *et al*, 1994). If patients have been involved in road traffic accidents phobic travel anxiety can develop (Mayou, 1992).

The severity of the physical injury is not a particular risk factor for developing PTSD (Feinstein & Dolan, 1991), although the nature of the trauma may have some effect (Curran *et al*, 1990). Premorbid factors, however, such as a neurotic personality or previous history of psychiatric illness have been implicated (McFarlane, 1989).

Debriefing techniques immediately after the traumatic event can be helpful in reducing the risk of PTSD, but some patients may be too badly injured to undergo this. There is usually no shortage of counsellors or other workers available to provide debriefing to victims if national disasters occur. There is little or no help available, however, for most patients admitted to hospital routinely after a road traffic accident or a serious personal assault. Mayou (1992) has argued that the psychological and social consequences of such incidents deserve greater attention and more psychological resources.

Abnormal illness behaviour

Abnormal illness behaviour is not a psychiatric diagnosis but a behavioural response to physical symptoms. It has already been discussed in Chapters 2 and 3. It is included here to emphasise that abnormal illness behaviour occurs in patients with organic physical illness. The management of abnormal illness behaviour is predominantly behavioural and is discussed in Chapter 5.

Managing difficult situations

In addition to treating psychiatric illness in the physically unwell, the liaison psychiatrist is often asked for advice by physicians about how to manage difficult situations. This section suggests ways of handling certain situations that may be encountered in the liaison setting.

Managing uncertainty

The psychiatrist may be asked how much information the physician should give a patient who has a serious recurrent illness and who is terrified of the condition returning. The physician may be tempted to falsely reassure the patient to shield him from distress, however, the psychiatrist should be able to help the physician acknowledge and legitimise the patient's concern.

> Dr: You're right, I don't know how long you have. That's the trouble, it is uncertain. I guess this uncertainty is making it hard for you.
> Patient: Yes it is. I wish I knew where I was in terms of when my illness is going to come back.
> The psychiatrist should advise the doctor to check if the patient would like to know what signs and symptoms would indicate a recurrence before taking things further.
> Dr: What I can do, but only if you wish, is to tell you what changes would indicate that your illness is back.
> Pt: I would find that helpful.
> Dr: I think you'll start feeling very weak again. You may go off your food and find that you are getting breathless.
> Pt: As before then?
> Dr: Yes, but of course you are clear of disease at the moment. As long as these signs are absent you should be alright.

The patient should then be asked how often he would like to be checked to see if he is disease free. The doctor should add that if any of these signs should occur or if anything else untoward happens between check-ups, the patient should get in touch directly. Few relatives or patients abuse this offer.

Sometimes uncertainty has several components, each of which should be teased out before giving any advice.

> Dr: You say it's the uncertainty of it all. What particularly are you concerned about?
> Pt: Dying in pain, dying alone and being a burden to you all.
> Dr: Any other worries?
> Pt: No.

> Dr: Well that's why you are here. So that we can improve your pain control and get you more active. We'll do our best to ensure that you won't be on your own when it comes to it.

Breaking collusion

Sometimes the medical team may ask the liaison psychiatrist for advice in a case where a relative has asked the doctors to withhold a diagnosis of a fatal illness from the patient. This usually occurs because the relative cannot bear to cause anguish to his loved one who he believes would not cope with the diagnosis. The physician should be advised to explore the relative's reasons and indicate that he respects these, as the relative could be right. It is then important to determine what effect the collusion is having on the relative's emotional state and relationship with the patient. This may reveal that the relative feels under great strain emotionally and is upset about not being close to the patient. When these costs of withholding information are clarified most relatives will see the sense of considering an alternative approach to collusion.

One such alternative (Maguire & Faulkner, 1988) involves asking the relative to allow the physician to talk alone with the patient on condition the physician will not tell the patient his diagnosis. Instead, the physician tries to establish the patient's awareness of his physical status ("how do you feel things are going?"). The patient's reply will indicate that he is aware or unaware of his predicament and is willing to talk about it ("I don't think things are going well at all – I don't think I'm going to get better from this so-called ulcer"). The physician can then acknowledge and clarify any cues that have been given. In this example this would mean clarifying the cue 'so-called ulcer':

> Dr: Why do you say 'so-called ulcer'?
> Pt: They've tried to kid me it's an ulcer but it's not, it's cancer.

This confirms that the patient is aware of the situation. The doctor should then confirm that the patient's perception is correct and explore his concerns, before seeking permission to convey this awareness to the patient's spouse. The physician can check if the couple are willing to discuss their resulting concerns with him. This is emotionally painful but allows a couple to identify key concerns and discuss possible solutions.

The psychiatrist may be asked to facilitate part of the above process if the physician feels unskilled or the relative or patient are particularly distressed. The psychiatrist must recognise that he has special skills to handle difficult feelings and emotions and should be willing to offer assistance even if there is no treatable psychiatric illness.

Stigma

When patients feel stigmatised by their disease it is important to check if their feelings are legitimate or represent an inappropriate response.

A mother of a child with leukaemia was ostracised by her next-door neighbours who also had young children. They refused to allow their children to have any contact with the young patient. In this case the mother's feeling that 'it was as though my daughter had leprosy' was valid. In other cases, however, the patient's views may arise from their own insecurity.

A woman with cervical cancer believed her illness had been caused by a virus and that everyone would shun her as they would think that she was contagious. Although there is a social stigma attached to cervical cancer this woman's fears were irrational and it was possible to discuss current viral theories with her and reassure her that she was not contagious. Her worry about other peoples' views of her was tackled using a cognitive approach in which her inappropriate attitudes, their antecedents, cognitive and behavioural consequences were analysed and challenged. She was then invited to substitute a positive view, "If I talk to my friends I will find that they are sympathetic" and given encouragement to test this out with a second positive cognition, for example, "If one person is unsympathetic they are in a minority – everyone else has been very supportive".

Search for meaning

Here, patients feel anguished because they cannot find an acceptable explanation for their disease or are wrongly implicating their personality, their inability to handle stress, or other people. Careful exploration of their beliefs and their origins should enable them to be challenged constructively. If no adequate explanation can be found, this should be acknowledged, for example, "No, I agree I can't explain why you have got cancer at this time" and the patient encouraged to express consequent feelings.

When a person's religious beliefs are threatened, they may benefit from talking with a priest or chaplain. Many hospital chaplains are skilled counsellors.

Loss of control

Some patients feel there is nothing they can do to help fight their disease and as a result they become 'helpless'. They should be helped to adopt more constructive responses, such as a healthier diet, taking more exercise and learning self-help techniques, such as positive imaging, relaxation and meditation (Bridge *et al*, 1988).

Information giving and breaking bad news

The liaison psychiatrist is unlikely to have to inform patients that they have a life-threatening physical illness or break bad news to them. Nurses and doctors, however, in the general hospital do this frequently, and may turn to the liaison psychiatrist for advice, particularly if the patient is also suffering from psychological distress.

The key is to determine how much information each patient wants to know about his illness and treatment. If the initial history has been conducted sensitively, the doctor should have elicited the patient's perceptions about his physical symptoms, and awareness of the possibility of serious illness. If the patient has considered this, the doctor's task is to confirm that the patient's suspicions are correct. When the patient does not realise or suspect that he has a serious illness the health professional faces the problem of how to break the bad news without disorganising the patient psychologically or provoking strong denial.

In either case the psychiatrist should advise the doctor to see the patient in a private place, and arrange for a relative or close friend to be present which often helps adaptation when bad news is broken (Fallowfield *et al*, 1986). The doctor should first fire a warning shot ("You will remember that I said the pain in your abdomen could be due to an infection. I'm sorry to say I now think it is more serious"). The doctor should then pause to allow the patient time to take this in and respond. The patient's response will indicate if he wishes to know more ("What do you mean you think it's more serious?") or prefers denial ("I don't want all the details. I'll leave the treatment in your hands, you're the expert"). In the latter case the doctor is being given a clear message not to bombard the patient with too much information – in such a case it would be advisable for the doctor to use a euphemism in further dialogue ("We'll need to operate to remove the abdominal mass"). In the former case, where the patient indicated that he wanted more information, the doctor should give him another clue ("You know we X-rayed your bowel. Well the films have shown an abnormal area"). The patient can still pull out ("Don't tell me any more. I'd like to see you next week when my partner can come with me – you can tell me more then"). Alternatively he can pursue it ("What do you mean abnormal?") and this would be followed by further clarification ("I think it's cancer").

In this way, the doctor can tailor what he says to what the patient indicates he wishes to know. Even when patients want to know everything this approach of approaching the diagnosis gradually allows patients to prepare themselves and facilitates psychological adjustment. Occasionally a patient will ask outright about his diagnosis ("Is it MS?"). Such questions should be reflected back to check why the patient is asking. Is he looking for confirmation or denial?

> Pt: Am I dying?
> Dr: Why do you ask?
> Pt: I have lost so much weight, I feel so weak, I'm no longer getting any more treatment.
> Dr: Any other reasons?
> Pt: No.
> Dr: Yes, I'm afraid you're right.

The doctor should then give the patient an opportunity to express his feelings. This signals to the patient that the doctor is interested in his emotions and this should facilitate later disclosure of concerns. For example:

> Dr: I imagine this has been a great shock.
> Pt: Yes, it's devastating, but I had expected it.

Giving patients audiotapes of bad news consultations also facilitates adaptation and is surprisingly acceptable to most patients (Fallowfield & Hogbin, 1989). It allows patients to go over information that they have been given but cannot assimilate at the time of the initial consultation.

Hidden psychological morbidity

Only 20–40% of the patients who develop psychological and psychiatric morbidity are detected by those involved in their care (see Chapter 2). Yet, these problems usually respond well to treatment. Both patients and health professionals contribute to this hidden morbidity (Maguire, 1985).

Patient-led barriers

Patients may not disclose emotional problems for several reasons:

(1) *Somatisation.*   Patients who are not psychologically minded or who find it difficult to express feelings may not verbalise psychological distress. Instead they may report somatic symptoms, for example, lethargy, insomnia, headaches or palpitations.

(2) *Misconceptions about psychological problems.*   Patients may not mention psychological problems because they believe that psychological problems are an inevitable consequence of having a serious illness and being treated for it. Hence, nothing can be done to relieve these problems and so there is no point in mentioning them. Others may

be aware that emotional problems can be treated, but the stigma of 'mental illness' prevents them from disclosing problems.

(3) *Supposed effect on health care professionals.*   Patients may not disclose emotional concerns because they worry that disclosure may lead to them being viewed as ungrateful, inadequate, or unco-operative. It may also give their doctor less time to attend to their physical problems. Moreover, patients realise that doctors and nurses are busy and have many patients to look after. Hence, they do not want to burden them further.

Patients may worry that it is not legitimate to mention psychological concerns since they perceive that few doctors and nurses ask about these directly. They claim that when they disclose psychological problems like a change in mood ("Since my operation I have felt increasingly low"), body image problems ("I can't stand my stoma") or sexual difficulties ("Things are no longer the same between us") these are ignored or dealt with superficially.

Professional-led barriers

In-depth interviews with doctors and nurses and direct observation of their consultations with cancer patients and relatives through audio and video recordings have confirmed two main findings. Firstly, questions which focus directly on psychological aspects such as, "How have you been feeling since your mastectomy" are asked rarely. Consequently, patients and relatives try to give verbal and non-verbal cues about psychological problems ("I'm worried about the future" or "I don't think I'll ever get used to this stoma"). Doctors and nurses then try to move the dialogue into neutral areas by using distancing tactics. Common distancing tactics include:

(1) *Normalisation.*   Here the distress of a patient or relative is explained away by the health professional as an inevitable and normal response.

> Pt: I'm very upset about having to have a mastectomy.
> Surgeon: I can see you are upset. You are bound to be. Everybody is when they have this kind of surgery.

(2) *Premature reassurance.*   The professional offers reassurance immediately after the patient voices a concern.

> Pt: I'm worried about the operation.
> Surgeon: Don't worry I am sure it will be fine

The reassurance is premature because the reasons for the patient's distress have not been established and will block subsequent dialogue. The consultation should have proceeded as follows:

> Pt: I'm worried about the operation.
> Surgeon: Why is that?
> Pt: My aunt had a similar operation. She got a clot on her leg and was on anticoagulants for months.
> Surgeon: How old was your relative?
> Pt: 50-years-old.
> Surgeon: Getting a clot on the leg is a complication after an operation but it is uncommon. Older people, like your relative, are more at risk. The chance of a young person like yourself getting a clot is very small.

(3) *Premature advice.* Health professionals are prone to move into 'advice mode' the moment that a patient voices a concern. There are two reasons for this; first, they think that providing information will resolve concerns, and second, that giving information is a safe activity.

> Dr: I have explained to you that you have a form of cancer of the lymph glands, that is a lymphoma. I am confident that it will respond to treatment with strong drugs, that is chemotherapy.
> Male Pt: Yes but.....
> Dr: I think we should get on with the chemotherapy straight away so that we can get the best response. Is that all right?
> Pt: I am not....
> Dr: Let me tell you exactly what this chemotherapy will involve.

In this example the patient did not take in what was being said because he had important concerns. These would have emerged had the doctor acknowledged and explored the basis of his distress. The interview should have been conducted as follows:

> Dr: I have explained to you that you have a form of cancer of the lymph glands, that is a lymphoma. I am confident that it will respond to treatment with strong drugs, that is chemotherapy.
> Male Pt: Yes, but.....
> Dr: But?
> Pt: I'm terrified of chemotherapy.
> Dr: Why?
> Pt: I have heard that it can make you so sick and sterile. My wife and I are desperate to have a child.

The doctor can now discuss what he can do to minimise the risk of sickness and sterility. For example, employing effective anti-emetics and banking sperm.

(4) *Switching.*   When a patient indicates that he wants to discuss a distressing problem, the health professional switches the topic to safer ground.

> Dr: How have you been getting on since your mastectomy?
> Pt: Getting on, I haven't. It's been awful. I just can't bear to look at myself.
> Dr: How has the pain in your arm been?

This patient wanted to discuss her reaction to her mastectomy. If the doctor had allowed her to do so he could have showed sympathy and offered support. In addition, there may have been help he could have offered, for example, supplying a prosthesis, discussing the possibility of breast reconstruction or identifying an associated sexual, affective or body image problem and offering treatment.

(5) *False reassurance.*   When doctors and nurses realise that the outcome of disease or treatment is poor they may be tempted to soften this by giving false reassurances.

> Pt: I am not going to get better am I? (newly admitted to hospice)
> Dr: Of course you are. You must stop being so pessimistic.

If the doctor had responded by asking, "Why do you think that?" a proper dialogue would have developed. It would have become clear that the patient was aware of how imminent her death was and was reconciled to it.

(6) *Jollying along.*   When health professionals sense that a patient or relative is feeling depressed or anxious they may react by advising, "Come on, there's no need to be so gloomy, let's see a smile".

Reasons for distancing

Distancing is not due to a lack of concern or ignorance of psychological problems. Instead, it stems from doctors and nurses feeling unequipped with the relevant interviewing skills. Moreover, they see the patient as fragile and worry that probing psychologically will cause harm and actual damage by unleashing strong emotions. They could be faced with difficult questions and may get too close to the patient's suffering and predicament. This would be painful emotionally and could lead them to question the value of medicine in general and their own role in particular. They may also worry that getting involved in psychological issues is too time consuming. So, the key issue is how to improve the ability of doctors and nurses to recognise psychological and psychiatric morbidity.

Improving recognition

Nursing and medical staff need to improve their communication skills if they are to identify psychological and psychiatric disorders and make appropriate psychiatric referrals. Psychiatrists need these same skills to ensure that their assessments are accurate.

Integrating physical and psychological enquiry promotes rapid disclosure. This involves taking a history of the presenting complaint, for example, a breast lump but asking the patient about her perceptions of it, ("What did you think the lump was at that time?") and about her feelings ("How did you feel?"). The use of open directive questions with a psychological focus ("How have you been feeling about your chemotherapy?"), summarising, the use of empathy and educated guesses about how the doctor thinks the patient is feeling at a particular point also enhance disclosure. The willingness to clarify any cues (e.g. "I have been feeling very upset") demonstrates to the patient that the doctor is willing to get alongside their experience thereby encouraging disclosure of concerns as well as the expressions of associated feelings.

Patients withhold information about the extent of any adverse effects of treatment on their lives unless appropriate questions are asked. Doctors and nurses worry that discussing psychological issues will overwhelm the patient. So, the first step is to negotiate with patients whether they are willing to talk about something that is potentially painful. If they are willing to do so it is important to talk for as much time as it takes for patients to feel that the doctor has established and understood the nature and intensity of their experiences. The patient will then move on to another topic or the doctor can check that the issue has been covered adequately before requesting permission to move on.

The use of precision and clarification, that is asking the patient to say exactly what they have been experiencing, promotes the disclosure and expression of feelings. It is also helpful to focus on the patients' agenda, i.e. the problems they wish to talk about rather than moving immediately to a review of systems or the symptom referred to in a referral letter.

Patient disclosure of problems is also greater if the doctor or nurse shows an interest in how the patient has responded to the diagnosis and proposed treatment. They can best do this by asking the following open directive questions.

How do you see the future working out? (uncertainty)
Have you come up with any explanation as to why you became ill? (searching for meaning)
Have you been able to do anything yourself to combat your illness? (loss of control)
Has becoming ill affected your view of yourself as a person? (sense of failure, stigma)

What have you said to other people about your illness? (secretiveness)
How have friends and relatives reacted? (isolation).

Reducing key concerns

The following approaches can be used to reduce psychiatric morbidity
in the liaison setting.

Identifying key concerns

Resultant distress that is evident during consultations should be
acknowledged ("I can see this has upset you") and the doctor should use
a style of negotiation ("Would you mind telling me just what is upsetting
you?"). This moves the patient on from feeling overwhelmed by their
predicament to identifying the contributing concerns which can be
resolved in part or whole.

> Dr: You seem very upset (acknowledgement).
> Pt: I am.
> Dr: Can you bear to say what is distressing you? (negotiation)
> Pt: I am shattered. I have heard that melanoma can spread and
> cause havoc.
> Dr: How did you hear this (exploration).
> Pt: I had a neighbour who had it and died. It went to her brain and
> she ended up in a coma.
> Dr: No wonder you are so upset. Are there any other things
> worrying you? (screening question).
> Pt: No, it's just the thought it will get me quickly and horribly.

The doctor can now reassure the patient that her melanoma is likely
to be more controllable and that he will make every effort to prevent
such complications.

The key concerns should be elicited before giving information or advice,
otherwise, they will remain hidden and hamper the patient's ability to
take in what you say. When focusing upon each concern it is important
to pitch comments appropriately. Thus, for a patient concerned about
dying in pain it is best to say, "I am hopeful that we can help you with
your pain" rather than "I can guarantee you will have no pain".

Whenever possible, the doctor should let the patient indicate what he
wants to know rather than relying on a relative's opinion. Withholding
information from patients who want it is as damaging psychologically as
giving it to patients who wish to remain in ignorance.

Providing patients with information

It is important that medical staff check if patients wish to have additional information about investigations and treatments. Patients' questions should be answered honestly. Possible adverse effects of treatment should be acknowledged rather than minimised. If patients have serious worries about treatment the reasons should be explored. They are often rooted in adverse experiences of physical illness of others.

It has been suggested that information packages about particular illnesses, e.g. Crohn's disease or cancer, may be helpful. Indeed many patient-run organisations and charities provide information sheets and so do some hospital departments. Although in many cases this information can be very helpful it does not allow for the variation between patients in their need for information, and how they like it presented. The doctor should not assume that the patient is knowledgeable about his illness even if he has received an information pack.

Treatment options

Some patients can be offered options or choices about treatment. For example, cancer patients may be given a choice between radiotherapy or chemotherapy. When choice is possible it seems that offering it can reduce subsequent psychiatric morbidity (Ashcroft *et al*, 1985; Morris & Royle, 1988). What is not clear is that these early advantages of choice may be offset by problems if recurrence occurs and a patient blames him or herself for making the wrong decision.

Staff training

A key question is how to help those already involved in caring for patients with physical illnesses improve their interviewing, assessment and counselling skills. Short intensive residential and multidisciplinary workshops which utilise videotape demonstrations, enable participants to practice these tasks under controlled conditions, and provide feedback and discussion of performance, have been shown to increase these skills in the short term (Maguire & Faulkner, 1988). Workshops can also improve attitudes to psychological aspects of care (Razavi *et al*, 1988). But further research is needed to determine the extent to which this learning is maintained or applied.

Use of volunteers

Other patients are important sources of information, advice and practical and emotional support. If they are to facilitate rather than hinder psychological adaptation they need to belong to a creditable volunteer organisation. Credibility should be judged on the group's willingness to select and train volunteers, audit their work, and cooperate with health professionals. Training should focus on basic listening and responding skills but avoid the trap of changing volunteers into professionals. Fortunately some major volunteer organisations now meet these criteria. Although there are many anecdotal reports of the value of face-to-face contact between volunteers there has been little study of their effectiveness.

Support groups

Only 10–20% of patients with cancer utilise self-help groups. Groups have an important role in facilitating sharing of experiences and concerns, giving support and reducing isolation. When they are led by, or in cooperation with, leaders who have a professional knowledge of group dynamics they appear effective in alleviating distress. This partly reflects the ability of such leaders to facilitate discussion even when it is between people with different prognoses. They are also able to maintain discussion at a safe but constructive level (Yalom & Grieves, 1977; Spiegel *et al*, 1981; Van den Borne *et al*, 1986). Groups that meet once a month and include patients, relatives and staff also appear effective (Plant *et al*, 1987).

Specialist workers

Many specialist services such as cancer and diabetic centres have appointed specialist nurses or social workers to provide information and advice as well as practical and emotional support to individual patients or groups. It has been hoped that this will reduce psychological and social morbidity, but there is no clear proof as yet that such initiatives will have a preventative effect (Watson, 1983). In the field of cancer, however, it has been established that specialist workers can achieve a marked reduction in psychiatric morbidity by not treating patients themselves, but by early recognition and psychiatric referral of those whom they detect as having a problem (Maguire *et al*, 1980). This can only be achieved if such nurses and counsellors are trained in the relevant interviewing, assessment and counselling skills.

Ongoing support from a nurse manager and the provision of regular supervision and clinical backup by a clinical psychologist or psychiatrist are necessary for such schemes to be fully effective. Unfortunately, specialist workers are often put into posts without relevant training, support or supervision. They then distance themselves from psychological aspects of care and focus on physical issues like the provision of a breast prosthesis or stoma bag. Alternatively, they may get over involved emotionally and/ or carry too large a case load. Both factors put them at risk of becoming psychological casualties. Some workers become too autonomous and give little feedback to the treating clinician about psychological aspects of care, increasing the likelihood that clinicians will leave psychological care to the specialist worker.

In a healthy system, the specialist worker gives regular feedback to the clinical team about problems patients are experiencing and discusses the actions to be taken. He involves a clinical psychologist, psychiatrist and/ or GP when appropriate. Such specialist workers can make effective links with, and encourage the development of, volunteer organisations and self-help groups. They can also play a vital role in helping upgrade the psychological assessment and counselling skills of non-specialist nurses involved in cancer care. This can free them to concentrate on those who have more complex difficulties.

Identifying at-risk groups

Worden (1983) pioneered this approach. At-risk patients were characterised by suppression of feelings, passivity, stoic acceptance, reducing tension through cigarette smoking or alcohol consumption, social withdrawal, blaming themselves or others for their predicament and being unduly irritable. When they tested this predictive model prospectively 80% of the at-risk group were identified correctly but only a minority accepted and completed the offered interventions. This highlights a major problem in such at-risk approaches. Few of those at-risk accept that they need help.

Alternatively, those people who are not coping could be identified before they become anxious or depressed. Promising markers include a past history of psychiatric illness, perceiving that friends and relatives are not supportive, finding it difficult to adapt to the loss of a body part or function, adverse effects of treatment and feeling helpless (Thomas *et al*, 1977*b*; Maguire, 1982; Dean, 1987). Preventative schemes aimed at patients who show one or more of these markers have still to be evaluated.

Psychological factors and survival

Linking psychological coping strategies to survival in patients with severe physical illness is a fascinating area and has only really been explored in relation to cancer. Greer *et al* (1979) found that patients who responded to their diagnosis of cancer by 'denial' or 'fighting spirit' survived longer than those who reacted with 'stoic acceptance' or 'helplessness'. Later work by other researchers (Dean & Surtees, 1989) did not find such a strong association between coping styles and outcome, although there is mounting evidence from a series of different studies that women who express psychological distress at the time of mastectomy have better long-term survival than women who repress their feelings (Levy *et al*, 1985; Jensen, 1987).

Recently, Ramirez *et al* (1989) have found a link between experience of a major life event and subsequent recurrence of breast cancer. If this link was replicated in a larger study, an intervention study aimed to target and help cancer patients who experienced life events would be justified.

In patients with advanced disease the provision of support through regular group meetings appears to lengthen survival (Spiegel *et al*, 1989). More intensive individual psychotherapy has been claimed to have a greater effect (Grossarth-Maticek *et al*, 1982). Concerns have been expressed about both studies because there was insufficient matching of key biological and treatment variables between the index and control groups. A long-term multi-centre trial of psychological intervention is required in order to allow adequately for all the key variables that could influence survival. A similar rigorous scrutiny is required of the counselling offered by cancer help centres. The case for improving psychological care would be even stronger if it improved the length as well as the quality of survival.

Summary

Psychological distress is common in patients with physical illness, but it is often unrecognised by medical and surgical staff. Individuals react in different ways to the knowledge that they have a serious illness and medical teams require education, help and support so that they themselves can help patients cope better with their illness. In acute illness, early intervention aimed at facilitating a natural adjustment to the illness can prevent the later development of psychological distress. In chronic illness the detection of psychiatric illness with subsequent appropriate treatment can also dramatically reduce the degree of long-term psychiatric morbidity.

The liaison psychiatrist needs to have a deep understanding of the effect of physical illness on psychological health and also needs the skills to be able to teach non-mental health workers to cope with difficult and upsetting emotions in patients with life-threatening or life-disabling conditions.

The work that has been pioneered in the field of cancer in terms of developing psychological services for cancer patients can be used as a template for developing services in other medical and surgical specialities.

References

Ashcroft, J. J., Leinster, S. J. & Slade, P. D. (1985) Breast cancer – patient choice of treatment: preliminary communication. *Journal of the Royal Society of Medicine*, **78**, 43–46.

Bancroft, J. H. J. (1989) *Human Sexuality and its Problems* (2nd edn). Edinburgh: Churchill Livingstone.

Bos Branolte, G., Rijshouwer, Y. M., Zielstra, E. M., *et al* (1988) Psychological morbidity in survivors of gynaecological cancers. *European Journal of Gynaecological Oncology*, **9**, 168–177.

Bridge, L. R., Benson, P., Petroni, P. C., *et al* (1988) Relaxation and imagery in the treatment of breast cancer. *British Medical Journal*, **297**, 1169–1172.

Burton, M. V., Parker, R. W. & Wollner, J. M. (1991) The psychotherapeutic value of a "chat": a verbal response modes study of a placebo attention control with breast cancer patients. *Psychotherapy Research*, **1**, 39–61.

Curran, P. S., Bell, P., Murray, A., *et al* (1990) Psychological consequences of the Enniskillen bombing. *British Journal of Psychiatry*, **156**, 479–482.

Dean, C. (1987) Psychiatric morbidity following mastectomy: pre-operative predictors and type of illness. *Journal of Psychosomatic Research*, **31**, 385–392.

—— & Surtees, P. G. (1989) Do psychological factors predict survival in breast cancer? *Journal of Psychosomatic Research*, **33**, 561–569.

Devlen, J., Maguire, P., Phillips, P., *et al* (1987) Psychological problems associated with diagnosis and treatment of lymphomas. II: prospective study. *British Medical Journal*, **295**, 955–957.

Fallowfield, L. J., Baum, M. & Maguire, G. P. (1986) Effects of breast conservation on psychological morbidity associated with diagnosis and treatment of early breast cancer. *British Medical Journal*, **293**, 1331–1334.

—— & Hogbin, B. (1989) Getting it taped – "bad news". Consultation with cancer patients. *British Journal of Hospital Medicine*, **41**, 330–334.

Feinstein, A. & Dolan, R. (1991) Predictors of post–traumatic stress disorder following physical trauma: an examination of the stressor criterion. *Psychological Medicine*, **21**, 85–91.

Greer, S., Morris, T. & Pettingdale, K. W. (1979) Psychological response to breast cancer: effect on outcome. *Lancet*, **2**, 785–787.

Grossarth-Maticek, Kanazin, D. I., Schmidt, P., *et al* (1982) Psychosomatic factors in the process of cancerogenesis. *Psychotherapy and Psychosomatics*, **38**, 284–302.

Gruen, W. (1975) Effects of brief psychotherapy during the hospitalization period on the recovery process in heart attacks. *Journal of Consulting and Clinical Psychology*, **43**, 223–232.

Hughson, A. V. M., Cooper, A. F., McArdle, C. S., *et al* (1986) Psychological impact of adjuvant chemotherapy in the first two years after mastectomy. *British Medical Journal*, **293**, 1268–1271.

Jensen, M. R. (1987) Psychobiological factors predicting the course of breast cancer. *Journal of Personality*, **55**, 317–342.

Langosch, W., Seer, P., Brodner, G., *et al* (1982) Behaviour therapy with coronary artery disease patients: results of a comparative study. *Journal of Psychosomatic Research*, **26**, 475–484.

Levy, S. M., Herberman, R. B., Maluish, A. M., *et al* (1985) Prognostic risk assessment in primary breast cancer by behavioural and immunological parameters. *Health Psychology*, **4**, 99–113.

Maguire, P. (1982) Psychiatric morbidity associated with mastectomy. In *Clinical Trials in Early Breast Cancer* (eds M. Baum, R. Kay & H. Scheurlen), pp. 373–380. Basle: Birkhauser Verlag.

—— (1985) Barriers to psychological care of the dying. *British Medical Journal*, **291**, 1711–1713.

——, Lee, E. G., Bevington, D. J., *et al* (1978) Psychiatric problems in the first year after mastectomy. *British Medical Journal*, **29**, 963–965.

——, Tait, A., Brooke, M., *et al* (1980) The effect of counselling on the psychiatric morbidity associated with mastectomy. *British Medical Journal*, **281**, 1454–1456.

——, ——, Tait, A., *et al* (1983) The effect of counselling on the physical disability and social recovery after mastectomy. *Clinical Oncology*, **9**, 319–324.

—— & Faulkner, A. (1988) How to improve the counselling skills of doctors and nurses in cancer care. *British Medical Journal*, **297**, 847–849.

Maunsell, E., Brisson, J. & Deschenes, L. (1989) Psychological distress after initial treatment for breast cancer: A comparison of partial and total mastectomy. *Journal of Clinical Epidemiology*, **42**, 765–771.

Masters, W. H. & Johnson, V. E. (1970) *Human Sexual Inadequacy*. London: Churchill.

Mayou, R. (1992) Psychiatric aspects of road traffic accidents. *International Review of Psychiatry*, 45–54.

McFarlane, A. C. (1989). The aetiology of post-traumatic morbidity: Predisposing, precipitating and perpetuating factors. *British Journal of Psychiatry*, **154**, 221–228

——, Atchison, M., Rafalowicz, E., *et al* (1994) Physical symptoms in post–traumatic stress disorder. *Journal of Psychosomatic Disorder*, **38**, 715–726.

Morris, J. & Royle, G. T. (1988) Offering patients a choice of surgery for early breast cancer: A reduction in anxiety and depression in patients and their husbands. *Social Science & Medicine*, **26**, 583–585.

Morrow, G. R. (1982) Prevalence and correlates of anticipatory nausea and vomiting in chemotherapy patients. *Journal of the National Cancer Institute*, **68**, 585–588.

Oldenburg, B., Perkins, R. J. & Andrews, G. (1985) Controlled trial of psychological intervention in myocardial infarction. *Journal of Consult Clinical Psycholology*, **53**, 852–859.

Plant, H., Richardson, J., Stubbs, L., *et al* (1987) Evaluation of a support group for cancer patients and their families and friends. *British Journal of Hospital Medicine*, **10**, 317–320.

Ramirez, A., Craig, T. K., Watson, J. P., *et al* (1989) Stress and relapse of breast cancer. *British Medical Journal*, **298**, 291–293.

Razavi, D., Delvaux, N., Farvacques, C., *et al* (1988) Immediate effectiveness of brief psychological training for health professionals dealing with terminally ill cancer patients: A controlled study. *Social Science and Medicine*, **27**, 386–375.

Schottenfeld, R. & Cullen, M. (1986) Recognition of occupational-induced PTSD. *Journal of Occupational Medicine*, **28**, 365–369.

Spiegel, D., Bloom, J. R. & Yalom, I. (1981) Group support for patients with metastatic cancer. *Archives of General Psychiatry*, **38**, 527–533.

—, —, Kraemer, H. C., *et al* (1989) Effect of psychological treatment on survival of patients with metastatic breast cancer. *Lancet*, **11**, 888–891.

Thomas, C., Madden, F. & Jehu, D. (1987*a*) Psychological effects of stomas: I. Psychosocial morbidity one year after surgery. *Journal of Psychosomatic Research*, **31**, 311–316.

—, — & — (1987*b*) Psychological effects of stomas: II. Factors influencing outcome. *Journal of Psychosomatic Research*, **31**, 317–324.

Thompson, D. R. & Meddis, R. (1990) A prospective evaluation of in-hospital counselling for first time myocardial infarction men. *Journal of Psychosomatic Research*, **34**, 237–248.

Van de Borne, H. W., Pruyn, J. F. A. & Van Dam de Mey (1986) Self-help in cancer patients: A review of studies on the effects of contacts between fellow patients. *Patient Education and Counselling*, **8**, 367–385.

Verres (1986) Krebs und Angst. Berlin: Springer-Verlag.

Watson, M. (1983) Psychosocial intervention with cancer patients: A review. *Psychological Medicine*, **13**, 839–846.

Whitehead, E., Shalet, S. M., Blackledge, G., *et al* (1982) The effects of Hodgkin's disease and combination chemotherapy on gonadal function in the adult male. *Cancer*, **49**, 418–422.

Williams, N. S. & Johnson, D. (1983) The quality of life after rectal excision for low rectal cancer. *British Journal of Surgery*, **70**, 460–462.

Wing, J. K., Cooper, J.E. & Sartorius N. (1974) *The Measurement and Classification of Psychiatric Symptoms*. London: Cambridge University Press.

Worden, W. (1983) Psychosocial screening of cancer patients. *Journal of Psychosocial Oncology*, **1**, 1–10.

Yalom, E. D. & Grieves, C. (1977) Group therapy with the terminally ill. *American Journal of Psychiatry*, **134**, 396–400.

7 Paediatric liaison psychiatry

Kate Klein & Bryan Lask

Like other areas of endeavour which defy precise definition, liaison psychiatry has invited many attempts at self-description. Much energy has been spent defining terms and arguing the relative merits of the terms 'liaison' and 'consultation', and child psychiatrists have been no more successful than their adult counterparts in reaching a consensus about terminology. For the purposes of this chapter, the term 'paediatric liaison work' will be used to describe all consultation, diagnostic, therapeutic, teaching, support and research activities carried out by psychiatrists and other mental health professionals in paediatric settings. Within this rubric the term 'consultation' will denote work with other professionals in relation to their direct work with clients, and/or the organisation of their clinical activities.

The principles of consultation work are in many ways similar in adult and in paediatric practice. In both situations the outcome of collaboration hinges on the psychiatrist's success in working effectively in different professional territories, and this requires carefully modulated and multifaceted communication. In paediatric work the problems of communication are further compounded by the number and variety of different professionals and family members involved, by their relative roles in the situation, and particularly by the hierarchy of responsibility which exists around the child. This means that much is both done and communicated on the child's behalf, and this can present difficulties where differences in opinion arise in relation to the best interests of the child. This chapter aims to describe the central elements of the work of paediatric liaison psychiatrists, and to outline the current knowledge base informing the management of childhood somatisation and of psychiatric disturbance associated with childhood illness.

Presentation of psychological problems in paediatrics

Indications for psychiatric consultation

Clinically, there are a number of situations in which the psychological problems of children or families may present primarily to paediatricians.

This may occur at the stage of initial presentation to paediatric services, or may arise in a child or family well known to the paediatrician, perhaps during long-term follow-up for a chronic physical illness.

Obvious emotional or behavioural disturbance in a child

This may be a new or long-standing problem, and the child may already be known to a psychiatric agency. Alternatively, evidence of disturbance may be picked up for the first time by paediatricians, paediatric nurses, play leaders or other staff during the course of a child's paediatric admission or out-patient assessment.

Obvious family dysfunction

This may present as extreme distress in a parent or other family member, obvious criticism of the child by either parent, apparent over-involvement or over-protection, or clear parental discord. These may prove to be long-standing, or may arise in the context of a change in the family's circumstances which seriously stretches their ability to cope. Examples of this would include parental unemployment, loss of housing, serious illness of another family member, and parental separation.

Suspected or proven learning difficulties or other evidence of developmental delay

In a younger child this may be picked up by the paediatrician or play leader, either because of clear delay in motor development, or markedly immature play or language. Any of these features may also be reported directly by the parents as specific concerns. In an older child, difficulties with school work, or behaviour problems or distress confined to the school setting may also justify suspicions of learning difficulties, although the latter presentation may also reflect other school-related problems such as bullying. A psychologist's opinion will certainly be needed in this situation, but consultation with a psychiatrist may also be helpful, depending on the degree of associated distress or functional impairment in the child and family.

Physical findings or behaviour in the child or parents raising concerns about possible child abuse

Poor physical care, unexplained bruising, or evidence of genital injury or infection may raise concerns at the stage of initial examination. The child's behaviour in relation to the parents may also raise questions at this stage, and these may be heightened during admission, with either subdued or fearful behaviour in the presence of a parent, or indiscriminate attachment to new adults. Occasionally, frankly sexualised behaviour or sexualised play outside the developmental expectations for a child's age may be displayed on the ward. In these cases the priority will be referral to a Child Protection Team, which should include a child psychiatrist. However, early consultation with a liaison psychiatrist may also be helpful in considering some of the difficult issues raised for the paediatric staff, and their relationships with the parents.

Parental psychiatric disorder

This may come to light because of a parent's disturbed behaviour, or, more commonly, the parent's general demeanour, care of their child and/or self-care may prompt concerns in the ward staff that they may be depressed or otherwise psychiatrically disturbed. Alternatively, a parent's psychiatric illness may be disclosed in the initial history. Where the illness is treated and controlled this may present no more than an additional vulnerability factor for the family at a time when they are presented with the stress of an ill child. At other times, it may explain the absence of a parent. The most important contact in this situation will be with the adult psychiatric services, but involvement of the paediatric liaison psychiatrist will be helpful in considering implications for the child. These may include impairment of parenting ability in general, and of the parent's role in managing the child's physical illness. The other parent or responsible adults may also need help in explaining the essential elements of the situation to the child in an age-appropriate way.

Undiagnosed physical symptoms

The presentation of physical symptoms of sufficient severity or persistence to reach the paediatric system, for which no sufficient organic aetiology is found, despite full examination and appropriate investigation. An example might be a child refusing to attend school because of recurrent abdominal pain without serious underlying cause.

Diagnosed physical illness, not sufficient to explain the child's distress

Different individuals have different levels of tolerance for physical discomfort, and very different reactions to it. Where the level of distress is high it is important to explore all possible ways of alleviating it, and this requires careful consideration of the relative contributions of possible perpetuating factors. These may include a 'constitutional' low pain tolerance, unacknowledged anxiety about the significance of the symptoms, other psychosocial factors undermining the child's coping strategies, or unrecognised secondary gain.

Poorly controlled illness, despite appropriate treatment

In some cases, poor control may reflect lability or intractability of the pathophysiological process in a particular child. However, full assessment may unearth psychosocial factors which may be operating to exacerbate the illness and/or undermine treatment compliance. Where this approach fails to suggest alternative strategies to improve control, it may still be possible to help the child and family to reinforce their own coping strategies, or consider other ways of dealing with the uncertainties and repercussions of the illness.

Diagnosis of a physical illness which is either fatal or seriously disabling

The diagnosis of physical illness will always rate as a significant life event, and hence a potentially powerful aetiological factor for the development of psychological disturbance. This may be the case even when the illness is self-limiting and expected to be followed by full recovery. Where the illness is more serious, involving unpleasant or distressing treatments, or significant functional disability, or where the prognosis is poor or uncertain, the impact on the child and family will be much greater. In some situations the illness may be a life event which stretches to the limit a system already strained by other factors; in others the stress presented by the illness may itself be sufficient to decompensate a previously adaptive, well-functioning family system.

It will be apparent that this range of presentations encompasses the entire workload of paediatricians. Some highly experienced and skilled paediatricians may feel able to proceed with further psychosocial assessment in some of these cases, but even the most psychologically oriented paediatrician will rarely be able to offer time-consuming treatments. Early consultation offers an opportunity to plan the most appropriate division of labour and expertise to meet the needs of the family, while matching available resources.

Epidemiology

Prevalence

Community samples

Data on the community prevalence of psychiatric disorder in physically ill children and on the rate of somatisation in childhood remains limited to the few large epidemiological studies to date. The Isle of Wight study of the 1960s (Rutter *et al*, 1970a) found a rate of psychiatric disorder in physically ill 10-year-olds of 13.3%, compared with 6.8% for the whole sample. Of those children with a neurological disorder, the rate was almost four times that of the general population (23.5%), while those children with other disorders had a more modestly increased rate of disturbance (10–11% cf. 6.8%). The Isle of Wight study did not collect data on the frequency of recurrent physical symptoms of the kind encountered in somatising children, and there have been only a few community studies looking at this problem over the last 35 years. Each of these has generally considered only one or two specific symptoms. Shapiro & Rosenfeld (1987) have reviewed this literature, and find prevalence rates for both abdominal pain and recurrent headache ranging from 10–25%. Rates are higher in girls, and this sex difference becomes more marked in older children. In contrast, the Ontario Child Health Study (Offord *et al,* 1987) gathered information on a whole range of unexplained physical symptoms, but only reported those of sufficient severity or persistence to meet DSM–III adult criteria for somatisation disorder. This reached a startling prevalence rate of almost 7%, almost all of this occurring among older children (aged 12–16), the rate for girls being much higher than that for boys (10.7% cf. 4.5%).

Clinical samples

In both in-patient and out-patient paediatric samples high rates of psychological disturbance have consistently been reported. Stocking *et al* (1972) found that almost two-thirds of children admitted to a paediatric ward would have benefited from psychiatric consultation. Awad & Poznanski (1975) also reported a high rate of psychopathology in hospitalised children, and noted that referral to child psychiatry was more likely to be made when the symptoms were of unknown aetiology, depression was suspected, or behaviour problems arose on the ward. In general paediatric out-patient clinics, Apley (1982) and Smithells (1982) found that half of the children seen had disorders in which psychological factors were felt to play a major aetiological role, and many of the remainder had significant emotional sequelae to their organic illness. Other studies have reported rates of between 28 and 36% (Fitzgerald, 1985; Cundall, 1987; Garralda & Bailey, 1989).

Outcome

Persistent physical illness seems likely to operate as a powerful perpetuating factor for psychological disturbance. However there are little data regarding the outcome of psychiatric disorder arising in association with physical illness, although Kokkonen & Kokkonen (1995) found that young adults who had suffered longterm physical illness since childhood were more likely to report persistent psychological symptoms than controls. The natural history of childhood somatisation is equally poorly documented, but Apley & Hale (1973) in their follow-up study of children with recurrent abdominal pain found that a third carried their original symptomatology into early adult life, a third continued to suffer from a variety of other functional complaints, and only one-third were completely free of any recurrent physical symptoms. This suggests that there may be considerable continuity between childhood and adult somatisation, but this is by no means clear, and is an area which needs further examination.

Aetiology

Contributory factors

Much is now known about the range of individual and environmental factors associated positively and negatively with the risk of developing psychiatric disorder. In childhood, these are conveniently organised into those factors primarily residing in the child (biological, developmental, psychological), those arising in the family (current relationships, family functioning, and the personal histories which are brought to bear on this), those arising in the outside world (school, peers, neighbourhood, professional agencies, wider society), and important life events, which may operate at any or all of these levels.

Child psychiatric assessment must take account of all these elements, which may operate as predisposing, precipitating, perpetuating or protective factors, and which often overlap to a considerable extent. These factors, which may reinforce or confound families' coping resources, can also be considered on a resilience–vulnerability continuum. Vulnerability factors are particularly useful in helping to understand the development of the problem, but identification of the child's and family's areas of strength and resilience is equally important, especially when considering treatment, since this is best planned to reinforce pre-existing strengths and coping mechanisms.

Psychophysiological mechanisms

The inextricable mutual relationship between psychological, physiological and pathological processes is now widely acknowledged, but not always readily remembered in clinical practice. The mechanisms underlying these relationships in children are essentially the same as for adults, including features of the physiology and perception of pain, the triggering and modulation of autonomic nervous system activation and the perception of the physiological changes associated with them, and the individual's genetically determined vulnerability to dysfunction in particular organ systems. In addition, the relationship between stress and the immune response is becoming increasingly clear in the adult literature, and although evidence for these mechanisms in children is lacking to date, it seems very likely that a similar relationship exists (Lask & Fosson, 1989).

However, there are important age-associated differences, particularly in the perception and communication of sensations and in the role of the parent as mediator in the child's understanding of experiences. Children are particularly poor at localising painful stimuli arising from internal organs, and young children are likely to refer all sorts of discomfort to the abdomen. In addition, children may lack the experience of similar sensations to help them judge significance, and the information which the child gathers in relation to the sensation is filtered through their current emotional state. When communicated to the child's parent the information is further filtered through the adult's own emotional state, attitudes, previous experience of physical symptoms and fears about illness. The presenting symptom is a result of all of these forces.

It is clear that physical symptoms can and do generate psychological distress. It is equally clear that 'stress' in its myriad forms begets 'distress'; that the normal physiological accompaniments of distress, such as tachycardia and sweating, are themselves distressing; and that where these physiological changes become persistent, the pathological changes of 'disease' may ensue or may be exacerbated in a vulnerable organ system, as in diabetes mellitus or asthma. Psychological and physical pathways are inextricably linked, and are never mutually exclusive. The fact that an episode of abdominal pain is self-limiting and not associated with demonstrable pathology does not necessarily mean that it had no physiological or even pathological basis, and certainly does not mean that the child was 'imagining' it. Where serious disease has been excluded, the salient question is not so much, "How 'real' is the symptom?" as "Why is this symptom causing so much distress in this child, and/or in this family? What is contributing to the distress, and how can we help alleviate it?". In order to understand this, we need to consider the components of the illness network.

The 'illness network'

All professionals involved in the care of sick children need to be aware of the 'illness network', not only because an understanding of this network is essential to assessment and treatment, but also because they form an integral part of it. The network consists of four interacting and interdependent components: the child, the illness, the family and environmental factors (Lask & Fosson, 1989).

The reciprocal relationships between illness and those experiencing it at different levels can exert a powerful influence on its course, and on the family's adaptation to it. The network can be thought of as being in a state of equilibrium, stable or otherwise, at any point in time, and each component has a number of variables which can affect the balance of the system. Child-related variables include age, temperament, intelligence, understanding of the illness and attitude to it, coping mechanisms, and emotional reactions. Illness-related variables include localisation, severity, chronicity, prognosis. Family variables include the quality of the marital relationship and of parenting, understanding of and attitudes to the illness, stability, cohesion and communication, and emotional reactions. Environmental variables include the medical, nursing and other staff involved in the child's care, the child's school and peer group, and friends and neighbours. To some extent these factors are the same as those which may operate to modify the course of illness at any age, but the developmental immaturity of children does warrant special emphasis, especially in relation to their understanding of illness.

Children's understanding of illness

Conceptualisation of disease in healthy children is age-dependent. The apparent sophistication of some articulate young children can belie the immaturity of their psychological constructs, and it is important to be aware of the ways in which they make sense of their experiences. Five and six-year-olds often consider illness to have magical causes, or to be the consequence of some transgression on their part. By 9–10 years the presence of germs is taken as sufficient to cause disease, and by 12–13 years children are able to understand that illness may be caused by a combination of factors (Bibace & Walsh, 1981). Children use a mixture of these ideas to speculate about cause and prognosis, and can sometimes generate frightening fantasies about what is happening to them. In addition, illness causes regression, and ill children may be using more primitive concepts than their age would suggest. Wherever possible children's fantasies about illness should be elicited and gently explored and discussed. The reality, simply explained, will often be less frightening than their fantasies, and this paves the way for a continuing dialogue with the child about their illness.

The role of the liaison child psychiatrist

A number of overlapping tasks can be distinguished within paediatric liaison work: consultation, assessment, treatment, support, teaching and research.

Consultation

A number of authors have discussed the principles underpinning consultation in child psychiatry. The diverse variety of professionals working with children bring differences in training, experience and conceptual frameworks which make this a particularly challenging task. Steinberg & Yule (1986) consider that the emphasis should be on helping consultees to make the most of their own experience, skills and resources. They have highlighted a number of important features of the relationship between consultant and consultee, and have stressed three points in particular:

(a) that the consultee should remain autonomous, and the consultant should not take over responsibility for the child
(b) that the consultant/consultee relationship should be one of mutual and equal collaboration
(c) related to these is the assumption that other professionals are competent, and are doing their best in a given situation.

The first of these points warrants further clarification, since it is important at the outset to be certain that the consultee wishes to remain autonomous, and is not asking the consultant to take over responsibility. Sturge (1989) has argued that problems can be avoided by clear agreement on what is required for each separate referral: assessment, consultation, joint work, parallel work or handover. Once it is established that the request is for consultation, it remains important to determine exactly what the consultees hope to gain from the process, since they may otherwise be left feeling dissatisfied, unsupported and misunderstood. However, the request for consultation may come in the wake of a crisis, and at this stage the consultees may not have fully formulated their own ideas and questions about the situation. The first priority at this stage is to help the consultees clarify their own ideas without appearing to challenge their competence, and this requires a sensitive approach. This is particularly true where professionals are struggling with negative feelings about the family. This territory is very familiar to psychiatrists, but may not be so to physicians and general trained nurses, and it may require considerable reassurance and non-judgemental listening to enable non-psychiatric workers to bring these issues clearly onto the agenda, and enable constructive discussion to follow.

The process of consultation

As in direct work with families, consultation with professionals may be prescriptive or facilitatory. The prescriptive mode is very familiar to those trained medically and involves a re-evaluation of the available information on the basis of the consultant's own experience, pooled experience gleaned from colleagues, and knowledge of the relevant empirical literature. It culminates in the consultant offering information or advice. The facilitatory mode requires an additional set of skills, and aims to help professionals to review the information they have gathered themselves, their assessment of it, and their own and the client's position in relation to treatment. The range of disciplines involved in paediatric work means that this process can potentially draw on a great variety of skills in different settings, for instance in hospital, school and play settings.

Communication of opinion

Ideally this should be done both verbally and in writing. The former allows for immediate discussion, while the latter enables further deliberation, and also provides a permanent record. In some cases the opinion will be provisional only, pending full assessment.

Assessment

The family's view of assessment

Although referral to general child psychiatry clinics is sometimes initiated by agencies other than the parents (e.g. school or social services), parents who attend are generally prepared for a psychological approach to the problem. In contrast, for many families presenting to paediatricians, psychiatric referral may be an unexpected, unwelcome and challenging turn of events. A prerequisite for successful engagement in these circumstances is an understanding of the expectations and reservations which the family bring to the assessment. Specifically it may be worth ventilating the 'mental illness' question. Parents may assume that psychiatric referral implies a view that they or their child are thought to be 'mad'. A brief explanation of what child psychiatrists do can be helpful, emphasising that the children and families seen are rarely mentally ill, and are more often families doing their best to cope with difficult circumstances. This can provide a convenient take-off point to consider physical illness and persistent symptoms as being particularly stressful for individuals and for families.

The first meeting

Both parents and the child should be seen as the minimum, and it is extremely helpful to see the whole family with whom the child lives. At later meetings it may also be useful to meet grandparents or other significant relatives. Usually the family will be seen together in the first instance, and it may also be helpful to see parents and child separately. The relative merits of each strategy will need to be decided in each situation. Inevitably the family will be anxious at this first meeting, and it is important to try to put them at ease, and to orientate them by carefully explaining how the session will proceed and how long it will last. If there is to be a break in the middle for consultation with colleagues this should be explained, and it is also important to introduce any special features in the room such as one-way mirrors and video equipment. The room should afford privacy and freedom from interruptions.

Children are sometimes uncertain whether or not they are expected to talk, so it is helpful to encourage them by asking about their school, hobbies or interests. A compliment or question about their clothing can also help to break the ice. There should always be age-appropriate drawing and play material, and this should be offered at an early stage. It is important to make it clear, however, that this is not intended simply as a diversionary tactic to keep the children busy, but rather that "Children often find it easier to listen to what's being said if they're occupied doing something". This is intended to give the children permission both to do something and to listen and participate, and signals to the adults in the room that the children are expected to be, and will be listening.

The agenda for the first meeting will vary enormously with the circumstances, and the family's order of priorities may be very different from that of the involved professionals. In addition, the family may be apprehensive about the issues which may be raised and the way they may be handled, and the parents need clear reassurance that the interviewer will respect and reinforce appropriate boundaries, and that separate meetings can be arranged to discuss issues inappropriate for a family meeting, such as marital problems.

The family's view of the problem

Both family and professional may feel that they are expected to reach a point of overt agreement to signal that 'engagement' has been reached or 'cooperation' achieved, and when each approaches the assessment with a different view, the covert agenda for each may be to reach this point by converting the other party to their own position. Certainly, where the psychiatrist has identified clear psychosocial components which the family deny, the transition towards treatment will be seen to require some adjustment of the parents' view. However, the parent is unlikely to be successfully persuaded of an alternative view without first feeling that their original view has received adequate consideration, and this requires more than peremptory dismissal by an 'expert'. Rather, it is important that the psychiatrist is at least able to demonstrate acknowledgement of their view, and hopefully also some understanding of it. While this is important to achieve full engagement, such an approach is far from being simply a public relations exercise. The family's own ideas and theories may prove to underpin the whole problem.

> Maria, a 15-year-old Italian girl, presented to casualty complaining of weakness; her parents appeared extremely worried, and lapsed into frequent agitated exchanges in Italian. Physical examination and investigations revealed no abnormality. The casualty officer became concerned that Maria might be depressed, and when she

disclosed thoughts about death, requested a psychiatric opinion. Examination of her mental state suggested that she was not clinically depressed, but she was initially reluctant to be drawn further on her preoccupation with thoughts of death. She was clearly extremely upset, and a number of potential contributory factors were identified, including a level of parental discord which all parties reported, and which was clearly apparent throughout the interview. However, it was not possible to make sufficient sense of the presenting picture until the family were asked for their own view of the problem. This question was initially met by much resistance and a further volley of exchanges in Italian, but ultimately both the parents and Maria separately disclosed their shared belief that a paternal aunt, living in Sicily, had placed a curse on Maria at the time of her birth. This had been taken to explain the run of poor health which Maria had suffered through her childhood, and was currently looming large, since the ultimate condition of the curse was that Maria would die before her 16th birthday, an anniversary then only 8 weeks away.

Gathering information

The information needed includes the details of the presenting problem, and its context – i.e. its current and its past context. The current context will include the following: the child's developmental and medical status and temperament; the family's composition, current functioning, and current acute stressors, including physical or psychiatric illness; and factors outside the family, including school, peer relationships and the family's support network. The past context will include the child's medical history and early experiences, and the social history of the nuclear family, including changing composition, relationships and life events. More distantly, it will include the parents' own personal histories, including their own childhood experiences of care from adults, their later relationships, experience of physical illness, and any history of psychiatric disorder or substance abuse. Finally, as highlighted above, the history is not complete without an account of the family's own beliefs and attitudes.

This range of information is never elicited at a single session, and indeed, some aspects of the parents' personal history are not appropriately sought in a family interview. The consultant may require several sessions of different composition to complete an assessment. It should also be remembered that parents are not themselves 'patients' in this context, and some important areas of questioning may seem intrusive, even when they are seen alone. Current family relationships and the parents' own family background may be particularly sensitive. However, much may be gleaned about these areas from detailed discussion of the presenting problem, particularly when this is broadened to consider how the problem is currently handled, its consequences for different family members, their beliefs about it, experiences of similar difficulties in the parents' own families, and their ways of coping.

The interviewer's reactions

As in all other situations in medical and psychiatric interviewing, the countertransference which emerges at the first meeting is a rich source of information about the family. Not only does it throw light on the emotional feelings which family members generate in each other, but also on those which are evoked in the family's dealings with the outside world.

Additional sources of information

In addition to this core of information from the family, further useful information may be obtained from other professional agencies who have had contact with them, particularly teachers, health visitors, GPs, Social Services, and any previously involved mental health professionals. Teachers can provide valuable information regarding the child's academic performance, classroom behaviour, and peer relationships, and this information can be particularly helpful in assessing the degree of functional impairment associated with the problem. Teachers can be interviewed directly, or can be asked either to provide a report or to complete a standardised questionnaire such as the Rutter B (Rutter *et al*, 1970*b*).

The potential importance of extended family members in understanding the problem has already been highlighted. In some cases meeting grandparents is like finding the last piece of a jig-saw.

> When Michael presented at the age of 7 with bouts of extreme irritability, the initial family and individual assessments revealed no obvious aetiological factors. He had suffered from moderately severe asthma since the age of 4, but this had been well controlled on regular sodium cromoglycate, and he only occasionally required the use of a bronchodilator. The episodes occurred two or three times a month, usually starting on a Sunday evening or Monday morning, and lasted for one or two days. In between, he was reported to be a good tempered and happy child, and these episodes remained unexplained until his grandmother by chance brought him to an out-patient appointment. She confided to the paediatrician that she was concerned about her daughter's tendency to restrict Michael's use of his medication. To compensate for this, when Michael stayed with her for weekends she would encourage him to use his bronchodilator four or five times a day. On reviewing the history, it became clear that his bouts of irritability did, indeed, follow visits to his grandmother, and were attributable to the excitatory effect of the Beta-2 agonist.

Observations

General observations.   The family's report of the problem may contrast markedly with the observations made. This is not necessarily the contradiction it appears, but rather a reflection that the family's own understanding of the situation will only encompass those factors of which they are consciously aware. The interviewers' observations are more organised around their professional experience of interaction between family members, and so will take account of patterns of communication and repetitive sequences which are usually beyond the family's immediate awareness. For example, the parents of a 9-year-old girl may complain that she gets headaches for no apparent reason, whereas an observer may notice that she complains of a headache when they start arguing. More commonly, a family may deny any problems in their relationships, but suggest a different picture from the positioning of their chairs in relation to each other, and their posture and non-verbal communication. Physical distance or proximity, and the amount of touching, eye-contact or referencing to each other are particularly easy to spot, but more subtle features, such as similarity or mirroring of posture are also worthy of note.

Parenting and family functioning.   There is no universally agreed consensus about the characteristics of a well-functioning family, but many would agree that the following components are important:

(1) the quality of parenting
(2) the ability to make decisions, solve problems and resolve conflicts
(3) the quality of communication – especially directness and clarity
(4) the expression of needs and emotions, and appropriate responsiveness
(5) mutual individual respect, and age-appropriate autonomy
(6) distinction between the 'roles' of parents and children, especially with respect to care-taking and decision-making.

Information about all of these features will be gathered during the assessment period by both report and observation, and particular features can sometimes be amplified by asking the family to discuss issues between themselves, allowing the interviewer to observe the ensuing interaction.

The clinically accessible features of parenting are the parents' behaviour in relation to the child, and their attitude toward the child. The interview situation offers only a snap-shot of parental behaviour, but the admission of children to hospital presents a range of stressful situations requiring skilful handling by parents. This affords the opportunity to observe their responsivity to the child, anticipation and containment of distress, and facilitation of difficult or unpleasant procedures, such as blood tests. In addition, the day-to-day routine enables observation of the parents' interest in the child's activities and awareness of the child's safety. Parental attitudes are more readily explored at interview, particularly warmth, expressed criticism, ability to consider the child's position empathically, and over-involvement or over-protection. Parents often volunteer information which clarifies this area, but if doubt remains it can be helpful to prompt them to talk more about their child, particularly describing his temperament or personality, and his usual way of coping with difficulties and frustrations. It can also be revealing to ask what parents feel is the most difficult aspect of the current situation, from their child's point of view.

Assessment of the child

This may be carried out entirely during the course of the family interview, or the child may also be seen alone. Some children find the latter threatening while others may be inhibited from talking freely in the presence of their parents, particularly older children and adolescents. In either situation the aim will be to assess the child's physical and neurodevelopmental status, social behaviour, mental state, self-esteem, and perceptions of their current situation.

Much can be learnt by simply watching the child, including observations on appearance and general demeanour, size and physical development, motor coordination, level of activity, attention span, and complexity of play or drawing, although it must be remembered that the child's attention to tasks will be affected by his monitoring of the conversation and other events in the room. Still more can be gleaned from the child's interaction with others in the room, including the frequency and type of approaches to parents, the child's behaviour towards the interviewer, and interactions with siblings. The child's mood, thoughts, and perceptions of the situation can be explored in a number of different ways depending on age, maturity, personality and willingness to participate.

Younger children can often be engaged using play or drawing as a fulcrum for conversation, and drawing can also be useful for older children, even up to adolescence. These approaches have the advantage that children can talk about characters in the drawings or play rather than directly about themselves, and can thereby maintain some control, keeping as much distance in the conversation as they wish. In addition, the interviewer can use the child's material as a basis for further enquiry, or can elaborate elements of it into simple metaphor. However, many children even at quite a young age are also able to talk in quite a direct way about their thoughts, ideas and feelings, and should be encouraged to do so, always with a clear regard for their level of understanding.

The importance of developmental assessment cannot be over-emphasised. Children with intellectual impairment, specific learning difficulties or other forms of developmental delay are very likely to have associated adjustment problems, and the likelihood of this is even greater when the difficulty has gone unrecognised. A rough assessment of intelligence, developmental level and reading skills should be made by whoever sees the child in the first instance. Referral should be made to a psychologist for formal psychometric assessment in any child where this raises a question about the child's development, or where a child presents with symptoms for which no other satisfactory explanation can be found.

Feedback to the family

The initial phase of contact is completed by communicating the professionals' view to the family, and this is a crucial stage which may secure or undermine engagement. Where the initial presentation was of obvious emotional or behavioural disturbance the parents may be well prepared for a psychological explanation, and may be only too willing for a psychiatrist to help them explore their difficulties further. Where the outcome of the assessment differs markedly from the parents' own theories, this task becomes a much more delicate one. If the child's symptomatology is physical the parents' working hypothesis may also be predominantly physical, and where no sufficient organic basis is found for the symptoms, parents will be forced to consider a range of alternative explanations. These may be outside their personal experience and may be considerably more distressing than their first line theories. A more comfortable immediate course may be for them to stick with their original position and to challenge the 'expert's' competence. Parents may need much support to reappraise the situation, and for some this will require a radical adjustment of perspective which may have distressing personal implications including feelings of being criticised or blamed, or of self-blame. The following example illustrates some of the issues which may arise.

> Susan was a 10-year-old only child, admitted with episodes of recurrent abdominal pain which had started one year before. These had steadily increased in frequency to once or twice a month, each episode leading to two or three days off school. On one occasion when her mother had sent her to school despite the pain, she was later sent home in great distress. Since then, although it transpired that the episodes usually settled in a day, Susan's mother insisted that she stay at home for a further one or two days "to be certain". Susan was doing well at school, and had a small circle of good friends. There was no family history of abdominal problems, and the parents denied any specific fears in relation to the symptoms. However, a favourite niece had become seriously ill with a brain tumour 2 years earlier, and the family felt this had been diagnosed late, after several months of increasing headache. This had left them anxious about any symptoms, and doubtful of professional competence. Susan's grandmother had died six months later, and in the wake of this bereavement her mother had become severely depressed, requiring a brief

psychiatric admission. Susan's mother had also suffered from intermittent migraine for many years, and this had worsened in the last year. Susan's father had a more pragmatic coping style, and although also upset by these events, thought it best to 'get on', and not dwell too much on distressing thoughts. Susan herself was described by both parents as sensitive but 'level-headed', and they reported that she had coped well with the family worries. Susan was well and active between the episodes of pain, and physical examination was entirely normal. However, in view of all these factors, the chronicity of the problem, and the significant functional impairment associated with it, the paediatricians had undertaken a full range of appropriate investigations, which were all normal.

This history highlights a number of important contributory factors including the family history of migraine, the recent family experience of illness and loss, and the mother's subsequent depressive illness. Her father's pragmatic coping style, and her mother's apparent vulnerability to both physical symptoms and psychological distress, may each have acted to inhibit Susan from expressing her own distress more directly, and her mother's over-anxious response to her symptoms may have heightened this effect still further. There may also have been a developmentally inappropriate expectation that Susan would 'cope', adding further to her responsibility to contain her own distress, especially in the face of her mother's. However, it may be too challenging to raise all of these issues with the family straight away, and it is important to pace the discussion sensitively, in the light of the family's immediate response.

Re-framing the issues

The initial feedback should be as clear and concise as possible, since it is difficult for anxious parents to absorb too much information at once. On the other hand, feedback should be unhurried, and it is particularly important to avoid appearing to diminish the severity of the presenting symptom or the distress associated with it. It is useful to begin with a brief recapitulation of the problem as a shared starting point, and it is helpful to refer back to the family's own original view, incorporating and emphasising those areas which are consonant with the clinical impression, and acknowledging their other ideas. An explanation can then follow of the physical findings and results of investigations, and the role of other factors in producing physical symptoms, including developmental, hereditary and psychosocial factors.

These are initially introduced in general terms, before suggesting how they may apply in the family's specific case. Care should be taken to explain the consultant's view in non-technical language using the family's own phrases wherever possible, and being ready to use metaphor or diagrams, and to draw parallels with psychophysiological reactions within the parents' own experience. A simple explanation from the paediatrician of psychophysiological processes can be very useful here, and it can also be helpful for both professionals to draw on their own personal experiences, both to help normalise the phenomena being described, and also to offer further evidence of empathic understanding. For instance "Everyone feels the physical effects of stress at times. I often get a headache when I've had a bad day." Questions should then be invited to encourage further discussion to develop along lines dictated by the parent's concerns, since their own agenda will need to be fully explored if they are to move on to consider alternatives.

This procedure will sometimes shift the discussion quickly onto the relevant issues, but in other cases ventilation of more sensitive areas may be best deferred until the family have had time to adjust to the initial formulation, when they may be more receptive to potentially more challenging ideas. It will be a matter of individual judgement whether to begin this process with the child and parents together, or initially to see the parents alone, and this will be dictated partly by the child's age and partly by the observations already made about the family's interaction. In either event, it will be important to offer both the child and parents additional time on their own for further discussion. In Susan's case the initial formulation of the problem was fed back to the family as follows:

> "These bouts of stomach pain have clearly been very distressing for Susan, and very worrying for all of you, especially after your niece's recent illness. She is very well otherwise, and that is very reassuring, but we have done a range of tests to be absolutely sure that there is no serious physical cause for these pains. We now have all of these results, and fortunately we have been able to exclude serious disease, so we can now be confident that there is no serious or dangerous physical problem causing Susan's pain. Nevertheless, her pain is very distressing, and is seriously disrupting her schooling, and we still need to be clear about what is causing it. In fact, stomach pains without any serious physical cause are quite common at Susan's age. As many as one in ten 10-year-olds have this problem, and it seems to be caused by the muscles of the abdomen going into spasm or a cramp. Like other sorts of muscle cramp, this sort of pain can at times be quite severe, and there are a number of different names for it, including 'spastic colon', 'periodic syndrome' or 'abdominal migraine'. It is, in fact, related to the migraine or tension headaches which adults get, and it also seems to run in families, so that we often find that one or other parent had a similar problem as a child, or has headaches as an adult. Like adult headaches, this sort of pain is most likely to happen when the child is under stress or upset. All 10-year-olds have some worries, and they sometimes find more serious worries hard to talk about, especially when the worries

are upsetting for everyone in the family, as with the recent illnesses in your family. Adults are often aware of increased muscle tension in themselves when they are anxious or upset, and may even describe themselves as 'tense'. In children who are prone to stomach cramps, 'locked-in' worries can cause stomach pain. Anxiety about the cause of the pain can make it worse, setting up a vicious cycle, and it is sometimes helpful just knowing that there is nothing serious causing it. But it can also be helpful to think about the sorts of things which may bring it on in a particular child, and how to make it easier to talk about worries and upsets."

After the parents' immediate concerns have been further explored, later discussion will need to be guided toward the responses of different family members, and their interaction. One way of approaching this area is to ask who Susan is most like in terms of her coping style, and what coping strategies other members of the family use. This is intended to signal in a non-judgemental way, firstly, that everyone has and needs coping strategies, and secondly, that there is no 'correct' strategy, and that a variety of responses are valid and understandable. In this way it is hoped to facilitate further discussion about the feelings which underlie individual responses to stress and distress.

The parents' response

There are three possible responses to the suggestion that further psychosocial assessment or treatment is indicated: acceptance, doubt or frank rejection. With the 'acceptance' group it is possible to move straight into further assessment and treatment. For the other two it is important to avoid conflict and over-zealous attempts to convince the parents that they are wrong; such confrontational strategies are most likely to lead to further entrenchment. It is preferable to continue exploring their doubts and convictions, which may arise from misunderstanding, lack of trust in doctors or mental health professionals, a history of previous errors, a fear of stigmatisation, a sense of guilt, or other forms of unrecognised distress.

It is sometimes helpful at this stage to ask parents what would convince them. If specific answers such as an X-ray or a biopsy are given, this may point to areas of misunderstanding arising from earlier explanations of the physical findings, or it may highlight a particular fear which has not previously emerged, or has not been adequately acknowledged and discussed. Further discussion with the paediatrician will be imperative at this stage. Some parents fear that a treatable physical illness may emerge at a later date, and these understandable anxieties need to be ventilated and acknowledged. It may be helpful to discuss in a very frank way the worst possible scenarios which might later emerge, at the same time explaining why these are felt to be unlikely, and also how they would be recognised. This helps demonstrate to the parents that their fears are not being dismissed, and, indeed, that the paediatricians have considered exactly these possibilities in their assessment, and have rejected them for sound reasons.

In some cases, however, parents remain intransigent. A number of courses can then be followed, but the most important aim is to keep channels of communication open, and to offer continuing, unconditional support. Failing all other strategies, it may be necessary to present the family with the 'chronic illness option', explaining that in the absence of a treatable physical explanation for the symptoms, it is very difficult to predict the outcome. It is possible that the symptoms may persist, perhaps indefinitely, and this will clearly be extremely distressing for the parents and child. An offer is then made to support the child and family through what will undoubtedly be a very difficult time. Occasionally parents are able to accept this form of help when they are not able to accept an overtly psychosocial approach.

Treatment

The whole range of therapeutic options used in general child psychiatry may be employed in paediatric liaison work. Treatment options include advising parents, behavioural approaches, parental counselling, family therapy, marital therapy, individual therapy, and drug treatments.

Advice and behaviour modification are essentially prescriptive treatments, the consultant directing the parent about what to do and how to do it. This can be very useful, especially for less entrenched problems, and may be all that is needed in some cases, especially where there are no major disturbances in parenting or family functioning. Parental counselling, in contrast, is clearly facilitatory, and is based on helping parents to explore their own feelings and difficulties, with a view to finding ways of solving problems using their own resources. The strategies available within this mode of therapy include ventilation of fears and feelings, clarification of issues and processes, recognition of existing skills and strengths, encouragement, and promotion of insight.

Any of the recognised approaches to family and marital therapy can be used in a paediatric setting (Lask, 1987; Gustaffson *et al*, 1989; John & Bradford, 1991), and a number of individual approaches can be used including play therapy, art therapy, role play and psychodrama, cognitive therapy, relaxation techniques and traditional psychoanalytic psycho-therapy. A number of specific indications are worthy of mention. Behavioural techniques have been used in the preparation for unpleasant or frightening procedures, for needle phobias, control of pain and vomiting and for the control of chronic, relapsing diseases including diabetes, asthma and epilepsy (Lask, 1994). Specific treatments used in these contexts have included relaxation and hypnotherapy, desensitisation, modelling, flooding, reinforcement, shaping and extinction.

A counselling approach similar to that used for parents may be useful in helping older children to cope with reality-based problems, such as those faced by children with chronic illness.

Support to staff

This element of liaison has been an issue of some contention, with a number of authors expressing anxieties about the boundaries of such work. Lipowski (1967) has reinforced this note of caution, suggesting that it is not the consultant's task to offer covert psychotherapy to the referring doctor. Few would disagree with these anxieties, but it remains a matter of concern that the inevitable tensions of working with sick children often go unrecognised and unresolved. Informal meetings with nursing and play staff can go some way toward acknowledging areas of stress, facilitating expressions of distress, and discovering or enhancing strategies for coping. Such groups are particularly valued on neonatal and paediatric intensive care units, and on other units where life and death issues are everyday events, such as cardiac, renal and oncology wards.

Staff caring for sick children regularly face distress, and they need and deserve support to help them recognise and acknowledge the feelings of sick children and of their parents, and also to recognise and cope with their own feelings. Peaks of distress are sometimes predictable, and the diagnosis of a seriously disabling or life-threatening illness is particularly stressful, both for the family and for those closely involved in their care. Families and individual family members react differently and with different intensities, but a common pattern is recognisable. Shock and disbelief is followed by denial, and then by varying mixtures of sadness and anger. The expression of these last, painful feelings depends on many factors, but sadness elicits more sympathy and comforting behaviour than anger, which may lead professionals to feel blamed and angry themselves. It is important to remember that both of these emotions are expressions of the same distress, and ward staff may need much support to help them negotiate these difficult interactions with appropriate sympathy.

Family members may vacillate between denial, anger and over-acceptance, and it is also important to recognise that individual family members may be at very different stages in their adjustment to the situation at any point in time. One parent may be plunging into the depths of despair while the other is swinging back towards denial and over-optimism. The inevitable swings between emotional synchrony and dissonance within the family can greatly exacerbate tensions, and sometimes leave the family members who are 'out of step' feeling very isolated. Acknowledgement of this process by members of staff can help the parents to tolerate some of their more temporary differences with greater understanding. In addition, the ward staff most intimately involved with the child are often quite junior nurses, who may themselves become emotionally involved with the child or family, and may for a time occupy a potent and potentially vulnerable position in the illness network. Such individuals need sympathetic support, and sometimes quite firm assistance in extricating themselves from the centre of the system.

Teaching

The child psychiatrist has an important educational role in paediatric liaison, both in the context of clinical work, and by involvement and interest in paediatric academic meetings and presentations. In the clinical arena, constructive use can be made of contacts with staff from all disciplines and at all levels, including consultant and trainee paediatricians, medical students, paediatric nurses, teachers, play leaders and other members of the clinical team. In addition, every aspect of paediatric liaison work should be educational for the psychiatrist, at whatever level in their training or career. Ideally, psychiatrists in liaison settings should be aiming to provide a conceptual framework and a perspective which others should find not only interesting, but also useful and useable.

Research

Little more than 10 years ago, a survey of paediatric liaison programmes found less than 50% reporting active research. Despite this slow start, liaison child psychiatrists have made a growing contribution to empirical knowledge relating to both the psychosocial antecedents of illness, and psychological reactions to it. A wide range of different disorders have been the focus for collaborative research (Graham, 1991).

Paediatric liaison in practice

Dulcan *et al* (1990) showed that paediatricians are likely to miss psychiatric disorder. Of 52 children who received a psychiatric diagnosis using relatively conservative criteria, only 17% were identified by the paediatrician as having a psychiatric disorder. These authors also noted that paediatricians have been found to identify psychopathology in only 4–7% of patients, in contrast to the much higher community estimates noted earlier. Stocking *et al* (1972) reported that emotional disorders are particularly likely to be overlooked in the presence of an acute treatable medical condition. In addition, the repercussions of illness for the family are frequently overlooked. A wide variety of psychosocial sequelae have been recognised, including marital conflict or separation, parental distress or illness, ill health in other family members, and family dysfunction (Garralda & Bailey, 1989; Dulcan *et al*, 1990). Research examining family variables has shown these to be influential in a wide range of chronic or recurrent illness, including asthma (Lask & Matthew, 1979), diabetes (Minuchin *et al*, 1978), epilepsy (Rutter *et al*, 1970*b*; Hoare, 1984), and malignant diseases (Greenberg *et al*, 1989; Mulhern *et al*, 1989; Morris & Craft, 1990). Similar observations have been made with regard to chronic disability (Palfrey *et al*, 1989).

Evaluation of liaison

Information is conspicuously lacking in respect of the efficacy of liaison, both in relation to the usefulness of consultation in general, and specific interventions and therapies in particular. However, a number of authors have investigated specific areas of liaison, and two studies have reported promising outcomes. Bingley *et al* (1980) found that of 95 children referred to a tertiary paediatric referral centre and treated by a multi-disciplinary team, 57 (60%) were rated as improved at 12–24 month follow-up. All of these had previously been unsuccessfully managed elsewhere. Dungar *et al* (1986) have demonstrated that use of a multi-disciplinary approach can facilitate the diagnosis of previously unexplained illness.

A number of other workers have investigated specific areas of paediatric practice. Phipps *et al* (1989) studied the mothers of 30 infants who had experienced an apnoeic episode and had been placed on an apnoea monitor. Transient, but high levels of mood disturbance were noted, and it was possible to predict persistent mood disturbance by monitoring levels of family resources and health locus of control beliefs. As a result, families at risk of maladaptive responses were identified and offered intensive psychosocial support. Jedlicka-Kohler & Gotz (1988) in their study of 65 children with cystic fibrosis noted that parents frequently over-estimated disease severity. Such differences between subjective and medical evaluation highlighted potential psychiatric disturbance, and identified a focus for treatment.

The importance of the multi-disciplinary team

The multi-disciplinary team is central to paediatric liaison work. Each team member brings knowledge and skills distinct from other team members, and each person has a special contribution, with some overlap of expertise. The strength of such work lies in the effective sharing of such skills and knowledge, to facilitate a more broadly-based understanding of problems. In paediatric liaison work the multi-disciplinary team usually consists of at least one paediatrician, nurse, play leader, teacher, social worker, psychologist and child psychiatrist. Other disciplines that may be involved with individual children include physiotherapy, speech therapy, dietetics, psychotherapy and the chaplaincy.

Strategies for paediatric liaison

Paediatric liason psychiatry can occur in many different forms and contexts. At the simplest level it may consist of a consultation service only, while at its most complex liason psychiatrists may participate as full and active members of the paediatric team. Models of liaison in highly specific contexts have been described, including surgical wards and intensive care units, but the principles and problems are similar whatever the situation. We have highlighted a number of the difficulties presented by liaison work, and the best solutions are probably offered by a flexible combination of all the possible modes of joint working, including psychosocial ward rounds, joint assessment, and apprenticeship of junior paediatricians on particular cases. The psychiatrist's role in supporting paediatric staff, and encouraging and sharing academic interests has already been discussed.

The psychosocial ward round

The central fulcrum of liaison work is the joint psychosocial ward round, a regular meeting of the multi-disciplinary team. The principal function of such meetings is to ensure that due consideration is given to the psychosocial aspects of the children and their families, but attention can also be paid to matters such as ward atmosphere and staff tensions and conflicts. The psychosocial round also offers a starting forum at which specific modes of liaison work can be discussed and negotiated in relation to individual cases. On smaller units it may be possible to discuss all the children in turn, but it is often necessary to prioritise cases. Either way the person chairing the meeting should ensure that adequate time is allocated to each case, and it is often helpful if these decisions are made in advance of the meeting so that key personnel can be adequately prepared. If it is clear that full assessment will be necessary, advance notification may enable at least part of the assessment to be made before the multi-disciplinary team meets.

Joint interviewing

Bingley *et al* (1980) have described a number of the benefits of joint interviewing. It enables greater expertise to be brought to bear on discussion of both organic and psychosocial factors, while actively demonstrating the emphasis which both psychiatrist and paediatrician place on both physical and psychological factors. This may help parents appreciate the inter-relatedness of body and mind. In addition, an effective working relationship between paediatrician and psychiatrist serves as a useful model of communication. Further, the paediatrician learns techniques of psychosocial assessment, and the psychiatrist gains more understanding of the problems faced by paediatricians.

Apprenticeship

Junior paediatricians in direct contact with children and families can themselves carry out some psychosocial assessments, under the joint supervision of the responsible paediatrician and liaison psychiatrist. The psychiatrist can become more actively involved at any stage if this is indicated, but the trainee will still be able to maintain contact and follow progress, and in this way learn more about the process of liaison work and the course which the family's difficulties may take. It is hoped that this experience may later inform their own practice, and also their understanding of how and when to make a referral for psychiatric assessment or treatment.

The pitfalls of paediatric liaison – predictable difficulties

We have already alluded to many of these difficulties in the relevant sections, but some points are worthy of further emphasis, in particular those relating to potential dissonance in philosophy or conceptual frameworks, and those relating to pitfalls in communication.

Conceptual frameworks

Differences in emphasis may lead the psychiatrist to feel critical of a medical approach which may appear limited or reductionist, and perhaps fixed in the dichotomous conflict of mind versus body, organ system versus child. However, it should be remembered that paediatricians can rarely devote the time which psychiatrists routinely spend with their clients, and so may be in a less advantaged position to appreciate the wider implications of illness for the child and family. In addition, the range of conceptual frameworks familiar to psychiatrists can seem abstruse and impenetrable to doctors primarily trained in the medical model, and mental health professionals have been justifiably criticised for their tendency to use "theories, speculations and unsettled controversies which tend to confuse rather than inform" (Rickards, 1978). On the other hand, some paediatricians complain about psychiatrists' preoccupation with epidemiology and statistics (Meadow, 1980), and it seems that psychiatrists are as likely to be criticised for using scientific methods as for practicing psychiatry as a purely clinical art. This emphasises further the different requirements which paediatricians may have, and the need for the psychiatrist to approach consultation with an open mind and a willingness to meet individual paediatricians on their own terms.

Communication

The issue of communication underpins the same areas of interdisciplinary work, but is perhaps even more likely to be implicated in the success or failure of a particular collaboration. No amount of psychodynamic speculation is helpful in a crisis when practical advice is sought; nor is the poor diagnostic precision of child psychiatry useful. The difference in conceptual frameworks need not necessarily present a problem in its own right, but communication may founder in the semantic quagmire presented by different terminologies. The liaison psychiatrist, trained in both disciplines and fluent in both languages, is in a unique position to bridge this gap, and enable the different varieties of expertise to be brought effectively to bear on the problems of children and their families.

References

Apley, J. (1982) One child. In *One Child* (eds J. Apley & C. Ounstead), pp. 23–47. London: Mackeith Press.

—— & Hale, B. (1973) Children with recurrent abdominal pain: how do they grow up? *British Medical Journal*, **3**, 7–9.

Awad, G. & Poznanski, E. (1975) Psychiatric consultations in a paediatric hospital. *American Journal of Psychiatry*, **132**, 915–918.

Bibace, R. & Walsh, M. (1981) *Children's Conceptions of Health, Illness and Bodily Functions*. Washington: Jossey-Bass.

Bingley, L., Leonard, J., Hensman, S., *et al* (1980) The comprehensive management of children on a paediatric ward: a family approach. *Archives of Disease in Childhood*, **55**, 555–561.

Cundall, D. (1987) Children and mothers at clinics: who is disturbed? *Archives of Disease in Childhood*, **62**, 820–824.

Dulcan, M., Costello, E., Costello, A., *et al* (1990) The paediatrician as gatekeeper to mental health care for children. *Journal of the American Academy of Child Psychiatry*, **29**, 453–458.

Dungar, D., Pritchard, J., Hensman, S., *et al* (1986) The investigation of atypical psychosomatic illness: a team approach to diagnosis. *Clinical Paediatrics*, **25**, 341–344.

Fitzgerald, M. (1985) Behavioural deviance and maternal depressive symptoms in paediatric out-patients. *Archives of Disease in Childhood*, **60**, 560–562.

Garralda, E. & Bailey, D. (1989) Psychiatric disorders in general paediatric referrals. *Archives of Disease in Chidhood*, **64**, 1727–1733.

Graham, P. (1991) *Child Psychiatry – A Developmental Approach* (2nd edn). Oxford: Oxford University Press.

Greenberg, H., Kazak, A. & Meadows, A. (1989) Psychological functioning in 8–16 year old cancer survivors. *Journal of Paediatrics*, **114**, 488–493.

Gustafsson, P., Kazak, A. & Meadows, A. (1989) Cost effectiveness: family therapy in a paediatric setting. *Family Systems Medicine*, **6**, 162–175.

Hoare, P. (1984) The development of psychiatric disorder among school children with epilepsy. *Developmental Medicine and Child Neurology*, **26**, 3–13.

Jedlicka-Kohler, I. & Gotz, M. (1988) Interventional assessment of physical and mental health in children and adolescents with cystic fibrosis. *Scandinavian Journal of Gastroenterology*, **23**, 34–37.

John, A. & Bradford, R. (1991) Integrating family therapy into in-patient paediatric settings: a model. *Journal of Family Therapy*, **13**, 207–224.

Kokkonen, J. & Kokkonen, E. R. (1995) Psychological and somatic symptoms in young adults with chronic physical diseases. *Psychotherapy and Psychosomatics*, **64**, 94–101.

Lask, B. (1987) Physical illness, the family and the setting. In *Family Therapy* (eds A. Bentovim, G. Gorell Barnes & A. Cooklin), pp. 319–344. London: Academic Press.

—— (1994) Paediatric liaison work. In *Child and Adolescent Psychiatry: Modern Approaches* (eds M. Rutter, L. Hersov & E. Taylor), pp. 996–1005. Oxford: Blackwell Scientific Publications.

—— & Matthew, D. (1979) Childhood asthma – a controlled trial of family therapy. *Archives of Disease in Childhood*, **54**, 116–119.

—— & Fosson, A. (1989) *Childhood Illness: The Psychosomatic Approach* (eds B. Lask & A. Fosson). Wiley Series in Family Psychology. Chichester: John Wiley.

Lipowski, Z. (1967) Review of consultation psychiatry and psychosomatic medicine. *Psychosomatic Medicine*, **29**, 153–171.

Meadow, R. (1980) Mammoth from a messiah. *British Medical Journal*, **19**, 1082–1083.

Minuchin, S. Rosman, B. & Baker, L. (1978) *Psychosomatic Families.* Cambridge, Mass: Harvard Press.

Morris, J. & Craft, A. (1990) Childhood cancer at what cost? *Archives of Disease in Childhood*, **65**, 638–640.

Mulhern, R., Wasserman, A., Friedman, A., *et al* (1989) Social competence and behavioural adjustment of children who are long-term survivors of cancer. *Paediatrics*, **88**, 18–25.

Offord, D. R., Boyle, M. H., Szatmari, P., *et al* (1987) Ontario child health study: II. Six-month prevalence of disorder and rates of service utilisation. *Archives of General Psychiatry*, **44**, 832–836.

Palfrey, J., Walker, D., Builer, J., *et al* (1989) Patterns of response in families of chronically disabled children. *American Journal of Orthopsychiatry*, **19**, 94–104.

Phipps, S., Drotar, D., Joseph, C., *et al* (1989) Home apnoeic monitoring. *Developmental and Behavioural Paediatrics*, **10**, 7–12.

Rickards, W. (1978) Patterns of collaboration between child psychiatrists and paediatricians. *Australian Paediatric Journal*, **14**, 66–68.

Rutter, M., Tizard, J. & Whitmore, K. (1970*a*) *Education, Health and Behaviour.* London: Longman.

——, Tizard, J. & Whitmore, K. (1970*b*) *A Neuropsychiatric Study in Childhood. Clinics in Developmental Medicine*, 35/36, London: Heinemann/Spastics International Medical Publications.

Shapiro, E. G. & Rosenfeld, A. A. (1987) Conversion and somatisation disorders in children: review of the literature. In *The Somatising Child* (eds E. G. Shapiro & A. A. Rosenfeld), pp. 29–51. New York: Springer-Verlag.

Smithells, R. (1982) In praise of out-patients: partnership in paediatrics. In *One Child* (eds J. Apley & C. Ounstead), pp. 135–146. London: Mackeith Press.

Steinberg, D. & Yule, W. (1986) Consultative work. In *Child and Adolescent Psychiatry: Modern Approaches* (eds M. Rutter & L. Hersov), pp. 914–926. Oxford: Blackwell Scientific Publications.

Stocking, M., Rothney, W., Grosser, A., *et al* (1972) Psychopathology in the paediatric hospital. *American Journal of Public Health*, **62**, 551–556.

Sturge, J. (1989) Joint work in paediatrics: a child psychiatry perspective. *Archives of Disease in Childhood*, **64**, 155–158.

8 Liaison in old age psychiatry

Susan M. Benbow & Gerald H. Dawson

*The context • Clinical problems presenting in liaison work •
Interventions in liaison psychiatry in late life • Models of liaison
between old age psychiatry and geriatric medicine*

Psychogeriatrics has been described, within the family of psychiatry, as married to geriatric medicine. This expresses the closeness of the relationship between psychiatrists and physicians who care for elderly people, and the close relationship between physical and psychiatric illness in late life, which has encouraged the development of various models of liaison.

The context

Ruskin (1985) wrote that 'hospitalised elderly patients with emotional problems present a unique diagnostic and therapeutic challenge'. What do we know about the challenge we face and how best to deal with it? Eastwood & Corbin (1985) have reported an increased prevalence of psychiatric problems with increasing age, but there is evidence that elderly people are under-represented in referrals for psychiatric consultation. Rabins *et al* (1983) found that patients aged over 60 occupied 28.5% of general hospital beds but only accounted for 21% of 651 consultations to the liaison psychiatry service, giving a consultation rate among over-60s which was only 61% of the rate among people aged under 45 years of age. Other authors in North America (Shevitz *et al*, 1976; Bustamente & Ford, 1981; Popkin *et al*, 1984; Folks & Ford, 1985; Ruskin, 1985; Mainprize & Rodin, 1987) have found a similar trend in people aged over 60; the older the patient, the less likely they are to be referred to a liaison psychiatrist.

Elderly patients tend to stay in hospital longer than younger patients, which might contribute to apparent (but not necessarily real) under-representation of elderly patients in studies of liaison referrals. Wise *et al* (1985) suggested that ageism and therapeutic nihilism might be factors in reluctance to refer, but also that potential referrers might fear the elderly patient's reaction to seeing a psychiatrist.

As with younger patients, psychiatric illness in elderly people in general hospital beds may be treatable, may affect the management of the physical illness, may cause distress, and may be an important factor in admission, delayed discharge, failure to cope after discharge or discharge to unnecessary institutional placements (Lichtenstein & Winograd, 1984).

Several authors have found that the predominant psychiatric diagnosis in physically ill people is depression (e.g. Shevitz *et al*, 1976); a treatable condition which carries substantial morbidity and mortality in late life. Almost 25% of elderly liaison referrals to Central Manchester Old Age Psychiatry service in 1984–85 were of people suffering from affective illnesses and a further third were suffering from dementing illnesses. Review of liaison referrals at that time (Benbow, 1987) established that they constituted a major part of the department's workload (35%), and that most were made by colleagues in geriatric medicine (58% of hospital doctor referrals). The remaining 42% of liaison referrals came from physicians and surgeons throughout the general hospital. Compared with GP referrals, liaison patients were more physically ill and more likely to come from outside the catchment area. Follow-up (of one sort or another) was offered to 43% of the liaison group.

Clinical problems presenting in liaison work

The following examples indicate that the presentations to an old age liaison psychiatry service differ from younger persons and cannot readily be placed in the categories according to the scheme outlined in Chapter 3 (p. 64; Thomas Classification, 1983).

Somatic presentation of psychological disorders

> Mrs ME, an 84-year-old widow, was admitted to a geriatric ward with vague abdominal pains, nausea, anorexia and constipation. Apart from the constipation, no physical cause for her symptoms was found on investigation. Her GP had been treating her for some time with a tricyclic antidepressant. On the ward, nursing staff noted low mood, worse in the mornings, early morning wakening, poor appetite and depressive speech e.g. 'I'm ill with worry', 'what will become of me?' The geriatric staff felt that the main problem might be depression and that her treatment needed review.
> The psychiatrist agreed with the geriatrician's diagnosis and suggested a change to an alternative antidepressant, and after discharge follow-up in the community by a community psychiatric nurse.

This case is similar to the somatic presentation of psychiatric disorders seen in younger people (Chapter 5), but admission to the geriatric ward may have been largely related to physical side-effects (predominantly constipation) of the tricyclic antidepressants. These may have exacerbated pre-existing somatic symptoms of depression.

Psychological reaction to physical illness

The following example illustrates the coexistence of physical and psychiatric disorders but is complicated as the latter leads to a marked psychological reaction to the physical illness.

> Mrs J, a 72-year-old widow with a long history of schizophrenia, fell at the nursing home where she lived and broke her femoral neck. She was admitted to an orthopaedic ward, and post-operatively became disruptive, shouting constantly and being verbally aggressive towards staff. She was referred as a consultation to the old age psychiatrist, who had been treating her previously in the nursing home. On assessment on the surgical ward she was not psychotic, but her behaviour was proving difficult to manage although she was starting to walk with the support of a frame. When the surgeons increased the dose of her major tranquilliser she had become drowsy and stopped walking.
> She was transferred to the old age psychiatry assessment ward, remobilised with a minimum of psychotropic medication, and subsequently discharged to the nursing home.

Here Mrs J's rehabilitation following her operation was adversely affected by her behaviour, which in turn related to her previous schizophrenic illness and its treatment. The rapid transfer of this patient from orthopaedic to psychiatric ward allowed speedy rehabilitation, with minimal sedation and confident psychiatric nursing.

Somatic presentation of psychiatric disorder

In late life referrals are often made when behaviour becomes disturbing, and the differential diagnosis between cerebral complications of physical illness and a primary psychotic disorder is difficult.

> Mrs W, a 73-year-old separated woman, was admitted from a rest home with a chest infection, but her behaviour became increasingly disturbed despite treatment of her physical illness. She was referred from a geriatric ward because of irritability, aggression and pacing. Very little information was available about her past history, but she was said to have had psychiatric problems in the past. When seen she was elated, irritable, disorientated and overactive, and a diagnosis of mania was made. Her memory was satisfactory. Despite her ongoing chest infection, it was agreed that she should be treated on the psychogeriatric assessment ward, since her behaviour was disrupting the geriatric medical ward. She was treated with a major tranquilliser, in addition to an antibiotic, and her mood gradually settled. When her previous psychiatric notes arrived, they revealed a long history of a bipolar affective illness.

It was not clear whether this is an example of an organic mood disorder (see p. 58), where the chest infection led to a manic episode or, more likely, that this patient had a manic episode triggered by the chest infection. In this case the patient was treated on the psychiatric ward. Another patient, who was less disturbed but with similar problems or who was on a less busy ward, might have been managed on the medical ward with ongoing advice from the psychiatrist. The basic requirement was that she should be able to access treatment from both specialities in whichever environment was best able to manage the practical problems. Negotiating management demands flexibility from both services.

Psychosocial factors complicating physical illness

Another situation, less common in young people, is where psychosocial difficulties exacerbate a physical illness.

> Mr R, a 76-year-old married man with Parkinson's disease, was referred for assessment while on a geriatric ward. He had been admitted with hypothermia and confusion. As his body temperature rose he had become increasingly confused and agitated, and haloperidol had been prescribed; this further impaired his mobility and put him at risk of falls. He was also described as having a 'social problem, in that he and his wife no longer wish to live together and he will be unable to look after himself at home'.
>
> His confusional state cleared when the haloperidol was stopped but he was discharged home before he could be fully reassessed by the psychiatrist. He was, however, readmitted to the geriatric ward, hypothermic again after a short while. It transpired that he and his wife had had an argument, which resulted in him being locked out of the house in the cold winter weather and subsequently being admitted to hospital with hypothermia. At interview, Mr R had a good grasp of the problems he faced, although he did have mild cognitive impairment. He could talk appropriately about his marriage, and the way he and his wife lived separately, though together. They had always had a conflictual marriage, and Mr R's cognitive impairment and increasing physical frailty had apparently unbalanced their relationship; the couple were referred on to the family therapy clinic.

This example indicates how hospital admission for mild physical illness (Parkinson's disease) is actually caused by psychosocial problems (marital conflict) rather than the illness itself.

Psychiatric disorder delaying discharge

It is recognised in people of all ages that psychiatric illness is likely to lengthen general hospital stay (Lipowski, 1983). Where psychiatric illness occurs in the elderly, organic causes tend to be over-rated and psychological and social factors are under-rated; drug treatments tend to be over-used and psychological and social approaches may be neglected (Krakowski, 1979). Psychotropic drugs bring the risk of side-effects and complications which, in themselves, might prolong hospital stay. The hospitalised elderly are therefore exposed to physical illness, its complications, psychiatric disorder and, possibly, side-effects from the drugs used to treat the psychiatric disorder. This may all lead to progressive functional disability which might affect recovery and/or discharge potential (Warshaw *et al*, 1982).

By recognising and treating psychiatric illness in elderly physically ill people, we would hope that length of stay (and bed-blocking) might be lower, care improved and that fewer people will be misplaced in institutions, when they could with help return to their own homes in the community (Levitan & Kornfeld, 1981). In elderly people undergoing surgery, Millar (1981) found that almost one-third had psychiatric problems before or after the operation. He pointed out that the identification of pre-operative intellectual impairment was important in order to allow correct diagnosis of acute confusional states following surgery. It may also be essential information in helping to discharge the patient home successfully. Pitt (1988) suggested that the prevalence of psychiatric disorder on general hospital wards might constitute a performance indicator for old age psychiatry services.

> Miss C, a 78-year-old single woman, was referred from the medical ward after being admitted with salicylate toxicity following an unintentional overdose. She was found on the ward to be forgetful and disorientated, and, when interviewed, relatives confirmed that she had gradually become increasingly forgetful over the previous six months. The medical staff felt that they could not discharge her in this confused state as she would be unable to cope on her own at home.
>
> Psychiatric assessment revealed a cheerfully disorientated woman with impaired recent memory, and no evidence of any mental illness other than probable Alzheimer's disease. Discharge home with appropriate support from social services following a home visit was advised. A home visit from the medical ward was unsuccessful so the patient was re-referred.
>
> After discussion with the medical team, the old age psychiatry team admitted the patient to the psychogeriatric day hospital, from which discharge home with support from home help, meals on wheels and daycare was successful.

This case illustrated to the old age psychiatric staff the difficulties of liaising closely with teams in the general hospital, and how misleading a dementia sufferer's performance in hospital can be. Medical and surgical teams see a person out of their usual surroundings in a strange and often hostile environment. Such staff may have little, if any, experience of home assessment and can find the proposed discharge of a cognitively impaired old person difficult and anxiety provoking. The liaison old age psychiatrist can perform a useful role in bridging the gap between hospital and home care, but, since beds may be blocked, rapid action is necessary. The psychogeriatric day hospital can be used to assess people from general hospital wards, provided places can readily be made available.

Failure to cope after discharge

Sometimes staff are reluctant to discharge someone for fear that they will be unable to cope. Other referrals follow a failed discharge, which may lead to rapid readmission. The case history below (Mr F) illustrates failure to cope after discharge and discharge to an unnecessary institutional placement.

> Mr F, an 83-year-old married man, was unable to walk following a stroke. He improved on the ward, but CT scan showed multiple infarcts, and he was noted to to be more forgetful, and have persistent personality change, tending to be irritable and aggressive when people approached him and he wanted to be left alone. His wife was told that she would be unable to care for him at home and a nursing home place was sought. No psychiatric referral was made.
>
> In the nursing home Mr F became increasingly withdrawn and aggressive. He refused to get out of bed or attend to his personal hygiene, when asked by the staff; he swore at them and threatened violence. When his wife came to visit he was more his usual self and would cooperate with her suggestions, with the result that the home insisted that she should spend almost all of every day with him, otherwise they were unable to cope with him.
>
> Mrs F then developed visual hallucinations of her husband when she was at home on her own and was referred for psychiatric assessment by the GP. She performed well on cognitive testing, was not depressed, but was distressed by her husband's absence and behaviour with home staff. As a result the psychiatrist arranged for Mr F to be admitted to the old age psychiatry assessment ward after discussion with his GP, and after assessment in hospital and at home, he was discharged home to live with his wife with social services and psychogeriatric support.

Neither of this couple was referred as a liaison consultation, although Mr F's physician had considered and rejected the idea, deciding instead that a nursing home placement would solve the problem. In fact, a liaison psychiatry referral would have been more appropriate from every point of view.

Question of mental capacity

Uncommonly people on medical or surgical wards are referred because of questions regarding their capacity to make decisions. One issue which may be raised is competency to make a will. Testators must be able to understand what assets they have at their disposal, who might be expected to benefit from them and what they are doing in making a will. Thus older adults with memory problems may be unable to make a will because of failure to recall what assets they have. However, people who have delusions may be capable, provided the delusions do not influence who might benefit, and those whose cognition fluctuates may also be capable provided they make the will in a lucid interval (Law Commission, 1991).

Interventions in liaison psychiatry in late life

Burstein (1984) suggested that elderly patients preferred medication follow-up in preference to psychotherapeutic treatments or a combined approach (psychotherapy plus medication). In central Manchester a clinical psychologist works closely with the geriatric physicians (Larner & Leeming, 1984) and has agreed to provide psychological treatments from within the geriatric medical team. This has proved a useful way of providing an intervention more acceptable to both staff and patients.

Blacher (1984) described psychotherapy for medical and surgical patients: two of his categories, which he labels confirmation of reality and speaking the unspeakable, are ones which are frequently encountered in clinical practice. These issues can be raised informally with medical and nursing staff during the course of consultation-based work and it is sometimes helpful, if staff identify particularly difficult issues, to offer to organise a teaching session or workshop on this topic: one example in our experience has been dealing with death and the dying patient.

It may be unclear which specialist is best placed to treat a person who suffers from concurrent physical and psychiatric illnesses, each of which would merit treatment in its own right. In practice it may not be easy to manage patients jointly, although various models have been developed to facilitate joint management. The *Bulletin of the Royal College of Psychiatrists* published guidelines for collaboration between geriatric physicians and psychiatrists in the care of the elderly in 1979 (Standing Joint Committee of the British Geriatrics Society and the Royal College of Psychiatrists, 1979). These stressed the need for services for elderly people to be a unity, but with explicit criteria for division of responsibility. Training reciprocity was regarded as necessary in order for mutual confidence to develop, and we will see later how this has developed. The guidelines asserted that "responsibility should be determined by the assessed needs of the patient", but that lack of resources does not redefine responsibility as lying within the province of the spousal service. It was recognised that patients might fall into the uncertain mid-zone between medicine and psychiatry, and that negotiation might be needed to decide on placement, but the basic principle of joint care was felt to be that patients assessed by one service as needing joint care should receive it and that past history should not prejudice future care needs.

Revised guidelines have been published (Standing Joint Committee of the British Geriatrics Society and the Royal College of Psychiatrists, 1992), but the basic principles have stood the test of time. The revised guidelines stress the applicability of principles of collaboration to patients in other hospital settings (i.e. not merely within psychiatric and geriatric wards and clinics), and the need for ongoing involvement of both specialities in joint service planning by health and social services. They also point out that goodwill and cooperation between colleagues is more important than specifically designated assessment units.

Thus there is, and has been for some years, agreement about some of the ground rules governing the relationship between geriatric medicine and geriatric psychiatry and both specialities are aware of the importance of joint working practices. An individual under the care of one service, is likely in many hospitals to be referred to the other specialist and seen as a ward consultation. Discussion between the two specialists in the light of both assessments will lead to agreement about how management should proceed. Ease and speed of communication is critical when very sick people are involved.

Effects of developing a liaison service for elderly mentally ill

The effect of establishing a liaison service in old age is similar to that of doing so for young age groups: it may increase referrals. Pauser *et al* (1987) found that their consultation rate doubled within one year when a liaison system was established in a university hospital old age psychiatry service.

Scott *et al* (1988) described the changes in referrals which occurred when a consultation service changed to a consultation–liaison service. Prior to the change only a small proportion of referrals were for functional illnesses (12% depression), but subsequently these referrals increased (28% depression) with a corresponding halving of referrals where the psychiatrist identified no mental illness (from 14 to 7%). The authors stressed the crucial role of their colleagues in geriatric medicine and identified 'secondary referrals', those people referred by physicians or surgeons to a geriatric physician who detected a psychiatric problem (with or without a 'geriatric' problem), and suggested referral on to an old age psychiatrist. Thus the geriatric physician's awareness of psychiatric morbidity had a knock-on effect, influencing practice on other hospital wards. The authors suggested that liaison contact with the geriatric service (attendance by a senior registrar at weekly multi-disciplinary ward round, case conferences and reviews) improved the knowledge of psychiatry among staff of the geriatric service, rather than helping solely in the treatment of individual patients. Anderson & Philpott (1991) have identified a similar effect in Liverpool, resulting from an active consultation service alone, so it may be that both models can have this effect.

Chandarana *et al* (1988) found that availability of a consultation service does not necessarily lead to increased utilisation and argued the need to forge specific links with other specialities. Old age psychiatrists benefit from focusing their liaison interests, as where an active geriatric medical service exists, most referrals will come from that source and it is easier to concentrate developments if one area contributes the majority of referrals. The Liverpool service, although relying on a consultation model, may have established other connections with the referrers which had an effect on their patterns of referrals, e.g. joint involvement in planning, in liaison with social services etc., and these too may facilitate the development of a cooperative and trusting relationship, which will enhance close working practices.

Models of liaison between old age psychiatry and geriatric medicine

It is clear that liaison between physicians and psychiatrists who care for older adults is important. There is, however, no preferred single model of how to effect liaison and different models have developed depending in part on resources, on the relative maturity of geriatric medical and psychiatric services and on the interest, energy and style of working of both psychiatrist and physician. We will describe some of these models, but would stress that none has universal applicability and that local interests and influences have always been powerful factors in the particular working models which have evolved. We will deal with the following models:

(1) consultation work
(2) joint out-patient clinics
(3) joint wards/departments
(4) reciprocal teaching and training.

Consultation work

In this model the physician and psychiatrist select referrals to make to their colleagues in the other speciality. Anderson & Philpott (1991) have pointed out that since psychiatric morbidity on non-psychiatric hospital wards greatly exceeds the capacity of a consultation service, an important objective within this model must be to help non-psychiatrists detect and manage most psychiatric illness in the medically ill without referral to a specialist. Referral will depend on each specialist recognising problems which might be helped by involving their colleagues. This is a widely used model and the one which we use in the old age psychiatry service in central Manchester and which Anderson & Philpott (1991) have described in Liverpool. Threshold of referral might be a problem, as might sensitivity to psychiatric problems and awareness (or unawareness) of the possible value of psychiatric treatment. Many geriatric physicians have much experience of people with mixed physical and psychiatric illness, in which case this model might work well.

Important practical issues

The psychiatrist will need to set aside sufficient time to assess patients and to confer with geriatric medical staff regarding their management. On a medical ward it can be difficult to find suitable undisturbed surroundings to conduct interviews. The psychiatrist needs to firmly resist the temptation to see patients on the ward amid a welter of distracting activity. For the patient who may be disorientated or forgetful, it would be unreasonable to expect them to function optimally with such competition, so an accurate assessment could not be made. For the patient who is distressed, it would be unreasonable to expect them to talk about sensitive topics when everyone on the ward might hear. More appropriate space can usually be found, although we have interviewed people in very strange places at times. Old age psychiatrists may have an advantage in that the majority of their referrals are probably from geriatric wards, and, with frequent contact, the staff will come to recognise the need for a private interview and will readily set it up.

It is important that referrals can be made easily, perhaps by telephone, and people do not have to wait long periods before being seen, since delays will tend to deter physicians from making referrals. The ability to offer a rapid assessment in the community following discharge can be useful to all concerned, provided that there is no uncertainty about arrangements for follow-up after discharge. Communication between teams can be difficult but is facilitated if people meet regularly, or at least speak frequently by telephone, rather than communicating in writing. It is important too for each to be clear of what the other can contribute to the care of a particular patient, and what the referrer wants from their colleague – openness and honesty are invaluable. Sometimes, with very complex problems, it can be helpful for psychiatrist and physician to arrange to see the patient together, despite the timetabling difficulties involved.

In addition to the value of consultations in the care of individual patients, they have an important role in education and in dispelling therapeutic nihilism (Duthie & Gambert, 1983). Over a period of years, referral practice has been shown to shift to more appropriate patient selection with fewer referrals of people who are not mentally ill, suggesting that there is an effect on education of the referrers (Anderson & Philpott, 1991).

Joint clinics

Some districts have made use of joint psychogeriatric/geriatric out-patient clinics. These primarily target elderly patients who do not need to be admitted to hospital but require further assessment. Such clinics are organised, among others, by both south Manchester (Jolley *et al*, 1980) and central Manchester old age psychiatry services. They take place weekly on a general hospital site. The clinic allows the opportunity for a detailed physical examination of patients who have initially been seen at home, and facilitates access to any investigative procedures, the majority of which take place at the time the patient attends the out-patient clinic. Both a geriatric physician and an old age psychiatrist attend, and either may refer to the clinic, although most referrals are, in practice, initiated by the psychiatrist. The expertise of the geriatric physician is available to help ensure that patients receive appropriate management for any physical disorders and the geriatrician can likewise tap into the expertise of the psychiatrist regarding the management of psychiatric disorders. The two specialists are also, through a process of mutual support and ongoing learning, able to deal with problems formerly seen as the province of one or the other, with increasing confidence and competence. As with other models of joint working, the opportunity for teaching and training within and between the specialities is an important additional benefit.

> A 79-year-old widow (Mrs A) was referred to the old age psychiatry service by her family doctor. She had been sleeping poorly, complaining about her neighbours and refusing any treatment which her GP suggested. Routine blood investigations carried out by her GP were within normal limits. She was assessed at home, and described a six month history of persecutory delusions and auditory hallucinations in the absence of any marked mood disorder or cognitive impairment. She also gave a history of recent weight loss in the absence of any past medical history or active known medical problems, other than bronchitis. Late-onset paraphrenia was provisionally diagnosed. Mrs B agreed to take small doses of thioridazine and to attend the joint clinic for more detailed assessment of her physical health.
> Physical examination in the clinic was basically unremarkable, but X-ray and other investigations revealed a probable lung cancer, which was discussed with the woman and her relatives. She was referred for bronchoscopy, but was reluctant to agree to invasive investigation, and follow-up in the clinic was continued.

The advantages of the joint involvement of physician and psychiatrist in the clinic were several. Firstly, the clinic provided a quick and efficient setting for physical examination and investigation without recourse to hospital admission. Secondly, once a probable physical disease was identified, the geriatric physician was able to advise on management, in the light of psychiatric information about the woman's mental state. Communication could not have been simpler, since both specialists were present in the clinic together. Thirdly communication with the patient and her relatives was facilitated and misunderstandings were prevented, as all parties contributed to the discussion about diagnosis and future care. This was particularly important since the probable diagnosis was cancer. Questions about treatment options for the cancer and its likely prognosis could be answered by the geriatric physician and the psychological reaction of the patient, together with the response of her psychotic illness to treatment, could be monitored by the psychiatrist. Thus the patient and her family received the expertise of both services, without having to be shunted from one to the other, and without delays or misunderstandings in communication between those involved.

Joint wards/departments

Pitt & Silver (1980) have outlined the nature and work of the joint unit established by the London unit. Admissions to this unit consist of both medically and psychiatrically ill elderly people; the former are typical of those traditionally taken to an acute geriatric ward and the latter are more selected. The mentally ill patients tend to be those with mixed physical and psychiatric disorders, acute confusional states, or non-specific symptoms which could point to either physical or psychiatric disorder and require assessment by both specialists as facilitated in this setting. The unit allows more appropriate targeting of the geriatric physician's and old age psychiatrist's expertise, as required to meet the needs of the elderly patient, and helps reduce duplication of work. A knock-on effect is also described whereby the presence of a psychiatrist in the joint unit influences other areas of the geriatric service and improves attitudes within geriatric medicine to psychiatric problems. However, it is emphasised that the joint unit is not a complete solution, and both geriatric and old age psychiatric services still require their own complementary services. The success of such a unit depends greatly upon the relationship between the partners and their ability to cooperate closely.

Arie & Jolley (1982) describe a different approach to joint working in Nottingham; old age psychiatrists and geriatric physicians are fellow members of a joint University Department of Health Care of the Elderly. In this case there is no shared ward but both services, although separately organised, are in close proximity which enables easy access to the partner service and its skills while still keeping the specialities distinct. Services which do not have joint ward facilities may still be able to manage people jointly with some negotiation, as illustrated by the next case history.

Mrs C, an 81-year-old widow, was admitted to an orthopaedic ward for treatment of severe generalised rheumatoid arthritis following a collapse. On the ward she was noted to be anxious and agitated, and was referred for psychiatric assessment after nursing staff found her putting a plastic bag over her head.

When seen on the ward, Mrs C gave a four year history of worsening depression with marked anxiety but had not previously seen a psychiatrist. After an overdose about 9 months previously she had moved to live in an elderly persons home. The diagnosis was a severe depressive illness with agitation and suicidal ideation. Treatment with an increasing dose of amitriptyline was commenced. One month later there had been no improvement despite compliance with the tricyclic antidepressant. Mrs C was advised to have ECT and the treatment was fully explained to her and her son. Pre-anaesthetic physical assessment was carried out by a consultant anaesthetist. She was treated with eight ECT as a day-patient in the psychiatric unit while remaining an in-patient on the orthopaedic ward. Following ECT she was much improved and appropriately concerned about where she would live after discharge. Her local social services department was involved to look at options, and she was discharged to an elderly persons home.

Reciprocal teaching and training

The development of joint working practices and closer cooperation between geriatric physicians and old age psychiatrists has led to consideration of the training needs of senior registrars in both specialities. Reciprocal training is one of the recommendations of a joint report of the Royal Colleges (Joint Working Party of the Royal Colleges of Physicians and Psychiatrists, 1989). It points out that the Joint Committee on Higher Medical Training recommends that senior registrars in geriatric medicine should receive six weeks training in old age psychiatry but that there is no such equivalent formal arrangement for senior registrars in old age psychiatry. It is unclear to what extent cross-training takes place at present. A minimum amount of training in the parallel service has been recommended as a condition of accreditation by the Report.

The importance of reciprocal training has also recently been highlighted by Forsyth (1992) who draws attention to the many vacant posts for consultant old age psychiatrists, which suggest that for some time to come geriatric physicians will have a heavy psychogeriatric workload. Effective liaison is therefore important. It is as important for old age psychiatrists to maintain their general medical skills as it is for geriatric physicians to be alert to psychiatric problems. There are three aspects to the medical skills necessary for an old age psychiatrist: firstly, the ability to perform a competent physical examination, secondly, the retention and acquisition of knowledge of relevant physical disorders and their treatment, and, thirdly, keeping up to date with the use of drugs in the treatment of physical disorders and, in particular, their side-effects and interactions with psychotropic medication.

A report has recently been prepared for the Liaison Committee of the British Geriatrics Society and the Royal College of Psychiatrists on the issue of training (Bagley, 1991). It considers the following two main areas:

(1) different models of joint training and associated difficulties
(2) current practice and future recommendations.

Different models of joint training and associated difficulties

Four types of model can be described. Firstly there is the joint training available when a joint ward or department has been developed. In the London unit (Pitt & Silver, 1980) the medical staff include junior doctors from both geriatric medicine and old age psychiatry. The opportunity exists in this model for ongoing training in each of the specialities, within the day-to-day work of the unit. The same advantage applies to the Nottingham University Department of Health Care of the Elderly, and the educational benefits to students, both undergraduate and postgraduate, of close working in this format have already been demonstrated (Arie *et al*, 1985).

Secondly there are 'block secondments', where senior registrars spend a period of time away from their usual duties, in the appropriate parallel service. This attachment may vary in duration from one week to six months. Thirdly, joint training may be based on sessions of variable frequency and content, perhaps involving attendance at a ward round, out-patient or joint clinic work, or working in a particular area of the service. For example, an old age psychiatry senior registrar might take an interest in a stroke rehabilitation ward or a geriatric medicine senior registrar an interest in ECT. Fourthly, in addition to another model or in isolation, there may be the opportunity to participate in joint academic meetings and/or joint case conferences.

Although fairly straightforward, in practice various problems can arise. Availability of experience in the parallel service is not consistent nationwide. There are a limited number of districts with joint wards and departments, and some districts have no psychogeriatric service at all (Wattis, 1988). It is therefore difficult for some senior registrars to set up joint training.

Another reason for this discrepancy is the potential conflict between training and service provision. Senior registrars who take up reciprocal training may find they are expected to use their specialist skills rather than being able to concentrate on gaining experience in and a greater understanding of the parallel service. There may also be a reluctance for the service commitment they are already providing in their own speciality to be lost, despite their supernumerary status. The Royal Colleges' report

(Joint Working Party of the Royal Colleges of Physicians and Psychiatrists, 1989) recommends supernumerary status as appropriate if it helps to develop the best training experience. A block secondment is regarded as more useful than a sessional commitment. There may, however, be drawbacks associated with this. Secondments are unlikely to be based on a direct exchange of senior registrars. It would be inappropriate for an old age psychiatry senior registrar to take on an equivalent level of clinical responsibility in geriatric medicine, since not all have had post-registration experience in geriatric medicine and most may have spent several years training in psychiatry. They may not have retained all the skills and knowledge required to perform at medical senior registrar level. A similar situation is likely with respect to geriatric medicine senior registrars in relation to psychiatry. A training post in the parallel speciality would inevitably be more junior, and, even then, may be purely observational.

Senior registrars who spend time in the parallel speciality may be regarded only as a specialist resource: psychiatry senior registrars in a geriatric medical setting may spend all their time seeing cases of suspected psychiatric illness in geriatric medicine patients, and geriatric medicine senior registrars in old age psychiatry may spend all their time seeing physically ill psychiatric patients. Although each service gains, training suffers. For trainees to be free to experience the parallel speciality liaison must take place independent of the trainees. The importance of crossover training to psychiatry is that future psychiatrists will gain experience of the mix of physical and psychiatric problems in both services and of differing approaches. Effective liaison requires a grasp of which problems are best assessed and treated within each speciality. Although there are guidelines, there are no hard and fast rules: a psychiatrist needs some understanding of what level of psychiatric awareness can be expected of a geriatric ward and what level of behaviour disturbance geriatric medical staff can manage. Similarly the psychiatrist needs some concept of what physical illnesses can be appropriately managed on a psychiatric ward, and how geriatric medical and psychiatric day hospitals differ in style and approach, so that decisions can be made of where individuals with mixed problems can best be helped. There are no fixed answers to these questions, as different services may show differing strengths and weaknesses, which can be tailored to the needs of different individuals. Trainees will benefit from experience of different styles of liaison between services.

Current practice and future recommendations

Bagley (1991) has confirmed that current practice is variable in availability and content of reciprocal training for senior registrars in both specialities. All senior registrars who responded to the questionnaire survey believed that they would need to liaise with consultants in the other speciality and most senior registrars in both specialities believed reciprocal training was necessary. Training inadequacies therefore need to be tackled, and the report makes seven recommendations, concluding that flexibility in training is important.

Increased joint working will also lead to greater opportunities for teaching, which is likely to enhance interest in collaboration between the two specialities and hence improve the quality of service provided to elderly people. The educational benefits of closer working have already been demonstrated in the Nottingham University Department of Health Care of the Elderly (Arie *et al*, 1985).

Other areas of liaison

Although the closest relationship is probably that between geriatric psychiatrists and physicians, links must be developed, among others, with social services, residential homes and voluntary organisations (such as Age Concern and the Alzheimer's Disease Society). Good liaison requires willingness to help, respect for colleagues and open communication. Flexibility, openness and respect are needed on all sides in order to evolve working practices tailored to individuals, rather than institutions.

Conclusions

Joint working between geriatric physicians and old age psychiatrists is clinically essential, and can be achieved in several ways. Setting up some form of a liaison service does have certain effects, in terms of referral patterns, expectations on behalf of staff and in demands on time and resources. It also has educational effects, which may alter the pattern of liaison referrals over time. Some practical problems can be anticipated, and difficulties of communication between specialities cannot be overestimated, but goodwill on both sides allows these to be overcome in various ways. It is essential that all trainees acquire the necessary skills to assess an old person who presents the need for psychiatric and geriatric medical assessment and to negotiate a management plan with their specialist colleagues.

References

Anderson, D. N. & Philpott, R. M. (1991) The changing pattern of referrals for psychogeriatric consultation in the general hospital: an eight-year study. *International Journal of Geriatric Psychiatry*, **6**, 801–807.

Arie, T. & Jolley, D. J. (1982) Making services work: organisation and style of psychogeriatric services. In *The Psychiatry of Late Life* (eds R. Levy & F. Post), pp. 222–251. Oxford: Blackwell.

——, Jones, R. & Smith, C. (1985) The educational potential of old age psychiatry services. In *Recent Advances in Psychogeriatrics* (ed T. Arie), pp. 197–207. Edinburgh: Churchill Livingstone.

Bagley, G. (1991) *Reciprocal Training for Senior Registrars in Geriatric Medicine and Old Age Psychiatry.* Report for the British Geriatrics Society/Royal College of Psychiatrists Liaison Committee.

Benbow, S. M. (1987) Liaison referrals to a department of psychiatry for the elderly. *International Journal of Geriatric Psychiatry,* **2**, 235–240.

Blacher, R. S. (1984) The briefest encounter: psychotherapy for medical and surgical patients. *General Hospital Psychiatry,* **6**, 226–232.

Burstein, A. (1984) Psychiatric consultations in a general hospital: compliance to follow-up. *General Hospital Psychiatry,* **6**, 139–141.

Bustamente, J. P. & Ford, C. V. (1981) Characteristics of general hospital patients referred for psychiatric consultation. *Journal of Clinical Psychiatry,* **42**, 338–341.

Chandarana, P. C., Conlon, P. & Steinberg, N. (1988) The evaluation of a consultation-liaison service. *General Hospital Psychiatry,* **10,** 378–381.

Duthie, E. H. & Gambert, S. R. (1983) Geriatrics consultation: implications for teaching and clinical care. *Gerontology and Geriatrics Education,* **4**, 59–66.

Eastwood, R. & Corbin, S. (1985) Epidemiology of mental disorders in old age. In *Recent Advances in Psychogeriatrics* (ed. T. Arie), pp. 17–32. Edinburgh: Churchill Livingstone.

Folks, D. G. & Ford, C. V. (1985) Psychiatric disorders in geriatric medical/ surgical patients. I: report of 195 consecutive consultations. *Southern Medical Journal,* **78**, 239–241.

Forsyth, D. R. (1992) Psychogeriatric training for senior registrars in geriatric medicine. *Psychiatric Bulletin,* **16**, 78–79.

Joint Working Party of the Royal Colleges of Physicians and Psychiatrists (1989) *Specialist Services and Medical Training for the Care of Elderly People with Mental Illness.* London: Royal College of Psychiatrists.

Jolley, D., Kondratowicz, T. & Brocklehurst, J. C. (1980) *Psychogeriatric Outpatient Clinic.* Paper presented to British Geriatrics Society Spring Conference: Isle of Man.

Krakowski, A. J. (1979) Psychiatric consultation for the geriatric population in the general hospital. *Bibliotheca Psychiatrica,* **159**, 163–185.

Larner, S. L. & Leeming, J. T. (1984) The work of a clinical psychologist in the care of the elderly. *Age and Ageing,* **13**, 29–33.

Law Commission (1991) *Mentally Incapacitated Adults and Decision Making; An Overview.* Consultation Paper 119. London: HMSO.

Levitan, S. J. & Kornfeld, D. S. (1981) Clinical and cost benefits of liaison psychiatry. *American Journal of Psychiatry,* **138**, 790–793.

Lichtenstein, H. & Winograd, C.H. (1984) Geriatric consultation: a functional approach. *Journal of the American Geriatrics Society,* **35**, 356–361.

Lipowski, Z. J. (1983) The need to integrate liaison psychiatry and geropsychiatry. *American Journal of Psychiatry,* **140**, 1003–1005.

Mainprize, E. & Rodin, G. (1987) Geriatric referrals to a psychiatric consultation-liaison service. *Canadian Journal of Psychiatry,* **32**, 5–9.

Millar, H. R. (1981) Psychiatric morbidity in elderly surgical patients. *British Journal of Psychiatry,* **138**, 17–20.

Pauser, H., Bergstrom, B. & Walinder, J. (1987) 294 psychiatric consultations involving in-patients above 70 years of age in somatic departments in a university hospital. *Acta Psychiatrica Scandinavica,* **76**, 152–157.

Pitt, B. (1988) Psychogeriatrics: miscellaneous papers. *Current Opinion in Psychiatry*, **1**, 499–504.

—— & Silver, C. P. (1980) The combined approach to geriatrics and psychiatry: evaluation of a joint unit in a teaching hospital district. *Age and Aging*, **9**, 33–37.

Popkin, M. K., Mackenzie, T. B. & Callies, A. L. (1984) Psychiatric consultation to geriatric medically ill in-patients in a university hospital. *Archives of General Psychiatry*, **41**, 703–707.

Rabins, P., Lucas, M. J., Teitelbaum, M., *et al* (1983) Utilization of psychiatric consultation for elderly patients. *Journal of the American Geriatrics Society*, **31**, 581–585.

Ruskin, P. E. (1985) Gero-psychiatric consultation in a university hospital: a report on 67 referrals. *American Journal of Psychiatry*, **142**, 333–336.

Scott, J., Fairbairn, A. & Woodhouse, K. (1988) Referrals to a psychogeriatric consultation-liaison service. *International Journal of Geriatric Psychiatry*, **3**, 131–135.

Shevitz, S. A., Silberfarb, P. M. & Lipowski, Z. J. (1976) Psychiatric consultations in a general hospital. A report on 1000 referrals. *Diseases of the Nervous System*, **37**, 295–304.

Standing Joint Committee of the British Geriatrics Society/Royal College of Psychiatrists (1979) Guidelines for collaboration between geriatric physicians and psychiatrists in the care of the elderly. *Bulletin of the Royal College of Psychiatrists*, November, 168–169.

—— & —— (1992) Revised guidelines for collaboration between physicians in geriatric medicine and psychiatrists of old age. *Psychiatric Bulletin*, **16**, 583–584.

Thomas, C. J. (1983) Referrals to a British liaison service. *Health Trends*, **15**, 61–64.

Warshaw, G. A., Moore, J. T., Friedman, S. W., *et al* (1982) Functional disability in the hospitalized elderly. *Journal of the American Medical Society*, **248**, 847–850.

Wattis, J. P. (1988) Senior registrar training in old age psychiatry in the United Kingdom. *Bulletin of the Royal College of Psychiatrists*, **12**, 233–234.

Wise, T. N., Mann, L. S., Dove, H. W., *et al* (1985) Patients' perceptions of psychiatric consultations. *Comprehensive Psychiatry*, **26**, 554–557.

9 Treatment methods and their effectiveness

Elspeth Guthrie & Francis Creed

The effectiveness of liaison psychiatry services • *Drug treatment in liaison psychiatry* • *Psychological treatment in the liaison setting* • *Managing complex situations*

This chapter provides a brief overview of treatment in liaison psychiatry, with sections on the use of psychotropic drugs and the adaptation of particular psychological treatments for use in the liaison psychiatry setting.

The effectiveness of liaison psychiatry services

The high prevalence of psychiatric disorders on general medical units means that the effects of intervention, with improved recognition and treatment of the psychiatric disorder should be considerable. The possible benefits include reduced use of medical resources (investigation and length of stay) and improved quality of life. In fact, the number of satisfactory studies are remarkably few. For a full review see the special section of *Psychosomatics* (Saravay & Strain, 1994).

Saravay & Lavin (1994) reviewed 26 outcome studies of the effect of psychiatric comorbidity on length of stay and associated health care utilisation. Only a few studies were prospective and controlled for severity of physical illness – the main predictor of length of stay. The principal conclusion, however, was that impaired cognition, depressed mood, substance misuse and other psychological variables contribute to prolonged hospital stay and greater utilisation of general medical health resources after discharge.

Cost-effectiveness studies

The classic study by Levitan & Kornfeld (1981) demonstrated the beneficial effects of a psychiatric liaison service provided for all patients over the age of 65 admitted to a female orthopaedic surgical unit for the emergency repair of a fractured femur. The intervention cost $10 000 but the reduced length of stay resulted in hospital savings of $55 000. This, together with home care, rather than nursing home placement, meant that the projected savings were $193 000 for an intervention cost of only $10 000.

This study was repeated by Strain *et al* (1991) using a more sophisticated design. The liaison psychiatrist assessed, and where necessary treated, every patient who consented and there were regular meetings with nursing staff and families to facilitate early discharge. The study was performed at two hospitals. Prior to the study, the consultation rate was 10% and 2% of all relevant patients; during the period of study this increased to 79% and 61% at the two hospitals. The majority of patients had organic mental disorders. The intervention led to a reduction of length of stay of two days; to some extent this could be related to significant improvement in mental state. At follow-up the experimental cohort had significantly fewer rehospitalisations, rehabilitation days and were significantly less burden on family carers. The cost savings were $80 000–140 000 at the two hospitals.

Smith *et al* (1986) conducted a randomised controlled trial to determine whether psychiatric consultation would reduce the medical costs of patients with multiple physical symptoms but no apparent physical disease. Thirty-eight patients were randomly assigned to treatment or control groups and studied for 18 months. After nine months the control group was crossed over to receive treatment with the same intervention.

Following the psychiatric consultation, the quarterly health care charges in the treatment group declined by 53%. In contrast the charges in the control group showed wide variations but no overall change. After the control group was crossed over to receive treatment, their quarterly charges significantly declined by 49%. No change, however, was produced in the patients' health care status.

More intensive specific psychological treatments such as dynamic or cognitive therapy have been shown to be helpful in treating patients with chronic fatigue (Butler *et al*, 1991), atypical chest pain (Klimes *et al*, 1990) and irritable bowel syndrome (Guthrie *et al*, 1991). These treatments have not been assessed in cost effectiveness studies. They will be discussed in more detail in the psychological intervention section later in this chapter.

Psychiatric intervention with general medical patients

In contrast to the studies mentioned above, studies which have examined the psychiatric and economic outcomes of consultation in general medical populations, rather than specific patient groups, have been disappointing. Levenson *et al* (1992) showed no differences on length of stay or medical utilisation rates in patients with psychiatric disorder on a medical unit seen by a liaison psychiatrist, compared to the control group. The authors stated that their study demonstrates that a very brief general psychiatric intervention, particularly one not requested by the primary physician, aimed at a very heterogeneous population is unlikely to produce cost savings. Similar conclusions have been drawn by Katon *et al* (1992). Both of these studies indicate that the patients who have depression in the general medical unit tend not to have this adequately treated, usually because antidepressant treatment is not continued after discharge (Mayou *et al*, 1988). These studies indicate that specific liaison psychiatry interventions are required for specific disorders and that consultation liaison psychiatry should not be regarded as a panacea for psychological problems in medical units. For fuller details see Katon & Gonzales (1994).

Drug treatment in liaison psychiatry

The liaison psychiatrist may be asked to advise about the treatment of patients who have either been taking psychotropic medication prior to hospital admission or require psychiatric treatment during their hospital stay. Extra care is required when prescribing psychotropic medication for patients who are physically unwell and the psychiatrist must be aware of potential interactions between psychotropic drugs and medical/surgical treatments.

In the next section the main uses of psychotropic medication in the liaison setting are reviewed. Medical disorders which may complicate psychotropic drug prescribing are discussed, and potential drug interactions highlighted. Not all conditions and drug interactions can be covered, and for further information see Bazire (1995) which is a useful pocket guide.

Antidepressant medication

Main uses

Antidepressant medication is used in two ways in liaison psychiatry. First, to treat anxiety and depression, and second as a treatment for chronic pain. Two reviews indicate the efficacy of antidepressants in general medical patients (Rodin & Voshart, 1986; Series, 1992). If used appropriately antidepressants double the chance of recovery from depression (from 30–60%) in the physically ill. Such recovery may be accompanied by improvement in the patient's physical condition. For example in stroke patients improvement of depression may be associated with improvement in activities of daily living (Lipsey *et al*, 1984; Reding *et al*, 1986).

The main reasons for failure of antidepressant treatment in the physically ill are inadequate dosage and poor compliance. Patients should be started on small amounts and the dose built up slowly. The long-term aim should be to stabilise patients on the maximum tolerable amount. The broader aspects of treatment of depression in the medically ill, including an explanation to be given to the patient, are discussed in Chapter 6.

Antidepressants are used for the treatment of chronic pain, both in patients with clear cut symptoms of depression and in those with no obvious symptoms. They have well recognised analgesic properties which are independent of their antidepressant action (Feinmann, 1985). There is no evidence of superiority of one type of antidepressant over others in respect to analgesia (reviewed by Onghena & Van Houdehove, 1992). In a randomised placebo controlled design, Feinmann *et al* (1984) demonstrated that tricyclic antidepressants reduced psychological morbidity and pain in patients with chronic atypical facial pain. Recent follow-up data suggests that this improvement is maintained (Feinmann, 1992).

Pilowsky & Barrow (1990) assessed amitriptyline, psychotherapy and combined treatment in a randomised controlled trial of patients in a pain clinic. This study showed that antidepressants reduced pain and led to increased levels of activity in chronic pain patients. Psychotherapy led to an increase in both activity and pain. This work emphasises the difficulty in engaging some groups of patients in psychiatric treatment whether it is drug treatment or psychotherapy or both. Unless considerable time and effort is spent in engaging patients in treatment the beneficial effects of antidepressants are unlikely to be achieved, as the following case illustrates.

> A 47-year-old woman with a 5 year history of chronic headaches had received a wide variety of different treatments and investigations including two CAT scans. In the last 2 years she had become severely disabled, spending many days in bed. Her physician spent 30 minutes with her (a long time in a busy neurology clinic) introducing the possibility of psychiatric referral. He emphasised the reality of her pain and explained that he did not think that she was 'mad or looney'. He told her that psychiatrists had particular expertise in treating pain and would also help her with her coexisting depression. Although she initially felt affronted by the suggestion of seeing a psychiatrist, she eventually agreed – probably because he had explained the referral in a detailed and sensitive way.
>
> Psychiatric assessment indicated that her sleep was poor, she had little energy, felt miserable and had little interest in her family and her usual activities. She believed that the pain had caused her to feel this way and that she would not improve until the pain was alleviated. She was very resistant to any psychological approach and dismissed antidepressants as they had not helped her in the past. The antidepressant medication, however, had been prescribed at low dosages and for inadequate periods of time.
>
> The psychiatrist concentrated on building up a trusting relationship with Mrs A and patiently explained the potential benefits of antidepressant medication. She emphasised the importance of taking the medication for several months and

building up the dose slowly; the patient eventually agreed. Within 3 months her mood had improved and her pain had diminished. She said that she felt 'like her old self' and that she was able to enjoy things once again. She still experienced headaches once or twice a week, but never had to take to her bed, and was able to control the pain with simple analgesics.

This case highlights the importance of persuading a reluctant patient to take antidepressants when necessary – the time spent is worthwhile in terms of the benefits. Without such time and effort the patient would not have agreed to take antidepressant medication and would have remained chronically unwell. This helps to explain the failure of studies such as Katon *et al* (1992) mentioned above.

Use of antidepressants in the medically ill

Antidepressant drugs differ in their side-effects. Serotonin specific reuptake inhibitors (SSRIs) have fewer side-effects than the tricyclic antidepressants, whose anticholinergic side-effects are particularly problematic in the physically ill (Series, 1992). Patients with organic brain syndromes and the elderly are especially susceptible to tricyclics which have strong anticholinergic side-effects (e.g. amitriptyline, imipramine, clomipramine); studies have shown 15% may develop delirium (Lipsey *et al*, 1984; Popkin *et al*, 1985). All SSRIs are free of anticholinergic effects but can cause increased sweating and insomnia. Some patients experience nausea, muscle tightness or leg cramps with fluoxetine. A recent study by Huyse *et al* (1994) suggests that fluoxetine is well tolerated by a wide range of severely ill medical in-patients.

Antidepressants are absorbed from the small intestine and therefore patients with Crohn's disease or those who have undergone bowel resection may experience malabsorption. Particular care must be taken when prescribing antidepressants for patients with the following physical conditions: cardiovascular disorders, renal disease, hepatic disease, diabetes, epilepsy and pregnancy (Table 9.1).

Cardiovascular disorders.   In general, SSRIs should always be used as the treatment of choice in depressed patients with cardiovascular disorders. Tricyclic antidepressants should be avoided as they inhibit re-uptake of peripheral biogenic amines which may increase myocardial norepinephrine levels and in conjunction with their anticholinergic and quinidine-like effects cause cardiac arrhythmias (Hale, 1993). Tricyclics can also depress the myocardium with resultant decreased contractility which can exacerbate congestive cardiac failure. Tricyclics produce a variety of ECG changes including ST segment depression and decreased-voltage, inverted or biphasic T waves.

Table 9.1 Brief guide to prescribing of antidepressant medication in patients who are physically unwell

Physical disorder	First line drug	Second line drug	Particular dangers
Cardiovascular disease	SSRI	RIMA Lofepramine	Avoid drugs for 2 months post MI
Renal disease	TCAD	SSRI	Avoid lithium
Hepatic disease	SSRI (low dosage)	TCAD (low dosage)	Avoid lithium Avoid lofepramine
Diabetes	TCAD	SSRI	
Epilepsy	RIMA	SSRI	Avoid lithium

TCAD, Tricyclic antidepressants; SSRI, Specific serotonin re-uptake inhibitors; RIMA, Reversible inhibitors of monoamine oxidase-A

If a patient is unable to tolerate an SSRI, lofepramine or moclobemide can be considered; the latter does not require dietary restrictions and is comparable in efficacy to the tricyclic antidepressants but is usually better tolerated (Versiani *et al*, 1989; Freeman, 1993). Lofepramine has fewer anticholinergic side-effects and is less cardiotoxic than the other tricyclic antidepressants. Depression is common following a myocardial infarction but it is advisable to avoid all antidepressants for the first two months. SSRIs can be used if necessary. Tricyclic antidepressants should not be used in patients with a history of cardiac arrythmias, unless there is a pacemaker.

Renal disease.   In patients with renal failure tricyclic antidepressants can be used in normal dosages but care must be taken with SSRIs. Reduced dosage levels of these drugs are recommended if serum creatinine rises to above 150 μmol/l. The use of antidepressants in patients undergoing renal dialysis needs to be carefully monitored (Lieberman *et al*, 1985).

Hepatic disease.   Tricyclic antidepressants, SSRIs and moclobemide can be used with caution at lower than usual dosages. Tricyclics cause increased sedation and in rare cases cholestatic jaundice. Lofepramine is contraindicated.

Diabetes.   Tricyclic antidepressants should be used in preference to SSRIs, unless there is a high risk of suicide, as some SSRIs may induce hypoglycaemic episodes.

Epilepsy.   Up to 30% of patients with epilepsy may require treatment for concurrent depression (Robertson & Trimble, 1983). As all tricyclics lower the fit threshold, moclobemide or the SSRIs should be used preferentially. SSRIs do have some epileptogenic activity with paroxetine probably being the safest drug to use in this class (Sedgewick *et al*, 1987).

If the patient is taking carbamazepine, levels should be closely monitored as levels can rise with associated use of some of the SSRIs (e.g. fluvoxamine). The older MAOIs had no epileptic adverse effects (Edwards & Wheal, 1992), and there are none recorded to date for moclobemide.

Pregnancy.   All drugs should be avoided during the first trimester of pregnancy if at all possible. There are, as yet, no reports of SSRIs causing foetal abnormalities when prescribed during pregnancy. Tricyclic antidepressants also appear reasonably safe. There are a small number of reports of tricyclic drugs causing teratogenic effects when prescribed throughout pregnancy but no conclusive evidence. Tricyclics can be safely prescribed during breast feeding. A tiny proportion of the adult dosage is passed to the baby. Tricyclic antidepressants with longer half-lives (such as maprotiline) should be avoided, as drowsiness and respiratory depression in the infant can occur. SSRIs should be avoided if the patient is breast feeding (Oates, 1995).

Other conditions.   Development of SSRIs has meant that depressed patients with conditions such as glaucoma, prostatism, and constipation, can be treated safely without exacerbation of their physical status.

Drug interactions with antidepressants

The psychiatrist should be fully aware of potential drug interactions between antidepressants and drugs used commonly in medicine and surgery (Table 9.2).

Analgesics.   Tricyclic antidepressants potentiate the analgesic properties of opioids. The older MAOIs should not be used in conjunction with opiates because of potential fatality. Care should be taken with the combined use of moclobemide and opioids. (Amreid *et al*, 1992). Pethidine, which has some 5–HT uptake inhibition, should be particularly avoided.

Drugs used in cardiovascular disease.   There is little evidence of any serious interaction between moclobemide or SSRIs and digoxin. Tricyclics should not be used because of the risk of arrythmias; hypotensive reactions can occur with a vasodilator and some antihypertensive medications. When tricyclics are given to patients receiving guanethidine, clonidine, bethanidine or debrisoquin, the antihypertensive action of these drugs is inhibited resulting in an elevation of blood pressure.

Moclobemide potentiates betablockers and further lowers blood pressure, but there is no evidence to date that orthostatic hypotension occurs. Concurrent use of SSRIs and propranolol increases the bio-availability of propranolol resulting in substantially higher propranolol serum levels. Propranolol dosage may therefore have to be lowered if concurrently administered with SSRIs.

Gastrointestinal drugs.   Cimetidine and moclobemide compete for metabolism by the liver thus, if used in combination, moclobemide should be started at the lowest possible dose and adjusted accordingly. If cimetidine is commenced after the start of moclobemide treatment, it is advisable to reduce the dosage of moclobemide by 50% and then adjust accordingly. The serum levels of most tricyclics are also raised when prescribed in combination with cimetidine and lower dosages should be used. The levels of SSRIs if used with cimetidine are not greatly affected. Fibre when prescribed as part of a high fibre diet can reduce levels of tricyclic antidepressants by one-third.

Anticoagulants.   Fluvoxamine when prescribed concurrently with anticoagulants, such as warfarin or nicoumalone, results in increased serum anticoagulant levels and longer prothrombin times. The anticoagulant dosage may, therefore, have to be adjusted.

Sympathomimetics.   At high doses of moclobemide there is a slight increase of the hypertensive effect of sympathomimetics. Tricyclic antidepressants should be used with caution with sympathomimetics, as there is a high risk of hypertension and cardiac arrythmias.

Oral contraceptives.   Decreased effects and increased toxicity have been reported when tricyclics are used in combination with oral contraceptives.

Anti-epileptics.   Moclobemide has little effect on the serum levels of anti-epileptic drugs. Some tricyclic antidepressants and SSRIs, however, can effect the levels of carbamazepine or sodium valproate and vice versa. Patients taking combinations of these drugs need to be monitored closely.

Anti-Parkinsonian drugs.   Selegiline is a MAO-B inhibitor used in the treatment of Parkinson's disease. Caution is required if it is used with moclobemide (an MAO-A inhibitor) as full MAO inhibition is likely to occur. The same dietary restrictions usually employed for the older MAOIs should be implemented.Toxic reactions have also been reported when selegiline has been used in combination with SSRIs.

Lithium

Lithium may be used as an adjunct to antidepressant treatment in patients with resistant depression or to stabilise mood in patients with recurrent

Table 9.2 Possible drug interactions when antidepressants are used in combination with drugs in the general medical setting

	Tricyclics	SSRI	RIMA
Digoxin	Do not use	Safe	Safe
B-blockers	Risk of toxicity	Lower dose of B-blocker required	Enhances lowering of BP
Cimetidine	Lower dose of TCADs required	Safe	Lower dose of RIMAs required
Anticoagulants	Safe (caution with lofepramine)	Anti-coagulant may need reducing	Safe
Sympatho-mimetics	Risk of hyperten-sion and arrythmias	Safe	Hypertension with high doses
Anti-epileptics	Serum levels may alter	Fluoxetine alters serum levels	Safe
Selegiline (Parkinson's disease)	Risk of toxicity	Risk of toxicity	Hypertensive reaction

TCAD, Tricyclic antidepressants; SSRI, Specific serotonin re-uptake inhibitors; RIMA, Reversible inhibitors of monoamine oxidase-A.

mood disorders. It has also been used to help treat L-dopa induced psychosis in patients with Parkinson's disease; neuroleptics usually exacerbate parkinsonian symptoms. Lithium should not be prescribed for patients with renal impairment. It is relatively safe, however, to prescribe for patients with hepatic disease or cardiovascular disease. Lithium lowers the fit threshold so it is best avoided in patients with epilepsy, but can be used with caution. It is safe to use in diabetes provided there are no diabetic, renal complications.

Lithium should not be prescribed during pregnancy but it can be reinstated immediately following delivery (Oates, 1995). Mothers taking lithium should be advised not to breastfeed as large quantities of the drug are passed to the infant in breast milk.

Lithium interacts with a wide range of drugs that are commonly prescribed in the general medical setting. If a patient is prescribed lithium in conjunction with any other drug, potential interactions should be carefully checked. Lithium is safe to use in conjunction with digoxin, oral hypoglycaemics and L-dopa. There is a risk of toxicity with all diuretics currently in use (Griffin *et al*, 1988) although frusemide is safer than the thiazide diuretics. Patients receiving stable diuretic regimens can generally tolerate lithium therapy without ill effects, although lithium levels, and electrolytes, particularly potassium, should be monitored regularly. Those who are seriously ill and require vigorous diuretic treatment may require temporary discontinuation of lithium treatment until their physical status is more stable. Most of the non-steroidal anti-inflammatory drugs interact with lithium resulting in increased levels and toxic effects. Aspirin is a possible alternative.

Several cases of severe toxicity have been reported when methyldopa has been prescribed for the treatment of hypertension in patients taking lithium. Other newer drugs such as captopril can also result in toxity when combined with lithium, so beta-blockers are therefore preferable for the treatment of hypertension. Clonidine can also be used but its hypertensive action is reduced by lithium so regular monitoring of blood pressure should be undertaken.

Other drugs which may interact with lithium to produce adverse effects include baclofen, verapamil, co-trimoxazole, metoclopramide, phenytoin, and tetracyclines. Drugs reported to reduce the serum levels of lithium include aminophylline and theophylline; bran fibre also may.

Anxiolytics

Anxiolytics are rarely used in liaison psychiatry because of the risk of dependence. Anxiety can be reduced by the judicious use of either low dosages of antidepressants or neuroleptics. Some patients are unable to tolerate these drugs, however, and short courses of anxiolytics can be very useful in patients who are either too anxious or too ill to learn relaxation techniques and anxiety management (see Chapter 6). Shorter lasting benzodiazepines should be used, such as oxazepam which has a half life of 5–15 hours. Lorazepam should be avoided because of its greater potential to create dependence compared with other benzodiazepines. Benzodiazepines should not be used in patients with severe respiratory difficulties.

Neuroleptics

Neuroleptics are usually used in liaison psychiatry in two situations. First, to treat patients who have coexisting physical and psychiatric disorders and secondly, to treat patients who become acutely psychotic on the medical or surgical wards. Neuroleptics are usually tolerated well in most physical conditions, however, it is advisable to begin with a small dose which is built up slowly. Low doses of neuroleptics should be prescribed in patients with renal problems.

Sulpiride has fewer side-effects than most other neuroleptics, but it cannot be given intramuscularly which may be required if the patient is agitated. It is also mainly cleared by the kidneys so particularly low doses are required in renal disease. As a general rule, haloperidol should be the drug of choice if a patient requires intramuscular medication. It has fewer anticholinergic side-effects than other neuroleptics and is less likely to cause severe hypotension. Extrapyramidal side-effects can usually be controlled with small amounts of anti-Parkinsonian medication.

The association between phenothiazines and hepatocellular jaundice is well documented although rare. Onset usually occurs within the first 4 weeks of commencing medication. Chlorpromazine should be avoided in patients with hepatic disease as it appears to be particularly hepatotoxic. Clozapine is also contraindicated in patients with severe disease.

Most neuroleptics have some effect on the fit threshold in patients with epilepsy. Chlorpromazine and loxapine should be avoided and it is best to use drugs with a less sedative action. Pimozide, thioridazine and fluphenazine are the safest. When prescribing a neuroleptic the dose should be built up slowly with additional anticonvulsant cover if necessary. In some physically ill patients very small doses of neuroleptics are sufficient to control psychotic symptoms, as the following example demonstrates.

> Mrs J had advanced multiple sclerosis. She was incontinent and had lost all power in her arms and legs and had deteriorating cognitive function. She was looked after by her husband and parents who were extremely supportive and caring. Despite being severely disabled the quality of her life was good and it was important to her and her family that she was cared for at home. She had developed persecutory delusions, with auditory and visual hallucinations, believing, at times, that communists had stolen all her clothes and that the police were watching her home. She was unable to tolerate any kind of neuroleptic medication all of which, even at small doses, resulted in severe side-effects. Benzodiazepines were used in small amounts to reduce distress resulting from her psychotic state.
>
> Her family were able to look after her until she began to incorporate them into her delusional system. She started to believe that her husband was trying to poison her and refused all food and drink. Unless her psychotic condition was treated it was clear that she would die. A special dilute suspension of haloperidol was prepared and administered to her intramuscularly by district nurses using a diabetic syringe (0.025mg of haloperidol twice a day). Her symptoms responded and she was untroubled by side-effects. She remained psychotic but was less distressed and no longer believed that her family were against her, so they could care for her at home until she died peacefully.

This case not only illustrates the extreme sensitivity that some patients have to psychotropic drug treatment, but also the deleterious effect of a psychiatric condition on the care and management of the patient's physical status.

Drug induced psychiatric disorders

There are numerous reports of drug induced psychiatric states. For more detailed information see Bazire (1995). Box 9.1 gives a brief list of drugs commonly used in the general medical setting that may cause psychiatric problems. If the offending drug is withdrawn, the patient's mental state usually returns to normal within a short period of time. If the drug cannot be withdrawn or changed to one less likely to provoke psychiatric disturbance, treatment of the psychiatric condition itself should be undertaken. Careful consideration of the patient's underlying physical status is required so that the most appropriate psychotropic drug is chosen.

Psychological treatment in the liaison setting

The use of psychological interventions in liaison psychiatry is best discussed in relation to patients with physical illness and for patients with functional somatic symptoms.

Psychological treatment in patients with physical illness

There is good evidence that brief psychological interventions can help reduce the psychological sequelae of acute physical illness and this has already been discussed in Chapter 6. Evidence, however, for the efficacy

---

Box 9.1 Drugs commonly prescribed in the general medical setting that can precipitate psychiatric disorder

Depression
Anti-Parkinsonian drugs: L-dopa; amantidine
Cardiovascular drugs: beta-blockers; clonidine; methyldopa; calcium channel blockers (e.g. nifedipine)
Gastrointestinal: H_2-receptor antagonists (e.g. cimetidine); metoclopramide
Non-steroidal anti-inflammatory drugs: indomethacin
Respiratory: aminophylline; theophylline
Steroids
Oral contraceptives

Anxiety and agitation
Anti-Parkinsonian drugs: L-dopa
Non-steroidal anti-inflammatory drugs: ibuprofen
Thyroxine
Respiratory drugs: salbutamol; theophylline

Psychosis
Anti-Parkinsonian drugs: L-dopa; pergolide
Cardiovascular drugs: digoxin; beta-blockers; clonidine; methyldopa
Steroids
CNS stimulants: ephedrine; phenylephrine

of psychological treatment in chronic physical disorders is less clear. In these conditions the prevalence of psychological distress is not particularly high but when present can lead to more severe physical symptoms and greater health care utilisation.

Most work has centred upon the traditional 'psychosomatic disorders', such as diabetes, peptic ulcer, asthma, ulcerative colitis etc. Psychosocial conflicts were thought to be the underlying cause of these conditions, but modern understandings emphasise pathophysiological mechanisms. Recently, psychological interventions have focused upon bringing about better physiological control or alleviating coexisting emotional distress, rather than attempting cure.

Diabetes

Diabetes has received the most attention and psychodynamic, cognitive–behavioural, a variety of different group interventions, and family therapies have all been tried. There are many case reports of psychoanalytic or psychodynamic treatment in diabetic patients resulting in more favourable control (Nathan, 1985; Boehnert & Popkin, 1986). Milton (1989) graphically described the treatment of six diabetic patients with poor compliance using brief focused cognitive–analytical psychotherapy (Ryle, 1982). In this kind of therapy the therapist helps the patient to identify underlying conflicts, usually called snags, traps or dilemmas, which result in maladaptive behaviours or difficulties in interpersonal relationships. In one patient, Miss A, a young woman in her twenties with an impeccable character and compliant manner, Milton was able to identify two underlying conflicts which contributed to her poor diabetic control. The first was: "If I don't continue to be openly compliant but secretly rebellious I feel I would become totally rebellious and let things go completely" and the second was: "If I acknowledge diabetes I feel immature and dependent. If I deny it I neglect my self-care". Although, as Milton pointed out, in such a brief therapy many issues were left unresolved at the end, Miss A's diabetic control improved and was maintained over the following 6 months. In later work by the same team more elaborate sequential diagrams have been developed to understand the complex interactions between patients' diabetic control and underlying psychological conflicts (Ryle *et al*, 1993). The outcome of this work is currently being evaluated.

A more intense dynamic approach with poorly controlled teenage diabetics has been described by Moran & Fonagy (1993). An in-patient programme of combined psychoanalytic psychotherapy and ward management was compared with admission to a medical ward with no psychoanalytic treatment or ward management programme. Patients in the psychoanalytic group received therapy 3–5 times a week for between 5–28 weeks. Parental involvement varied but most parents were seen and given help to cope with their child's condition.

Glycosylated haemoglobin (HbA) values decreased significantly in the psychotherapy treatment group and remained low at follow-up one year later, reflecting better diabetic control than the control group. This study may reflect the other aspects of intervention as well as the psychotherapy but it is one of the few attempts to evaluate systematically a psychoanalytic treatment using a 'hard' outcome measure.

A wide variety of different behavioural interventions have been described. Progressive muscle relaxation and electromyographic feedback have been described as reducing serum glucose levels in two small studies, each of five diabetic patients (Lammers *et al*, 1984; Landis *et al*, 1985). Other workers have reported similar improvement with non-insulin dependent diabetics (Surwit & Feinglos, 1983) but less success with diabetic patients selected for their poor control and emotional disorder (Feinglos *et al*, 1987).

Cognitive therapy has been described as being effective in patients with a combined problem of diabetes and an eating disorder (Peveler & Fairburn, 1989). This approach has been modified from the cognitive–behavioural treatment developed for patients with bulimia nervosa (Fairburn *et al*, 1991) and consists of two stages. The first stage focuses on weight gain and during this period the patient is seen weekly for 24 weeks. In addition to the normal monitoring of thoughts and eating behaviour, the effects of changes in eating habits on glycaemic control are noted and appropriate adjustments in the insulin dose discussed. Once weight gain is proceeding satisfactorily, more intensive use of cognitive techniques are employed, but meetings are reduced to fortnightly. In this second stage, specific thoughts associated with weight, shape and diabetes are elicited. For example, "How dare you eat if your sugar level isn't perfect?" or "This hypo serves you right for not managing your diabetes properly". In addition, the patient is encouraged to be less rigid in her diabetic control, helping to reduce unnecessary episodes of hypoglycaemia. This second stage lasts for a further 24 weeks within which the target weight is usually reached and maintained.

There have been a number of influential case reports and studies in the literature evaluating the role of group and family work in patients with diabetes. Supportive groups for young adults with diabetes have been described and reported to improve compliance (Warren-Boulton *et al*, 1981). Minuchin's pioneering work using family therapy with children whose diabetes was poorly controlled, and who required repeated hospital admissions is well documented (Minuchin *et al*, 1975). Minuchin's group suggested that poor diabetic control was related to a particular family constellation involving enmeshment, rigidity, and lack of conflict resolution. Working with the families resulted in fewer hospital admissions.

Many brittle diabetics perceive their difficulties primarily as being physical in origin, and do not welcome psychological treatment. The patients described in the above studies represent a small subgroup where engagement is possible – no randomised controlled trial has been performed.

Other chronic physical disorders

Psychological interventions in patients with other chronic diseases are mostly case reports – there are only a few accounts of controlled evaluations (Table 9.3). Rosser *et al* (1983) studied dynamic psychotherapy in patients with chronic bronchitis and emphysema; this was compared with supportive psychotherapy, treatment from an experienced nurse with no psychotherapeutic training and a treatment as usual group. Only the supportive psychotherapy group showed evidence of sustained improvement; the nurse group became less breathless but more depressed. This was a careful study using both psychological and physical outcome measures. The findings suggested that patients with severe chronic physical illness are too ill to be able to function in dynamic psychotherapy: many of the patients were elderly, severely ill and hypoxic.

A recent, large (*n*=174) randomised controlled trial of cognitive therapy in patients with cancer demonstrated more favourable results (Greer *et al*, 1992). Patients in the therapy group developed more 'fighting spirit' and became less helpless than controls. At four months follow-up, they had significantly lower scores than controls on measures of anxiety, psychological symptoms and psychological distress. This well controlled study suggests that psychological treatment may be helpful in selected patients with cancer. Only patients with a life expectancy of 12 months survival were recruited; they were younger and probably slightly less physically disabled than the patients in the Rosser study.

Sjodin's (1983) study of dynamic psychotherapy in peptic ulcer disease suggests that patients with chronic disease which is not physically severely disabling may respond to psychological approaches. Over 100 patients were randomised to either medical treatment plus 12 sessions of therapy versus medical treatment alone. The physical and psychological outcome of patients in the psychotherapy group was significantly better than controls at the end of the trial and at follow-up one year later.

Hypertension does not appear to be amenable to psychological intervention. Two well conducted studies, using relaxation (Van Montfrans *et al*, 1990) or stress management (Johnston *et al*, 1993) found that psychological treatment was ineffective in lowering blood pressure in patients with mild hypertension.

In summary, there is some evidence that brief, well-timed psychological interventions during the initial stage of an acute illness may have a protective effect against the subsequent development of psychological disorder (see Chapter 6). The evidence that psychotherapy is helpful in more chronic conditions or those that carry a long-term threat to life is less convincing. Further research in this area may help to clarify which

Table 9.3 Controlled evaluations of psychotherapeutic interventions in patients with physical disease

Authors and type of illness	Type of therapy	No. of patients	Study length[1]	Follow-up[2]	Outcome
Rosser *et al* (1983) Chronic bronchitis	Dynamic therapy *v.* support *v.* control	65	8	no	Nurse group less breathless/support group less psychological distress
Moran *et al* (1991) Brittle diabetes	Psychoanalysis *v.* routine care	22	26	no	Treatment group significantly better diabetic control
Ewer & Stewart (1986) Asthma	Hypnosis: low *v.* high susceptibility	39	6	no	High susceptibility group improved Respiratory Function Tests, low susceptibility group no change
Oldenburg *et al* (1985) Myocardial infarction	Counselling *v.* education *v.* routine treatment	46	1	12	Both treatment groups better than controls for psychosocial functioning
Van Montfrans *et al* (1990) Mild hypertension	Relaxation training *v.* controls	42	8	12	No significant difference between groups
Sjodin (1983) Peptic ulcer disease	Dynamic therapy + routine treatment *v.* routine treatment alone	101	12	12	Therapy significantly better than control: on both psychological and GI symptoms
Johnston *et al* (1993) Hypertension	Stress management *v.* controls	96	10	no	No difference between groups
Greer *et al* (1992) Cancer	CBT + routine *v.* routine alone	174	8	4	CBT group less anxious and depressed than controls

1. Length of study in weeks.
2. length of follow-up in months.

groups of patients with chronic illness would benefit most from a psychological treatment approach.

Psychological treatment in patients with functional somatic symptoms

The somatic manifestation of psychological distress is extremely common. Various terms have been used in recent years to describe this phenomenon, including 'medically unexplained symptoms', 'somatisation' or 'functional somatic symptoms' (Chapter 5). The most common symptoms are pain (in various sites) and tiredness or fatigue. In the majority of cases the symptoms are transient but in a significant minority are persistent, associated with distress, disability and tenacious health care seeking. In severe cases patients may receive extensive investigations and treatment, with little relief of symptoms.

It is for this group of patients that an intensive psychological intervention is most appropriate but psychological symptoms are more responsive to such treatment than pain (Malone & Strube, 1988). These authors conducted a meta-analysis of non-medical treatments for chronic pain. They included 109 published studies, but only had enough information to calculate effect sizes on 48 of them. Types of pain included migraine, back pain, joint pain, and facial pain. Techniques evaluated included relaxation, stress management packages, biofeedback, hypnosis, cognitive therapy and operant behavioural interventions. They concluded that effect sizes were, generally, positive and of modest magnitude. Mood and the number of subjective symptoms consistently showed greater responses to treatment than did pain intensity, pain duration, or frequency of pain.

The main kinds of psychological treatment that have been employed over the last 15 years to treat patients with chronic somatic symptoms can be grouped into five areas: cognitive–behavioural, hypnosis, dynamic psychotherapy, 'pain clinic packages', and couple and family work. The main randomised controlled trials of psychological treatment in patients with chronic somatic symptoms are summarised in Table 9.4.

Cognitive–behavioural interventions

The principles of this approach and its adaptation for patients with chronic physical symptoms have been described by Sharpe *et al* (1992). The therapy is conducted on an out-patient basis with individuals, although family members may be involved at some stage to help with the treatment. Sessions usually last for one hour and number between 10–20 over a course of treatment. Assessment focuses on the patient's symptoms and associated cognitions and behaviour. The aetiological model takes into account both psychological and physiological mechanisms (Sharpe & Bass, 1992). The patient may be asked to keep a diary of these and then

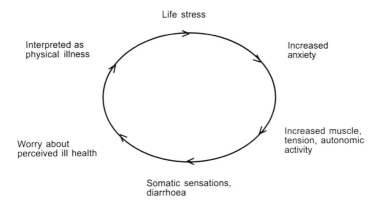

Fig. 9.1 Diagrammatic model of the aetiological factors involved in the development of a patient's symptoms. Functional bowel symptoms are used as an example (after Sharpe & Bass, 1992).

a formulation is constructed about how the patient's thoughts, behaviour and physiological responses are interlinked to perpetuate his/her symptoms, distress and disability. Figure 9.1 gives an example of a diagrammatic representation of the aetiology of one patient's symptoms. The therapist is particularly vigilant in helping the patient to be aware of and to re-examine catastrophic cognitions (e.g. "This chest pain means I am going to have a heart attack") and avoidant behaviour (e.g. not doing any physical activity for fear of provoking further symptoms).

This approach has now been evaluated in a variety of different somatic conditions (Table 9.4). Klimes *et al* (1990) have demonstrated its effectiveness with patients with atypical chest pain referred either from GPs or hospital out-patient clinics. Wessely *et al* (1989) have reported encouraging results using a more behaviourally orientated approach in patients with chronic fatigue, and a systematic evaluation of this intervention is now being undertaken. Bennett & Wilkinson (1985) found cognitive–behavioural therapy (CBT) was as effective as routine medical care in newly referred out-patients with irritable bowel syndrome (IBS), but psychological treatment was more cost-effective. This study was notable for including an economic evaluation. A recent study by Corney *et al* (1991), however, failed to show any difference between behavioural treatment and routine treatment in consecutive out-patients with IBS. Although there is evidence that CBT may be helpful in patients with mild to moderate somatic symptoms its effectiveness with patients with chronic and severe symptoms needs to be evaluated.

Table 9.4 Controlled evaluations of psychotherapeutic interventions in patients with functional somatic symptoms

Authors and type of illness	Type of therapy	No of patients	Study length[1]	Follow-up [2]	Outcome
Svedlund (1983) IBS	Dynamic therapy + routine v. treatment alone	101	12	12	Therapy group significantly better than controls for psychological and GI symptoms
Guthrie et al (1991) Refractory IBS	Dynamic therapy + routine v. support + routine care	102	12	12	Therapy group significantly better than controls for psychological and GI symptoms
Whorwell et al (1984) Refractory IBS	Hypnosis v. support	30	6	no	Hypnosis group significantly better than controls for GI symptoms
Corney et al (1991) IBS	Behavioural therapy v. routine medical treatment	42	6–15	9	Both groups mild improvement, no difference between them
Saarjarvi et al (1992) Low back pain	Couple therapy v. controls	28	12	60	Psychological symptoms less in therapy group; no difference on disability scores
Pilowsky & Barrrow (1990) Chronic pain	AMI + therapy v. AMI + support v. placebo + therapy v. placebo + support	102	12	no	AMI reduced pain, therapy increased pain but improved productivity
Klimes et al (1990) Atypical chest pain	CBT v. assessment only	31	4–11	6	Treatment group better than controls for chest pain
Harvey et al (1989) IBS	Individual v. group hypnosis	33	7	3	Both groups improved, no difference between them

AMI, amitriptyline; IBS, Irritable bowel syndrome.

Hypnosis

Hypnosis has been a widely used and popular treatment for over 100 years. Its usefulness in alleviating somatic symptomatology has, however, rarely been evaluated. There have been several recent publications describing striking effects using hypnosis to treat IBS (Whorwell *et al*, 1984; Harvey *et al*, 1989) and it has also been found to be of help in patients with mild breathlessness (Ewer & Stewart, 1986).

When used to treat functional bowel symptoms, the kind of hypnosis employed focuses entirely on the problematic symptom, and does not involve exploration of the patient's state of mind. A deep trance-like state is induced, following which, attention is directed towards the control of intestinal smooth muscle. The patient is asked to place his/her hand on the abdomen, feel a sense of warmth and relate this to asserting control over gut function. Patients are also given an auto-hypnosis tape to practise techniques at home (Whorwell, 1987).

Hypnosis has been demonstrated to relieve symptoms in patients with refractory IBS, previously unresponsive to a variety of different treatments. It seems to be less effective in patients who complain of severe pain, those with coexisting psychological problems, and in elderly subjects (Whorwell *et al*, 1987). It is usually conducted on an individual basis over 10–12 sessions but can be carried out in a group format (Harvey *et al*, 1989).

The impressive results achieved by using hypnosis are interesting. The work has often been carried out by physicians or non-clinically trained psychologists in medical clinics. The patients never have to see a psychiatrist or other psychological health professional and there is no discussion about psychological matters. The hypnosis is administered almost like a drug. The trials carried out to date have included only small numbers of patients, and the rates of psychiatric morbidity in the trial groups have been lower than expected. None of the studies recruited patients on a consecutive basis, suggesting they may have been selected on the grounds of suitability for hypnosis. Another difficulty in evaluating the findings of these studies, is the absence of a detailed psychological assessment at the beginning and end of the treatment intervention.

In summary, hypnosis appears to produce marked beneficial change in certain groups of patients with functional somatic symptoms. Unlike other psychological interventions, the treatment is conducted in the setting of the medical clinic and the patient is discouraged from exploring psychological issues.

Dynamic psychotherapy

As with the other kinds of psychological interventions there are a plethora of case reports suggesting dynamic therapy can be helpful in patients with somatic symptoms, but few randomised controlled evaluations. As an example of the former, Whale (1992) treated patients in a pain clinic with six sessions of brief dynamic therapy, which helped several patients. Whale discovered a striking association between the development of the pain and unresolved difficulties with grieving and loss; the therapy helped the patient to become aware of a psychological problem that had previously been denied so the pain was perceived from a different perspective.

There have been two controlled trials of dynamic therapy in patients with chronic pain; in both studies recruitment was difficult. Bassett & Pilowsky (1985) first compared 12 sessions of dynamic psychotherapy with six sessions of supportive therapy in 26 patients attending a pain clinic but the study was too small to show a significant difference. In the second study (Pilowsky & Barrow, 1990), four different treatment interventions were compared: (antidepressant plus psychotherapy *v.* antidepressant plus support *v.* placebo plus psychotherapy *v.* placebo plus support) in 102 patients with chronic pain. The antidepressant medication was effective in both reducing pain and increasing the patients' activity level; psychotherapy appeared to improve patients' productivity but increase their reports of pain.

The difficulty of recruiting patients in the pain clinic to psychotherapy (only a quarter of patients were successfully recruited) means that it cannot be recommended as a general treatment because most pain patients would refuse it. Specific treatment packages for pain patients will be discussed in the next section.

Dynamic therapy, however, has been demonstrated to be both acceptable and effective in patients with refractory IBS. Two randomised controlled trials, both with over 100 patients, have shown that brief dynamic therapy is superior to either routine medical treatment (Svedlund, 1983), or support plus routine treatment (Guthrie *et al*, 1991). In the second study, out of 113 consecutive patients only four refused to enter the trial. Recruitment of patients was made easier by the therapist's presence in the gastrointestinal clinic, and by an initial emphasis on the patient's physical as opposed to psychological problems. Patients with overt symptoms of depression or anxiety did particularly well and improvement in the psychological symptoms was correlated with improved bowel symptomatology. Patients with more chronic and constant symptoms were less likely to respond; they resembled patients with chronic pain.

The individual psychotherapy consisted of a long first session (up to 3 hours) followed by six sessions of 45 minutes each. The main approach followed the conversational model of Hobson (1985). This model was specifically chosen for patients presenting with somatic symptoms because of its emphasis on metaphor and the development of a mutual relationship between therapist and patient through conversation. The therapist helped generate a 'feeling language' by the explicit use of bowel symptoms as metaphors for the patient's emotional state, e.g. 'you're a bit bunged up', or 'you feel all churned up inside'.

The long first session contributed to the development of a strong therapeutic alliance, and helped to allay the patient's fears of psychiatry and psychological approaches. It also facilitated the early emergence of transference material. Key components of the therapy were: allowing the patient to acknowledge psychological distress; moving the patient from a physical aetiological model of their symptoms to a model which accommodates psychological factors; helping the patient, through the transference relationship, to recognise difficulties or deficiencies in relationships outside therapy; making a link between symptom development and relationship difficulties; and finally, the patient making changes to his/her relationships which resulted in symptom reduction.

> A 35-year-old woman had suffered from abdominal pain and distension for the previous 18 months. There were no obvious adverse life events before the onset of her symptoms but she had commenced a new relationship with a man several months previously. She described this relationship as being very happy, remarking that her boyfriend was caring, supportive and understanding. Five years previously her marriage had broken up. She had thought that the marriage was happy and stable only to be told one evening by her husband that he had been having an affair for the previous 2 years and intended to leave her for another woman. She described feeling utterly shattered by this and unable to comprehend how she could have been unaware of her husband's infidelity.
>
> She revealed that her father had also had an affair, when she was a little girl, which had resulted in the break-up of her parent's marriage. In the long first psychotherapy session, she described this in detail, mentioning her surprise at being met from school one day by her father, sitting in his car outside the school gates, and being told by him that he would no longer be living at home. She was able, in the session, to make a link for the first time between her feelings then and her feelings when her husband told her of his affair. When the therapist wondered about any fears she may have about her new boyfriend, she initially affirmed how wonderful her relationship was, but then in the silence that ensued became more and more distressed. From this point, it became possible for her to acknowledge that although her new relationship was 'wonderful', underneath she had terrible fears that her boyfriend would desert her as her father and husband had previously done. She was also able to acknowledge a possible link between the development of her bowel symptoms and the deepening of her emotional attachment to this new man. A focus was agreed in which her feelings and fears about rejection would be explored and her tendency to idealise relationships and deny difficulties would be examined.

Further case examples are described by Guthrie (1991). Brief dynamic therapy is clearly a helpful intervention for patients with moderate/severe symptoms. The treatment is conducted on an individual, out-patient basis. Patients with very severe symptoms with deeply ingrained maladaptive patterns of abnormal illness behaviour are less likely to respond to a brief dynamic approach.

Pain clinic packages

Patients with chronic and disabling symptoms usually require more intensive treatment (Benjamin, 1989) (see Box 9.2). One group of therapies is based on the theoretical concept of operant conditioning (Fordyce *et al*, 1973) which suggests that the experience of, and behaviour related to, pain can be positively reinforced by certain consequences such as increased attention and care, and avoidance of responsibility or work. Treatment involves identifying the reinforcers then changing environmental contingencies to stop reinforcing learnt pain behaviours and reward alternative positive behaviours.

The second group of therapies uses a cognitive–behavioural approach. Negative and inappropriate beliefs and expectations about pain are identified and challenged (Pearce, 1983). Specific cognitive skills are used to replace the negative cognitions with more appropriate ideas and coping strategies.

Pain programmes can result in significant improvements in physical and work activity and reductions in analgesic consumption and demand,

---

Box 9.2 Common components of pain packages (after Benjamin, 1989)

Identification of specific goals

Signed contract giving details of agreed goals and commitments

Operant based activity programmes aimed at encouraging appropriate behaviours and reducing inappropriate behaviours

Physical exercise and activity

Marital and family interventions to obliterate relatives' inappropriate reinforcing of abnormal behaviour and to foster relatives' positive reinforcement of appropriate behaviour

Close liaison with other involved agencies (medical, social, voluntary)

Cognitive–behavioural strategies to challenge inappropriate cognitions about pain and illness

Relaxation training

Problem solving

---

though efficacy in relieving pain is variable (Linton, 1986). In-patient treatment is expensive; results from out-patients-based CBT treatment for patients with chronic pain are encouraging (Skinner *et al*, 1990). Patients with severe and chronic symptoms made significant improvement after treatment in measures of analgesic consumption, anxiety, depression, physical disability and coping skills. By coping skills, the researchers meant that after treatment, when patients experienced pain, they were more likely to "think of something pleasant rather than concentrate on the pain" or "think of things to do to distract from the pain".

Similar programmes to this have developed sporadically in parts of the UK, although the general availability is still limited. The programmes are not suitable for all patients with chronic pain. Many patients refuse to contemplate such an approach, so the patients who enter the programmes are a self-selected group. Treatment results in improvement, although whether this is maintained on a long-term basis remains to be established.

Couple therapy

Spouses of patients with chronic functional somatic symptoms often unwittingly collude with the patients' abnormal illness behaviour or reinforce maladaptive ways of coping with illness, but there are few reports evaluating the efficacy of couple intervention (Roy, 1989).

In one controlled study of an out-patient group receiving treatment for chronic pain, spouse involvement was not found to enhance the immediate outcome of the treatment (Moore & Chaney, 1985). Saarijarvi *et al* (1992) also reported disappointing results of five monthly sessions of structured couple therapy in patients with chronic back pain. The psychological distress in the couple group gradually decreased over time whereas it gradually increased in the control group but there was no difference between the groups, after treatment, or at follow-up 5 years later, in scores of marital adjustment and communication or pain and disability scores.

Although the results of this study suggest psychological distress may be reduced by a couple intervention, the overall outcome in terms of disability was disappointing. Couple therapy, however, would seem a fruitful avenue to explore in individual patients where spouse involvement in the patient's disability and health beliefs is marked.

Summary

A variety of different therapeutic approaches have been tried in patients with chronic physical illness, but there is little evidence of benefit for the effectiveness of psychotherapy in patients with chronic physical illness, with the possible exception of diabetes accompanied by emotional difficulties contributing to poor diabetic control. Patients who have severe physical symptoms and are debilitated by their illness respond poorly to psychotherapy. For patients with functional somatic symptoms, on the other hand, there is now substantial evidence suggesting that a wide variety of different psychological interventions are helpful, including dynamic psychotherapy and behaviour therapy – there seems little difference between these on the evidence to date.

An important methodological point is the matching of the intensity of the treatment to the severity of the symptoms. Some studies failed because of inattention to this point. An example of an inappropriately intensive intervention is that employed by Blanchard *et al* (1992) in patients with IBS. In this study up to 22 sessions of cognitive–behavioural therapy were employed in an unselected group of patients with IBS; such patients are known to have a high placebo rate (Klein, 1988). Not surprisingly, the results indicated that the placebo group did as well as the intervention group. A massive study would have been required to demonstrate a potential difference between the two groups. If the study had been better designed, patients with recent-onset IBS who have a high placebo response rate, would have been excluded.

Intensive psychological treatment is warranted if the patient group studied has chronic or severe symptoms which are unlikely to spontaneously remit. Whorwell *et al* (1984), Svedlund (1983) and Guthrie *et al* (1991) used selected patients with refractory IBS. These patients have a placebo response rate of less than 20% and have a high prevalence of depression/anxiety. The resulting psychological treatment trials were all able to test successfully whether or not the particular psychological treatment being evaluated was effective.

Managing complex situations

Patients who are psychiatrically disturbed in the general hospital often provoke great anxiety in hospital staff. Such situations are sometimes quite difficult to manage, but the liaison psychiatrist may well be asked to advise. In the following section some case examples of complex situations are described and their management discussed. It is not possible to anticipate every conceivable situation that may arise but general principles of management can be extrapolated from the following cases to other situations which the trainee may encounter. The importance of receiving supervision from a senior psychiatrist should once again be emphasised.

Factitious disorder

> A 27-year-old woman was admitted to an obstetric ward with a history of vaginal bleeding. Ms A was 22 weeks pregnant and had

been suffering from abdominal pain throughout the pregnancy. Placenta praevia was considered the most likely diagnosis but an ultrasound scan was normal.

After one week of bed rest Ms A suddenly collapsed with profuse vaginal bleeding. A placental abruption was suspected and she was rushed to theatre. A Caesarian section was performed and her baby son was successfully delivered but no cause for the bleeding could be found. Ms A continued to lose profuse amounts of blood *per vagina* engendering great anxiety in the obstetricians caring for her. Eventually vaginal examination revealed two large lacerations high up in the vaginal fornix. These were sutured which curtailed the bleeding and Ms A was transferred back to the ward. She was groggy after the operation for 24–36 hours, during which time her son, due to his prematurity, suffered a cerebral bleed causing severe brain damage.

Psychiatric advice was sought at this stage. The nursing staff looking after her were extremely shocked and frightened that she could potentially harm herself or other babies on the ward. The obstetric team felt anxious and guilty as they felt their intervention had lead indirectly to her son's severe brain damage. They did not know how to broach the self-inflicted injury with her and feared confrontation might precipitate further injury.

The liaison psychiatrist is expected to advise in this situation of uncertainty and anxiety but the following questions regarding management are pertinent: how would one assess Ms A's mental state? What advice would one give to staff? Would one admit her to a psychiatric ward? What advice would you give regarding her contact with her son?

Even before seeing Ms A, simple telephone advice based on issues of safety may help to provide a containing structure for the nursing staff and reduce anxiety. The psychiatrist could recommend that the patient should not leave the ward unaccompanied; should be nursed in a room where she can be easily and regularly observed by nursing staff; and a nurse should always supervise any visits to her son.

After discussion with surgical and nursing staff it was decided not to confront Ms A because so little was known about her psychologically, and her reaction would have been difficult to predict. Instead, the obstetricians gently discussed the lacerations with her and professed puzzlement as to how they could have occurred. She initially denied all knowledge but later the same day confided to one of the nurses that she had stabbed herself. She agreed to see a psychiatrist. If she had not confessed, a psychiatric consultation would still have been required because of the potential harm to the patient and/or her baby.

At the initial assessment, the psychiatrist was able to establish that she was not suicidal and she was not harbouring any thoughts about harming her son or other infants on the ward. She was distressed and shocked about the consequences of her actions. There was no evidence of a depressive illness or psychotic state. On the basis of this it was decided that she should stay on the ward and be allowed to visit her son. The level of nursing observation was discussed in detail and the psychiatrist spent approximately one hour with the nursing staff, providing clear information, guidelines, support and reassurance.

Box 9.3 provides a guide to the main areas that should be discussed. These areas also need to be discussed with the medical or surgical team. The psychiatrist should not assume that the nursing staff will automatically pass on his/her advice. Communication between medical and nursing staff is sometimes very poor.

The long-term management of Mrs A's case included a series of in-depth psychotherapeutic interviews which revealed that she had an extremely deprived childhood. Her mother was weak and unaffectionate and her father was aggressive and violent. When she was 5-years-old he had murdered her elder sister and was convicted and sent to prison. She had blanked out much of the violence and abuse of her childhood and developed a fragile and false persona. She had coped relatively well with life until the 'ordeal' of pregnancy precipitated unbearable thoughts and feelings from her past.

Compliance

Mr B was a 47-year-old man maintained on renal dialysis for the last 8 years; a prior kidney transplant had been unsuccessful. One morning he phoned the renal unit to tell them that he had 'had enough' and wished no further treatment. One of the experienced nursing sisters spent a long time on the phone with him and finally persuaded him to come down to the unit. In the meantime the liaison psychiatrist was called and asked to come to the renal unit to sign the section of the Mental Health Act so that dialysis could be enforced. The psychiatrist made clear that the Act cannot be used in this way and insisted on a detailed assessment.

Mr B lived by himself and had very little social support; he had been unemployed for five years because of his illness. He had lived with his mother until her death 2 years previously, which he found very difficult. The failed transplant, two burglaries and the death of his cat all led to marked depression with biological symptoms and feelings of hopelessness and worthlessness: he felt he was an evil person and was being punished by God. He refused voluntary admission but was eventually admitted to the psychiatric unit under Section 2 of the Mental Health Act, where he agreed to take antidepressant medication and re-start dialysis. Had he continued to refuse, a contingency plan had been discussed.

Box 9.3 Example of guidelines for general nursing staff in relation to the management of 'complex cases'

Provide a clear summary of the psychiatric assessment
Give specific advice about suicidal risk or risk to others
Stipulate how closely the patient needs to be observed
Discuss contingency plans should the patient decide to leave or take his/her discharge
Provide an emergency contact number (if this is the duty psychiatrist, make sure the on-call psychiatrist knows about the situation)
State clearly how often you will visit the ward
Elicit concerns and provide support and advice
If anxiety remains high after all of the above, consider the involvement of an experienced psychiatric nurse to provide additional advice and support

---

In this case the psychiatrist could be clear that Mr B's judgement was affected by the depression and he could not make an appropriate judgement regarding compliance with renal dialysis, without which his life was in danger. The psychiatrist explained to the renal team that under common law they should continue to provide treatment. Had he refused treatment, the assessment order would be converted to a treatment order and ECT instituted, on the basis that Mr B's life was at risk, unless a quick improvement in his mental state could be achieved and the illness would be expected to respond to this treatment.

The management difficulties raised by this case are not uncommon but they may be more complex if the patient was not so severely depressed. The psychiatrist would have to try to understand the reasons underlying the patient's refusal to accept treatment and may have to work with the staff and the patient to overcome the patient's ambivalent feelings about his illness, anger with the staff (often projected anger for his hopelessness) as well as the staff's feelings.

Some of the most common reasons for poor compliance are listed in Box 9.4. It is helpful to have this checklist in the back of one's mind when trying to understand why some patients on some occasions do not comply with treatment.

Demanding behaviour

Ms C was a 26-year-old student who was admitted to an orthopaedic ward following a serious suicide attempt. She had jumped in front of a moving train and had sustained severe injuries including a shattered pelvis. She had been admitted to a psychiatric hospital 4 weeks prior to the attempt but took her own discharge on the day of the incident. The psychiatrists responsible for her care had not considered her to be severely depressed and suicidal, her diagnosis had been 'personality disorder'.

On psychiatric assessment on the ward she appeared to be depressed and was extremely tearful and agitated. She was disappointed that the attempt had not been successful and wanted to die. The actual risk of suicide was low, however, as she was immobile. She was started on antidepressant medication and the nursing staff were given advice about her management. She was not allowed any sharp implements and she was regularly monitored. Her mood improved with antidepressant treatment, her suicidal wishes disappeared but she began demanding more and more attention from the nursing staff. She hated being in hospital and said that she was surrounded by 'old people' whom she 'loathed'. She wanted the curtains drawn round her bed on a permanent basis so that she didn't have to look at "the old bags" on the ward. She accused the staff of not liking her and ignoring her, particularly if they did not respond immediately to her demands.

The psychiatrist spent some time with Ms C trying to understand possible causes of this behaviour. Her childhood was privileged but unhappy and she described her parents as distant and disinterested in her, often 'palming her off' onto other relatives for lengthy periods of time; their expensive presents did not compensate for this behaviour. An illegitimate pregnancy four years previously further complicated the relationship; after she decided against a termination she eventually allowed her own parents and the child's father to take over her daughter's care leaving Ms C feeling guilty. Ms C admitted to the psychiatrist that she was 'selfish' and 'spoilt'; she had some insight into her behaviour on the ward but said she felt so angry at times she just wanted to scream. She felt that she had made a mess of everything in her life, sabotaging relationships at the point when she began to feel involved with someone.

Box 9.4 Common reasons for poor compliance

Side-effects of treatment
Miscommunication between doctor and patient
Forgetfulness/ confusion
Lack of understanding why the treatment is necessary
Ambivalence re physical illness
Anger re physicians/surgeons
Fear and denial of illness
Relative disagrees with treatment and persuades patient to stop
Alcohol problems
Depressive illness
Psychotic symptoms
Philosophical choice of alternative approach or no treatment

After consultation with the nursing staff the psychiatrist made three suggestions:

(1) the psychiatrist would visit the ward on a weekly basis to advise about her drug treatment, monitor her mental state and allow her to ventilate angry and resentful feelings

(2) a nurse from the department of psychiatry would visit to advise staff about management

(3) the nursing staff should allocate a specific amount of time per day (30 minutes) to sit with her and listen to her frustration. This time should be towards the end of the afternoon. If she demanded time before this, the nurses were to ask her to wait until the allotted time. The nurse or nurses who took on this task would receive support and back-up from the psychiatric nurse advisor.

This carefully laid plan failed in the first week as the nursing staff on the ward appointed the most junior nurse (a student nurse) to spend time with Ms C. This nurse panicked at the responsibility and found it impossible to cope with Ms C. The whole plan had to be re-thought and re-negotiated. One of the main reasons the plan faltered was related to the attitude of the nurses to psychiatric problems. They felt that their job did not entail 'talking to patients' and despite the considerable support offered by the psychiatric team the ward nurses felt that the psychiatric team should be the ones seeing Ms C on a daily basis and not themselves. They had therefore pushed the responsibility onto the lowest nurse in the nursing hierarchy: the student.

The situation was partially resolved by persuading the nursing staff to try the scheme again, but with more experienced nurses. The psychiatric nurse provided greater support and the house surgeon was also invited to become involved. Ms C's behaviour settled quite quickly although she still had the occasional unpredictable outburst. The psychiatric team remained in close contact until she was discharged and transferred back to her local psychiatric service.

Polypharmacy

A 49-year-old man was referred to the liaison team for psychiatric assessment prior to neurosurgical excision of occipital nerve to relieve severe right-sided temporo-occipital pain. Nine months previously, Mr E had undergone coronary artery bypass surgery and during the period of time he was in hospital he suffered a grand mal convulsion. Investigation revealed he had a meningioma. Two months later he underwent a right craniotomy and the meningioma was debulked. Not all of it could be removed because of its proximity to the occipital nerve. Following the operation Mr E developed sharp, extremely painful right-sided pain which radiated from the top of his head to both occipital and frontal regions. Large quantities of opiates were required to control the pain and local anaethesic infiltration and phenol injections only provided slight temporary relief.

Four months later he required further surgery as the meningioma had surprisingly regrown. Once again it could not be completely removed and he was sent to the regional cancer hospital for radiotherapy. The pain continued and as a last resort, the neurosurgeons decided to remove his occipital nerve. His regular medication at this point was aspirin 300mg daily, Gaviscon 10 ml q.d.s., ranitidine 150mg b.d., lactulose 10 ml b.d., morphine sulphate 30 mg b.d., Oramorph 20 mg prn, Tylex x2 prn, carbamazepine 400 mg b.d., amitriptyline 50 mg b.d., phenytoin 450mg nocte, temazepam 10 mg nocte and cyclizine 50 mg prn. The amitriptyline had been prescribed for pain relief.

On psychiatric assessment, it became clear that Mr E had marked symptoms of depression and anxiety which had been largely undetected by the surgical team. His mother, with whom he had been very close, had died 2 years previously. He was solitary, found it difficult to talk about his feelings and during the interview with the psychiatrist, it was notable that his pain became much worse when he became anxious and distressed. The psychiatrist demonstrated that his pain could be brought on by anxiety by getting Mr E to hyperventilate. When Mr E relaxed and began to breath deeply his pain became less severe.

Physical treatment of this patient's illness included dealing with the polypharmacy. This commonly occurs as one drug after another is added to try to control a patient's pain. A first step would therefore be the rationalisation of his medication. The physical treatment would also involve antidepressants – he had no evidence of arrthymias so treatment with tricyclic antidepressants was satisfactory.

Psychological treatment involved further explanation and reassurance (so far as it could be given) about the nature of his condition, including an explanation that some of his symptoms were related to depression. The psychiatrist also had to liaise carefully with the neurosurgeons to advise them to postpone further surgery and encourage them to provide him with regular detailed information about his physical status. Social treatment involved working with the patient to establish some form of social network after discharge.

Summary

This chapter outlines the care which must be taken in prescribing psychotropics in liaison psychiatry and understanding drug interactions. Particular emphasis has been placed on psychological treatment; the last few complex management situations indicate that a combination of drug treatment and psychological treatment is often required.

Psychiatric liaison services have been demonstrated not only to reduce psychological morbidity but also to reduce the cost of hospital treatment. Close liaison with the referring physician or surgeon is essential as otherwise recommendations are unlikely to be acted upon. Patients who are severely physically ill may not necessarily recover, but a psychiatric intervention may still provide relief from unnecessary psychological suffering in some cases.

The liaison psychiatrist must have a detailed knowledge of psychotropic drug interactions and confidence when prescribing psychotropic drug treatment in the physically ill. Knowledge of different psychological treatments which can be helpful in the liaison setting is important, as is the realisation that many psychological treatments have to be adapted for use with patients who may not think they will be beneficial.

Further reading

House, A. (1995) Psychiatric disorders, inappropriate health service utilisation and the role of consultation–liaison psychiatry. *Editorial Journal of Psychosomatic Research,* **39**, 799–802.

Mayou, R., Bass, C. & Sharpe, M. (1995) *Treatment of Functional Somatic Symptoms.* Oxford: Oxford University Press.

Rodin, G., Craven, J. & Littlefield, C. (1991) *Depression in the Medically Ill. An Integrated Approach.* New York: Brunner-Mazel.

References

Amreid, R., Guntert, T. W., Dingemanse, T., *et al* (1992) Interactions of moclobemide with concomitantly administered medication: evidence from pharmacological and clinical studies. *Psychopharmacology,* **106**, S24–31.

Bassett, D. & Pilowsky, I. (1985) A study of brief psychotherapy for chronic pain. *Journal of Psychosomatic Research,* **29**, 259–264.

Bazire (1994) *Psychotropic Drug Directory: The Professionals' Pocket Handbook and Aide Memoire.* Wiltshire: Mark Allen.

Benjamin, S. (1989) Psychological treatment of chronic pain: A selective review. *Journal of Psychosomatic Research,* **33**, 121–131.

Bennett, P. & Wilkinson, S. (1985) A comparison of psychological and medical treatment of the irritable bowel syndrome. *British Journal of Clinical Psychology,* **24**, 215–216.

Blanchard, E. B., Schwarz, S. P., Suls, J. M., *et al* (1992) Two controlled evaluations of multicomponent psychological treatments of irritable bowel syndrome. *Behaviour Research and Treatment,* **30**, 175–189.

Boehnert, C. E. & Popkin, M. K. (1986) Psychological issues in treatment of severely non-compliant diabetics. *Psychosomatics,* **26**, 11–20.

Butler, S., Chalder, T., Ron, M., *et al* (1991) Cognitive behaviour therapy in chronic fatigue syndrome. *Journal of Neurology, Neurosurgery and Psychiatry*, **54**, 153–158.

Corney, R. H., Stanton, R., Newe, R., *et al* (1991) Behavioural psychotherapy in the treatment of irritable bowel syndrome. *Journal of Psychosomatic Research*, **35**, 461–469.

Edwards, J. G. & Wheal, H. V. (1992) Assessment of epileptogenic potential: experimental, clinical and epidemiological approaches. *Journal of Psychopharmacology*, **6**, 204–213.

Ewer, T. C. & Stewart, D. E. (1986) Improvement in bronchial hyper-responsiveness in patients with moderate asthma after treatment with a hypnotic technique: a randomised controlled trial. *British Medical Journal*, **293**, 1129–1132.

Fairburn, C. G., Jones, R., Peveler, R. C., *et al* (1991) Three psychological treatments for bulimia nervosa. *Archives of General Psychiatry* , **48**, 463–469.

Feinglos, M. N., Hastedt, P. & Suwit, R. S. (1987) Effects of relaxation therapy on patients with type I diabetes mellitus. *Diabetes Care*, **10**, 72–75.

Feinmann, C. (1985) Pain relief by antidepressants: possible modes of action. *Pain*, **23**, 1–8.

—— (1992) Antidepressants and their role in chronic pain: an update. In *Medical Symptoms Not Explained by Organic Disease* (eds F. Creed, R. Mayou & A. Hopkins), pp. 85–90. London: Royal College of Psychiatrists and Royal College of Physicians.

——, Harris, M. & Cawley, R. (1984) Psychogenic facial pain: presentation and treatment. *British Medical Journal*, **288**, 436–438.

Fordyce, W. E., Fowler, R. S., Lehmann, J. F., *et al* (1973) Operant conditioning in the treatment of chronic pain. *Archives of Physical Medical Rehabilitation*, **54**, 399–408.

Freeman, H. (1993) Moclobemide. *Lancet*, *ii*, 1528–1532.

Greer, S., Moorey, S., Baruch, J. D., *et al* (1992) Adjuvant psychological therapy for patients with cancer: a prospective randomised trial. *British Medical Journal*, **304**, 675–680.

Griffin, J. P., D'Arcy, P. F. & Speirs, C. J. (1988) *A Manual of Adverse Drug Interactions* (4th edn). London: John Wright.

Guthrie, E. (1991) Brief psychotherapy with patients with refractory irritable bowel syndrome. *British Journal of Psychotherapy*, **8**, 175–188.

——, Creed, F. H., Dawson, D., *et al* (1991) A controlled trial of psychological treatment for the irritable bowel syndrome. *Gastroenterology*, **100**, 450–457.

Hale, A. S. (1993) New antidepressants: use in high-risk patients. *Journal of Clinical Psychiatry*, **54** (suppl), 61–70.

Harvey, R. F., Hinton, R. A., Gunary, R. M., *et al* (1989) Individual and group hypnotherapy in treatment of refractory irritable bowel syndrome. *Lancet*, *i*, 424–425.

Hebenstreit, G. F., Baumhack, U., Chan-Palay, V., *et al* (1991) The treatment of depression in geriatric depressed and demented patients by moclobemide: results from the international multicentre double-blind trial. In *Fifth Congress of IPA Abstracts* 31.

Hobson, R. (1985) *Forms of Feeling*. London: Tavistock.

Huyse, F. J., Zwaan, W. A. & Kupka, R. (1994) The applicability of antidepressants in the depressed medically ill: an open clinical trial with fluoxetine. *Journal of Psychosomatic Research*, **38**, 695–703.

Johnston, D. W., Gold, A., Kentish, J., *et al* (1993) Effect of stress management on blood pressure in mild primary hypertension. *British Medical Journal*, **306**, 963–966.

Katon, W., Von Korff, M., Lin, E. B., *et al* (1992) A randomised trial of psychiatric consultation with distressed high utilizers. *General Hospital Psychiatry*, **14**, 86–98.

—— & Gonzales, J. (1994) A review of randomised trials of consultation–liaison studies in primary care. *Psychosomatics*, **35**, 268–278.

Klein, K. B. (1988) Controlled treatment trials in the irritable bowel syndrome: a critique. *Gastroenterology*, **95**, 232–241.

Klimes, I., Mayou, R. A., Pearce, M. J., *et al* (1990) Psychological treatment for atypical non-cardiac chest pain: a controlled evaluation. *Psychological Medicine*, **20**, 605–611.

Lammers, C. A., Naliboff, B. D. & Straatneyer, A. J. (1984) The effects of progressive relaxation on stress and diabetic control. *Behaviour Research and Therapy*, **8**, 641–650.

Landis, B., Jovanovic, L., Landis, E., *et al* (1985) Effect of stress reduction on daily glucose range in previously stabilized insulin-dependent diabetic patients. *Diabetes Care*, **8**, 624–626.

Levenson, J., Hamer, R. & Rossiter, L. (1992) Randomized controlled study of psychiatric consultation guided by screening in general medical inpatients. *American Journal of Psychiatry*, **149**, 631–637.

Levitan, S. J. & Kornfeld, D. S. (1981) Clinical and cost benefits of liaison psychiatry. *American Journal of Psychiatry*, **138**, 790–793.

Lieberman, J.A., Cooper, T. B., Suckow, R. F., *et al* (1985) Tricyclic antidepressant and metabolite levels in chronic renal failure. *Clinical Pharmacology Therapy*, **37**, 301–307.

Linton, S. J. (1986) Behavioural remediation of chronic pain: a status report. *Pain*, **24**, 125–141.

Lipsey, J. R., Robinson, R. G., Pearlson, G. D., *et al* (1984) Nortriptyline treatment of post-stroke depression: a double-blind study. *Lancet*, *i*, 297–300.

Malone, M. D. & Strube, M. J. (1988) Meta-analysis of non-medical treatments for chronic pain. *Pain*, **34**, 231–244.

Mayou, R., Hawton, K. & Feldman, E. (1988) What happens to medical patients with psychiatric disorders? *Journal of Psychosomatic Research*, **32**, 541–549.

Milton, J. (1989) Brief psychotherapy with poorly controlled diabetics. *British Journal of Psychotherapy*, **5**, 532–543.

Minuchin, S., Baker, L. & Rosman, B. (1975) A conceptual model of psychosomatic illness in children. *Archives of General Psychiatry*, **32**, 1031–1038.

Moore, J. E. & Chaney, E. F. (1985) Outpatient group treatment of chronic pain. Effects of spouse involvement. *Journal of Consulting and Clinical Psychology*, **53**, 326–334.

Moran, G. S., Fonagy, P., Kurtz, A., *et al* (1991) A controlled study of the psychoanalytic treatment of brittle diabetes. *Journal of the American Academy of Child and Adolescent Psychiatry*, **30**, 926–935.

—— & —— (1993) A psychoanalytic approach to the treatment of brittle diabetes in children and adolescents. In *Psychological Treatment in Disease and Illness* (eds M. Hodes & S. Moorey), pp. 166–192. London: Gaskell.

Nathan, S. W. (1985) Psychological aspects of recurrent diabetic ketoacidosis in preadolescent boys. *American Journal of Psychotherapy*, **39**, 193–205.

Oates, M. (1995) Risk and childbirth in psychiatry. *Advances in Psychiatric Treatment*, **1**, 146–153.

Oldenburg, B., Perkins, R. J. & Andrews, G. (1985) Controlled trial of psychological intervention in myocardial infarction. *Journal of Consulting and Clinical Psychology*, **53**, 852–859.

Onghena, P. & Van Houdenhove, B. (1992) Antidepressant induced analgesia in chronic non-malignant pain: a meta-analysis of 39 placebo-controlled studies. *Pain*, **49**, 205–219.

Pearce, S. (1983) A review of cognitive–behavioural methods for the treatment of chronic pain. *Journal of Psychosomatic Research*, **27**, 431–440.

Peveler, R. C. & Fairburn, C. G. (1989) Anorexia nervosa in association with diabetes mellitus: a cognitive–behavioural approach to treatment. *Behaviour Research and Therapy*, **27**, 95–99.

Pilowsky, I. & Barrow, C. G. (1990) A controlled study of psychotherapy and amitriptyline used individually and in combination in the treatment of chronic intractable 'psychogenic' pain. *Pain*, **40**, 3–19.

Popkin, M. K., Callies, A. L. & Mackenzie, T. B. (1985) The outcome of antidepressant use in the medically ill. *Archives of General Psychology*, **42**, 1160–1163.

Reding, M. J., Orto, L. A., Winter, S. W., *et al* (1986) Antidepressant therapy after stroke: A double-blind study. *Archives of Neurology*, **43**, 763–765.

Robertson, M. M. & Trimble, M. R. (1983) Depressive illness in patients with epilepsy: a review. *Epilepsia*, **24** (suppl 2), 109–116.

Rodin, G. & Voshart, K. (1986) Depression in the medically ill: An overview. *American Journal of Psychiatry*, **143**, 696–705.

Rosser, R., Denford, J., Heslop, A., *et al* (1983) Breathlessness and psychiatric morbidity in chronic bronchitis and emphysema: a study of psychotherapeutic management. *Psychological Medicine*, **13**, 93–100.

Roy, R. (1989) *Chronic Pain and the Family. A Problem Centered Perspective.* New York: Human Sciences Press.

Ryle, A. (1982) *Psychotherapy: A Cognitive Integration of Theory and Practice.* London: Academic Press.

——, Boa, C. & Fosbury, J. (1993) Identifying the causes of poor self-management in insulin dependent diabetics: the use of cognitive-analytic therapy techniques. In *Psychological Treatment in Disease and Illness* (eds M. Hodes & S. Moorey), pp. 157–165. London: Gaskell.

Saarijarvi, S., Alanen, E., Rytokoski, U., *et al* (1992) Couple therapy improves mental well-being in chronic low back pain patients. A controlled, five year follow-up study. *Journal of Psychosomatic Research,* **36**, 651–656.

Saravay, S. & Lavin, M. (1994) Psychiatric comorbidity and length of stay in the general hospital: a critical review of outcome studies. *Psychosomatics*, **35**, 233–252.

—— & Strain, J. J. (1994) APM task force on funding implications of consultation-liaison outcome studies. Special series introduction: a review of outcome studies. *Psychosomatics*, **35**, 227–232.

Sedgewick, E. M., Cilasun, J. & Edwards, J. G. (1987) Paroxetine and the electroencephalogram. *Journal of Clinical Psychopharmacology*, **1**, 31–34.

Series, H. G. (1992) Drug treatment of depression in medically ill patients. *Journal of Psychosomatic Research*, **36**, 1–16.

Sharpe, M. & Bass, C. (1992) Pathophysiological mechanisms in somatization. *International Review of Psychiatry*, **4**, 81–97.

——, Peveler, R. & Mayou, R. (1992) The psychological treatment of patients with functional somatic symptoms: A practical guide. *Journal of Psychosomatic Research*, **36**, 515–529.

Sjodin, I. (1983) Psychotherapy in peptic ulcer disease: A controlled outcome study. *Acta Psychiatrica Scandinavica*, **67** (suppl 307), 1–90.

Skinner, J. B., Erskine, A., Pearce, S., *et al* (1990) The evaluation of a cognitive behavioural programme in outpatients with chronic pain. *Journal of Psychosomatic Research*, **34**, 13–19.

Smith, G. R., Monson, R. A. & Ray, D. C. (1986) Psychiatric consultation in somatization disorder: A randomized controlled study. *New England Journal of Medicine*, **314**, 1407–1413.

Strain, J., Lyons, J., Mariner, J. *et al* (1991) Cost offset from a psychiatric consultation-liaison intervention with elderly hip fracture patients. *American Journal of Psychiatry*, **148**, 1044–1049.

Surwit, R. S. & Feinglos, M. N. (1983) The effects of relaxation on glucose tolerance in non-insulin dependent diabetes. *Diabetes Care*, **6**, 176–179.

Svedlund, J. (1983) Psychotherapy in irritable bowel syndrome. A controlled outcome study. *Acta Psychiatrica Scandinavica*, **67** (suppl 306), 1–86.

Van Montfrans, G. A., Karemaker, J. M., Wieling, W., *et al* (1990) Relaxation therapy and continuous ambulatory blood pressure in mild hypertension: a controlled study. *British Medical Journal*, **300**, 1368–1372.

Versiani, M., Oggero, U., Alterwain, P., *et al* (1989) A double-blind comparative trial of moclobemide vs imipramine and placebo in major depressive episodes. *British Journal of Psychiatry*, **155** (Suppl. 6), 1–88.

Warren-Boulton, E., Anderson, B. J., Schwartz, N. L., *et al* (1981) A group approach to the management of diabetes in adolescents and young adults. *Diabetes Care*, **4**, 620–623.

Wessely, S., Butler, D. A. & Chalder, T. (1989) Management of chronic (post-viral) fatigue syndrome. *Journal of the Royal College of General Practitioners*, **39**, 26–29.

Whale, J. (1992) The use of brief focal psychotherapy in the treatment of chronic pain. *Psychoanalytic Psychotherapy*, **6**, 61–72.

Whorwell, P. J. (1987) Hypnotherapy in the irritable bowel syndrome. *Stress Medicine*, **3**, 5–7.

——, Prior, A. & Faragher, E. B. (1984) Controlled trial of hypnotherapy in the treatment of severe intractable irritable bowel syndrome. *Lancet, ii*, 1232–1234.

——, —— & Colgan, S. (1987) Hypnotherapy in severe irritable bowel syndrome: further experience. *Gut*, **28**, 423–425.

10 Research in liaison psychiatry

Francis Creed & Elspeth Guthrie

Effect of service development • Prevalence of psychiatric disorder in general medical settings • Psychophysiological relationships • Intervention and cost benefit studies

---

This chapter aims to provide the trainee with an overview of research in liaison psychiatry, emphasising specific aspects of research methods. This should equip the trainee to understand and evaluate published studies as well as to provide ideas for small research projects which might be performed by a senior registrar. For the purpose of this chapter, research in liaison psychiatry will be divided into four types of study:

(1) effect of service development
(2) studies of prevalence of psychiatric disorder in general medical settings
(3) psychophysiological relationships
(4) intervention and cost benefit studies.

This chapter will review each area in turn to establish the important methodological aspects of each and will indicate the possibilities for small and large scale projects. It is written on the assumption that each senior registrar in liaison psychiatry will expect to do one or two small research and/or audit projects but some may be interested in developing a larger research project, for which external funding might well be required.

Effect of service development

Referral rate

Numerous studies have demonstrated that increasing the availability of liaison psychiatrists leads to an increased rate of referrals. These studies may indicate the effect of a service to an overall hospital (e.g. Thomas, 1983; Brown & Cooper, 1987; Creed *et al*, 1993). Alternatively they may refer to individual units (Torem *et al*, 1979; Sensky *et al*, 1985).

Brown & Cooper (1987) compared the referrals for deliberate self-harm (DSH) and other cases in a newly developed psychiatric service. The results demonstrated that there was a similar increase in both DSH and other referrals. The former may have resulted from increased demand. The latter, increase of non-DSH referrals, was probably solely attributable to the increasingly available service.

The studies by Sensky *et al* (1985) and Creed *et al* (1993) excluded patients with deliberate self-harm. Both recorded the reason for referral for each patient. Sensky *et al* found that attachment of a liaison psychiatrist to a medical unit led to a three-fold increase in the number of referrals, with particular increases in the number of patients referred with somatic presentation of psychological disorder and with psychological reaction to physical illness. This study concluded that close liaison with ward staff led to more patients reaching appropriate psychiatric treatment. A similar American study showed a comparable result with as many as 20% of all medical in-patients being referred to the liaison psychiatrist (Torem *et al*, 1979). This is almost certainly too many but the correct proportion is unknown (see below).

The study by Creed *et al* (1993) also indicated a sharp (three-fold) increase in referrals with increasing availability of a liaison psychiatrist. The nature of the referrals was compared to those from a general practitioner. The results demonstrated that the overall severity of disorder (among the depressed patients) was similar between GP referrals and the general hospital referrals. There was, not surprisingly, a much greater proportion with physical illness in the liaison referrals; somatic presentation of psychiatric disorder and psychological reactions to physical disease were much more common among the liaison referrals than the GP referrals. This study drew attention to several aspects of service delivery that might be picked up in future research. One of the most important areas is that of classification of psychiatric disorder. The inadequacies of current psychiatric classification systems in liaison psychiatry have already been discussed in Chapters 2 and 3.

The relative importance of the following variables in accurately describing a sample of liaison referrals is still not clear: psychiatric diagnosis, severity and aetiology of the psychiatric disorder and classification of presenting problem according to the relationship with physical disorder.

Alternative ways of classifying patients (e.g. according to Thomas, 1983) need to be evaluated. For example, in the Creed *et al* (1992) study, the term 'psychological reaction to physical disease' was not entirely satisfactory as many of the patients in this category also had independent stressors (measured by DSM–III Axis V); so a patient may have had marital problems in addition to physical disability, where the time course suggested that the marital problems were more closely related to the psychiatric disorder than physical illness.

In the same study, the diagnostic categories in ICD–9 and DSM–III for psychiatric disorders most frequently encountered in the general hospital were reviewed: these have now been superseded by ICD–10 (for details see Chapter 3) but more work is needed to clarify the borderline between adjustment and depressive disorders in the general medical setting and between the different somatoform disorders. In addition, subclinical psychiatric disorders which do not warrant a formal diagnosis, are extremely important in liaison psychiatry and can often result in serious complications if a patient also has physical disease. There is no satisfactory system at present for recording such problems.

The term 'liaison' implies personal discussion between psychiatrist and general medical staff. This occurred in 86% of ward consultations in the Creed *et al* study (1993); further assessment of the time and expertise involved in such consultations is necessary as up to 10 hours of psychiatric time might be required in certain consultations (Lyons *et al*, 1988).

Unmet needs

There are numerous studies which indicate that 12–15% of medical in-patients have definite psychiatric disorder but less than 1% of all medical admissions are referred to the psychiatrist in most services (Bridges & Goldberg, 1984; Feldman *et al*, 1987). This means that there is a large potential pool of people who might be referred to the psychiatrist but for various reasons this does not happen. This situation is analogous to primary care, where many patients with significant psychiatric disorder, even when recognised by the GP, are not referred to psychiatrists. A system of 'levels and filters', borrowed from Goldberg and Huxley, has been proposed by Sensky for the liaison setting (Sensky, 1986). This is a stimulus to think of potential research questions in liaison psychiatry along the lines of the research previously performed in primary care. The key research questions, therefore, are familiar in terms of health services research:

    (1) Is there a large pool of unmet need among medical patients, in terms of mental health problems, not recognised and treated by the physicians and does referral to the psychiatrist reduce this unmet need?

    (2) Can we understand the factors which lead to referral or militate against it?

Does referral reduce unmet need?

The studies mentioned above suggest that provision of psychiatric services does meet needs that were previously unmet. However, more studies are required to clarify the unmet needs in general medical patients in the absence of referral to a psychiatrist; crucial to this debate is whether mild depression spontaneously resolves and does not need treatment. At least one study suggested that chronic depression remains untreated even after discharge, indicating that GPs also have difficulty in detecting and treating depression in the medically ill (Mayou *et al*, 1988).

Relevant to the study of unmet need in liaison psychiatry are those studies which have examined the proportion of all DSH patients who are not referred to the liaison psychiatry service. In fact, systematic studies have demonstrated that a considerable proportion of patients are not seen by a psychiatrist in the A & E department and leave the hospital with an inadequate assessment (Black & Creed, 1988; Owens *et al*, 1991). In this group of patients it has been policy for patients to be screened by physicians and for those who merit a further assessment, by a psychiatrist. There is very little systematic evidence to support the notion that there is a clear hierarchy of needs, with those patients who have the greater needs being referred to psychiatrists and the remainder being discharged.

An audit of case notes for DSH patients has indicated the paucity of information recorded by non-psychiatrists assessing many of these patients (Black & Creed, 1988). This study needs to be repeated in different hospitals at different times to ensure that the quality of care of patients with DSH improves (Ebbage *et al*, 1994; Hawton & James, 1995).

Reasons for referral

With regard to understanding the reason for referral, Maguire *et al* (1974) studied psychiatric disorder on medical wards. They found that factors such as disturbed behaviour and non-compliance were more likely to lead to referral than unremarkable depression. A similar approach was taken by Seltzer (1989), who studied a series of patients with psychiatric disorder not referred to the psychiatrist. He canvassed nursing opinion, using a questionnaire, to find out why these patients were not referred. It appears that nurses recognised the majority of psychological problems but deemed psychiatric intervention unnecessary in most, usually because the psychiatric disorder was not severe enough or did not present a management problem.

Both of these studies (Maguire *et al*, 1974; Selzer, 1989) used the classic method of screening with a GHQ and interviewing high scorers with a standardised psychiatric interview. This method might be used in future research in a variety of different medical and surgical settings to elicit the prevalence of psychiatric disorder. In addition, this approach could be used to examine differences between the ability of staff in different units to detect psychiatric disorder and make appropriate referrals. Such research could be modelled on the paradigm already developed to examine detection of psychiatric disorder by GPs (Goldberg & Huxley, 1980).

One set of studies in primary care has shown that each GP has a unique referral threshold (Wilkin & Smith, 1987). Presumably this is so of physicians and surgeons in the general hospital but it has been little studied. Other studies of patients referred by GPs to psychiatrists have shown that patients with severe disorders and men with suicidal ideas are most likely to be referred to the psychiatrist (Goldberg & Huxley, 1980); the factors which determine referral to the psychiatrist in the general hospital have not been studied.

Further studies are also required to extend the work of Maguire, whose work with cancer patients (Maguire & Selwood, 1982) suggests that much psychiatric morbidity is unlikely to be detected by surgeons and the training of cancer nurses is an effective way of detecting such disorder.

It may be worth emphasising the simple nature of the majority of these studies. A study relating referral rate of GPs to the psychiatrist was linked to quality of referral letter (Creed *et al*, 1990*b*). This can be repeated in the general hospital (Leonard *et al*, 1990). Such a project may be useful in itself to study a theoretical point. It may also be extremely useful in promoting a dialogue between the liaison psychiatrist and the physicians/ surgeons in the hospital about all aspects of delivery of the liaison psychiatry service.

Future studies of referral

A number of questions which might form the basis of further studies include the following: What factors determine referral? How does this vary between units? Is it related to severity of psychiatric disorder? How does the pattern in my own hospital compare to that in others? Does it change if the form of service delivery changes?

Three important variables need to be considered in relation to referral: severity of psychiatric disorder, detection of psychiatric illness by physicians/surgeons and the availability of liaison psychiatrists. These variables can be assessed through measures of referral rates, examination of case notes, and questionnaires to screen patients or to collect staff views.

All of this might be within the scope of a one year attachment of a senior registrar, who may wish to study the difference between referrals from two or three specific medical/surgical units or monitor his own workload and training experience.

Prevalence of psychiatric disorder in general medical settings

Methodological aspects of measuring prevalence

Two studies discussed in the previous section (Maguire *et al*, 1974; Seltzer, 1989) used the GHQ (Goldberg, 1972) to screen for psychiatric disorder, and a clinical interview as the secondary case finding method. Many studies, however, have been published which have used a self-administered questionnaire as the only criterion of definition of psychiatric disorder. Such studies (Mayou & Hawton, 1986) suggested unrealistically high rates of psychiatric disorder in general medical populations. Those studies which employed research interviews to determine the prevalence of psychiatric disorder have indicated much lower prevalence rates.

Table 10.1 Prevalence of anxiety, depressive and somatisation disorders

	GHQ Self-rating (%)	PSE Interview (%)
General population	19–30	7–11
General hospital, in-patients	43–60	15
General hospital, out-patients	46–52	25[1]

1. 12% for all patients with organic disorders and 37% for patients with no definite organic disorders (Van Hemert *et al*, 1993).

This discrepancy between estimated rates from self-administered questionnaires and rates ascertained by interview comes about because somatic symptoms, included in psychiatric screening questionnaires, may be due to the underlying physical illness, rather than depression and anxiety. Two examples will illustrate the point.

First, in rheumatoid arthritis, the most common measure for many years was the Minnesota Multidimensional Personality Index (MMPI; Graham, 1987) – more a personality measure than one of psychiatric disorder. A group of rheumatologists (Pincus *et al*, 1986) examined the questionnaire in detail and found four items which were included as indicators of depression (e.g. "I have been able to work as well as others, I have few or new pains") could be scored positively as a result of the arthritis. When these items were removed, the results obtained indicated that patients with rheumatoid arthritis had similar personality profiles to the normal population, thus destroying the prior concept of a 'rheumatoid personality' (see also Creed *et al*, 1990c).

The second example concerns the GHQ in a neurology ward. Bridges & Goldberg (1984) indicated that a cut off point of 11+ should be used, instead of 4/5, as this most closely approximated to a diagnosis made at clinical interview. It is important for trainees to realise that the originator of the GHQ has written that it cannot be used in the general medical setting as an alternative to clinical interview (Goldberg, 1986).

One attempt to overcome the problem of somatic symptoms is the development of the Hospital Anxiety and Depression Scale (HADS; Zigmond & Snaith, 1983), which specifically excludes somatic items. The resulting questionnaire is simple to use in a variety of settings. It has, however, been little validated and may not have any advantage over the GHQ with an adjusted score (Meakin, 1992).

Meakin (1992) reviewed the screening instruments used for depression in the medically ill and commented that the validation of these scales is patchy and "almost endless scope remains for continuing to compare rating scales and for selecting optimal cut-off levels in differing populations". This suggestion could readily be taken up by a senior registrar prepared to screen a particular medical population and perform second stage interviews to determine the appropriate cut off for that population.

Prevalence of psychiatric disorder using research interviews

The few studies that have employed research interviews on general medical in-patients have consistently shown a prevalence of around 15–20%, i.e. much lower than self-administered questionnaires. The most extensive UK study is that by Feldman *et al* (1987). This was a large study which demonstrated the following features:

(1) the prevalence rates are 2–3 times those in the general population but the usual sex difference is not apparent
(2) rather higher rates of psychiatric disorder were found in patients with severe cardiac disease, strokes and haematological cancers
(3) an expected higher rate of previous psychiatric disorder was associated with current psychiatric disorder
(4) approximately half of the patients with psychiatric disorder were detected by house physicians but only a tiny proportion were referred to the psychiatrist
(5) the rates of alcohol related problems were much higher in males than in females (see Table 3.1).

There is only one comparable study of medical out-patients (Van Hemert *et al*, 1993; see Chapter 3). The study was performed in the Netherlands and its findings cannot necessarily be applied elsewhere. Further studies are clearly needed. Van Hemert *et al* showed that there was a much higher prevalence of psychiatric disorder in patients with non-organic conditions. It also showed the relatively low prevalence of somatisation disorder.

There have been insufficient studies of this nature that have used a clinical interview to define psychiatric disorder and have also divided the patients into different groups according to the relationship between the physical and psychiatric disorders. The study by Moffic & Paykel (1975), discussed below, used a self-administered questionnaire but would merit repetition with a clinical research interview. Moffic & Paykel administered the Beck Depression Inventory (Beck *et al*, 1961) to general medical in-patients and used a score of 14 or more as an indicator of depression. The results indicated that two-thirds of these depressions were secondary to the physical illness. Only 14% of the depressed patients had a somatic presentation of depression (somatisation). For the remaining 20% the depression preceded the onset of physical illness; the majority of this group had experienced a severe life event which was followed first by depression and later by the onset of physical disorder.

Prevalence studies in particular patient groups

In contrast to studies of general medical units as a whole, there have been a number of studies which have examined the prevalence of psychiatric disorder in particular patient groups. The contrast between patients with non-organic and organic disorders is clear. This can be illustrated by a series of prevalence studies of psychiatric disorder in non-organic gastrointestinal disorders compared with patients with organic gastrointestinal disorders.

The strikingly consistent rate of 40–60% prevalence of psychiatric disorder in patients with functional gastrointestinal disorders is persuasive that this is a true finding. The variation may reflect the measuring instruments rather than different samples.

Are further prevalence studies required?

There are several ways in which such studies might provide useful information.

Particular subgroups

Firstly, particular subgroups of patients (especially those with a probable high prevalence) might merit further study. In this context the elderly, those with life threatening physical illness, those with chronic disabling illness and those without organic disorders are of great interest. In such subgroups, where the prevalence of psychiatric disorder is high, the relationship between predisposing factors (family history, past personal history of psychiatric disorder, childhood deprivation, etc.), personality disorders and severity of physical illness, in the development of psychiatric disorder, is of special interest.

An example of such a study was that of Ramirez (1989). The study included 50 patients referred to a liaison psychiatrist and indicated that lack of a confiding relationship and previous history of psychiatric illness were significantly associated with sustained intense episodes of psychological disturbance rather than transient distress. Such a distinction is useful in planning services. Similar studies need to be performed on consecutive series of patients in medical and surgical units rather than only patients referred to a liaison psychiatrist.

Other examples of such studies have compared the prevalence in different groups of patients. Possible comparisons include the following: a study of new out-patients and chronic attenders (Guthrie *et al*, 1990), a comparison of medical patients in rural and inner city areas (the prevalence of alcoholism in the latter has been shown to be much higher), prevalence of sexual disorders in mastectomy patients and functional or organic gastrointestinal disorders (Maguire *et al*, 1978; Guthrie *et al*, 1987).

Table 10.2 Prevalence of psychiatric disorder in functional bowel disorder/irritable bowel syndrome using standardised research psychiatric interviews

Author	No. of subjects	Instru- ment	Functional bowel dis- order (%)	Organic GI dis- order (%)	Healthy controls (%)
McDonald & Bouchier (1980)	32[1]	CIS[2]	53	20	–
Colgan *et al* (1988)	37[1]	CIS	57	6	–
Craig & Brown (1984)	79[1]	PSE[3]	42	18	–
Ford *et al* (1987)	48[4]	PSE	42	6	8
Toner et al (1990)	44[4]	DIS[5]	61	–	–
Blanchard *et al* (1990)	68[4]	DIS	56	25	18
Kingham & Dawson (1985)	22[1]	HRSD[6]	64	–	–

1. FBD, Functional bowel disorder (i.e. consecutive non-organic gastrointestinal disorders in the clinic).
2. CIS, Clinical Interview Schedule (Goldberg *et al*, 1970).
3. PSE, Present State Examination (Wing *et al*, 1974).
4. IBS, Irritable bowel syndrome patients.
5. DIS, Diagnostic Interview Schedule (Robins *et al*, 1981).
6. HRSD, Hamilton Rating Scale for Depression (Hamilton, 1967).

In this way a variety of different psychiatric disorders can be studied in different diagnostic groups.

Studies of severity of psychiatric illness

Additional useful data, helpful in planning services, will be collected in a prevalence study which also examines the severity of psychiatric disorder. As well as diagnosis, therefore, future studies should try and assess the need for care; this may be related to severity of psychiatric disorder but may also be complicated by the severity of physical disability. The combination of physical illness and chronic depression may be particularly disabling (Wells *et al*, 1989) and there may be a need for shared care (by both physician and psychiatrist). It is also known that depression and physical illness are associated with increased suicide risk. Few data have previously been collected regarding the potential suicidal risk of patients in medical units who have depression – these form a group of patients with undoubted need for specific psychological help.

Outcome of psychiatric disorders in medical setting

Too few studies have been performed concerning the factors related to outcome. It is known that serious physical illness and delirium are associated with high mortality. It is not known which patients with depression continue to be depressed and whether some adjustment disorders turn into major depression following discharge. The type of study performed by House *et al* (1990) with stroke patients, which was of a longitudinal nature, could be usefully repeated in different groups of patients.

Psychophysiological relationships

An exciting area of research, which tends to be rarely available to senior registrars is the opportunity of performing psychophysiological measurement on patients with somatic symptoms and psychological disorder. Some of the work in this area has been reviewed by Sharpe & Bass (1992).

In general the number of patients who can be studied is inversely proportional to the complexity of the technique. Thus the measurement of end tidal pCO_2 in patients who hyperventilate may reveal very considerable differences between patients and controls which can be identified with small numbers (Bass & Gardner, 1985). Similarly Spurrell & Creed (1993) were able to study lymphocyte response in a small number of patients and found an interesting difference between people who had recently been bereaved and those who had depressive illness.

There are many clinical projects which do not require sophisticated physiological measurement or special equipment. There is much to be learned concerning the relationship between somatic symptoms, psychiatric disorder, life events, abnormal illness behaviour and cognitive functioning, when detailed measures of each are used simultaneously. Examples of studies which have used one or more of these measures will be considered in turn. The reader is referred to the specific studies for details. It is intended that similar projects may be performed in other medical conditions.

Cognitive functioning.   This has been studied in multiple sclerosis and systemic lupus erythematosis (SLE) (Ron & Logsdail, 1989; Hay *et al*, 1992; Gilchrist & Creed,1994). It appears that mild abnormalities of cognitive functioning are more closely related to psychiatric disorder than cerebral damage resulting from these illnesses.

Relationship of psychiatric disorder to severity of physical illness.   Although it has been often stated that psychiatric disorder in physical disease is secondary to the disability or symptomatology of the physical illness, this has rarely been demonstrated. For example, in rheumatoid arthritis, there does not appear to be a clear correlation between severity of disability or activity in rheumatoid arthritis and a presence of psychiatric disorder

(Murphy *et al*, 1988). The same is true of SLE (Hay *et al*, 1992) and MS (Ron & Logsdail, 1989). Thus factors other than the severity of physical illness need to be measured to explain the depression; the predisposing factors mentioned above are likely to be most important in this respect.

Life events.   These are difficult to measure reliably but there is no reason why trainee psychiatrists cannot acquire skills in the use of the Life Events and Difficulties Schedule (Brown & Harris, 1978). This method has been applied successfully in a variety of projects concerning the onset of various physical/functional conditions: back pain (Crauford *et al*, 1990); rheumatoid arthritis (Conway *et al*, 1994); stroke (House *et al*, 1990); low birth weight babies (Mutale *et al*, 1991); miscarriages (O'Hare & Creed, 1995); overdoses (Creed, 1985, 1993).

Abnormal illness behaviour.   This has been studied in relation to a number of different conditions. These may be chronic painful conditions (Creed *et al*, 1990*a*), hysteria (Wilson-Barnett & Trimble, 1985) or organic conditions such as rheumatoid arthritis (Murphy *et al*, 1988). There is some interest in trying to discern abnormal illness behaviour which is separate from psychiatric disorder and there is much work to be done in this area. The work by Barsky on hypochondriasis (Barsky, 1981; Barsky *et al*, 1986) indicates the close relationship between patient beliefs in relation to hypochondriasis, cognitive mechanisms and a potential for therapy.

Other psychological measures

Type A personality is another measure which has been used in chronic fatigue syndrome and irritable bowel syndrome (Woods & Goldberg, 1991; Lewis *et al*, 1994). Coping mechanisms have been used in arthritis (Newman *et al*, 1990).

These are generally isolated studies and the use of the same measures across different populations may greatly increase our understanding. For example, type A personality was previously thought to be specific to heart disease but later was shown to be important in several conditions (Rime *et al*, 1989). There is considerable scope for further small scale projects assessing the relationship between severity of physical illness, presence of psychiatric disorder, abnormal illness behaviour, cognitive factors and personality. The relationship between these measures can be assessed on relatively small numbers of subjects, usually with a similar diagnosis. Such patients are therefore easy to collect.

Intervention and cost benefit studies

Intervention studies

Intervention studies have been described in Chapter 9. This section will illustrate some general principles in relation to this area of research. Intervention studies are generally beyond the scope of senior registrars in liaison psychiatry. However, much preliminary work needs to be done and a small project may be useful as a preliminary one on which a larger intervention study may be planned. Some intervention studies have been performed without adequate preliminary work. This may result in an inappropriate treatment being used which does not match the severity of the condition.

Studies are needed in which information is clearly communicated to the patient's doctor (physician or GP) and acted upon by that doctor. The effect of the psychiatric intervention could then be tested. The most frequently recommended intervention is prescription of antidepressants. Reasons cited in the current literature include failure to recognise the potential benefit from psychiatric intervention, physician resistance to any form of psychological intervention and being unfamiliar with antidepressant medication at the appropriate dose (Mayou & Smith, 1986). Further research is indicated to understand why these obstacles to patients receiving appropriate psychotropic drugs are not overcome.

Many senior registrars will suggest antidepressants but it would be useful to audit compliance with such recommendations and understand, if the drugs are not prescribed, why this is so. If such drugs are prescribed, it is necessary to follow-up patients and see whether they are effective.

Before undertaking a treatment trial, it is essential that power calculations are carried out to determine the number of patients that will be required to demonstrate a statistical difference between the trial groups, should the treatment under study be effective. In many areas of liaison psychiatry, there is little information regarding the effectiveness of psychological treatments, and it is difficult to do power calculations. A pilot study carried out by a senior registrar on a small number of patients may allow the effect size of a treatment to be calculated and hence provide invaluable information for a much larger project. For example, a survey of patients on a medical ward, or in a gastroenterology out-patient clinic, who have alcohol problems and who might be entered into an intervention trial would be sensible. The counselling for patients with alcohol problems can only be applied once it has been determined which patients are actually available and willing to undergo counselling. However, the counselling developed by Chick *et al* (1985) could usefully be repeated in other hospitals and in out-patient clinics.

Similarly, a prevalence study of marital or sexual problems among diabetic patients, for example, would indicate (a) the frequency of such sexual and marital problems; (b) the availability (and willingness) of patients to undergo treatment for these problems, and (c) the type of treatment (sexual, marital, individual psychological treatment) and the likely response rate. These data are essential to design a large intervention study but could be within the realm of a senior registrar attached to the diabetic unit over a period of time.

Effectiveness versus efficacy

Effectiveness is the therapeutic benefit of a treatment tested under research conditions. Efficacy is the therapeutic benefit of a treatment in the clinical setting. The two are not the same. For example, the amount of time and attention that patients receive in a trial of antidepressant treatment may far outweigh the time and attention patients receive when antidepressants are prescribed in the clinical setting. Trial groups are often 'pure', i.e. only contain patients who meet stringent diagnostic criteria for the particular psychiatric disorder under scrutiny. Many patients in a clinical setting, however, have mixed problems which do not fit neatly into specific diagnostic categories. Some patients refuse to participate in treatment studies or drop-out before the end. Few treatment trials adequately describe the recruitment process, so it is often difficult to assess the acceptability of a treatment to the majority of patients for whom it is meant.

Thus, the effect of a well-proven treatment (such as antidepressant treatment for depression) may be different if that treatment is delivered in an unusual treatment setting (e.g. a neurology clinic) or is prescribed to patients with heterogeneous clinical problems (e.g. patients with mixed anxiety/depressive disorders plus physical illness).

More naturalistic studies are required, which attempt to address the extent to which particular treatments – drug or psychological – are appropriate in medical settings (e.g. Huyse *et al*, 1994). Although most of these projects may be beyond the scope of a senior registrar, a simple evaluation of a treatment delivered in a clinical setting may provide valuable feedback and lead to change of clinical practice.

Cost analysis and quality of life

There is an urgent demand for studies that examine the cost of treatment in the NHS. Because of the paucity of research in this area, small scale projects in liaison psychiatry may produce dramatic findings. Such small projects include; studies of health care utilisation before and after attending a neurologist (Grove *et al*, 1980; Fitzpatrick & Hopkins, 1981); a careful estimation of the cost to the NHS of the care of one patient with somatisation disorder (Bass & Murphy, 1991); and the study by Shaw & Creed (1991) which calculated the medical costs incurred by patients with somatic symptoms, before they were referred to a psychiatrist.

Further such projects could be undertaken in almost any medical speciality and are likely to yield interesting results. Such small projects obviously provide the impetus and rationale for more detailed and accurate larger scale studies.

An important component of outcome when comparing the costs of different treatment is the quality of life or health status of the patient after receiving treatment. Mental health status of the physically ill is an important component of quality of life and it is a determinant of social and occupational function after treatment (Wells *et al*, 1989). Strain and colleagues (1991) have demonstrated that treating psychiatric disorder in patients undergoing hip replacement can not only improve their health status but also reduce health costs.

Certain conditions, such as non-ulcer dyspepsia, are known to have a large psychological component and also incur enormous costs to health services for investigation and treatment (Nyren *et al*, 1985). Future evaluations of psychological interventions in such conditions should include an economic assessment.

Economic assessments should adopt a broad view of service utilisation and must include visits to GPs as well as to the hospital. For example, consultations with a GP for headaches are reduced after an expensive visit to the neurologist (Fitzpatrick & Hopkins, 1981). However, it has been shown that consultation with a GP during the year after consultation with the neurologist remains high in terms of all consultations, even though it is low for headaches (Grove *et al*, 1980).

Summary

Research in liaison psychiatry has been developing over the last 15 years. It is a huge field with wide ranging possibilities for future research. The high level of psychiatric morbidity in hospital patients has been established, but further work is required to identify subgroups of patients who are particularly at risk. Detection of psychiatric morbidity by general medical staff needs to be improved, better classification systems need to be developed, and more detailed study of the potential populations for intervention studies need to be determined. This chapter has identified some of the small projects which senior registrars might undertake during a one year liaison attachment.

Further reading

Huyse, F., Strain, J. J., Hengeveld, M. E., *et al* (1988) Interventions in consultation liaison psychiatry: the development of a schema and a checklist for operationalized interventions. *General Hospital Psychiatry*, **10**, 88–101.
—, — & Hammer, J. S. (1990) Interventions in consultation liaison psychiatry. II: Concordance. *General Hospital Psychiatry*, **12**, 221–231.

References

Barsky, A. J. (1981) Hidden reasons some patients visit doctors. *Annals of Internal Medicine*, **94**, 492.

——, Wyshak, G. & Klerman, G. L. (1986) Medical and psychiatric determinants of out-patients medical utilisation. *Medical Care*, **24**, 548–560.

Bass, C. & Gardner, W. N. (1985) Respiratory and psychiatric abnormalities in chronic symptomatic hyperventilation. *British Medical Journal*, **290**, 1387–1390.

—— & Murphy, M. (1991) The chronic somatiser and the Government White Paper. *Journal of the Royal Society of Medicine*, **83**, 203–204.

Beck, A. T., Ward, C. H., Mendelson, M., *et al* (1961) An inventory for measuring depression. *Archives of General Psychiatry*, **4**, 561–571.

Black, D. & Creed, F. (1988) Assessment of self-poisoning patients by psychiatrists and junior medical staff. *Journal of the Royal Society of Medicine*, **81**, 97–99.

Blanchard, E. B., Scharff, L., Schwarz, S. P., *et al* (1990) The role of anxiety and depression in the irritable bowel syndrome. *Behaviour Research and Therapy*, **28**, 401–405.

Bridges, K. W. & Goldberg, D. (1984) Psychiatric illness in in-patients with neurological disorders: patients' views on discussion of emotional problems with neurologists. *British Medical Journal*, **286**, 656–658.

Brown, A. & Cooper, A. F. (1987) The impact of a liaison psychiatry service on patterns of referral in a general hospital. *British Journal of Psychiatry*, **150**, 83–87.

Brown, G. W. & Harris, T. O. (1978) *Social Origins of Depression: A Study of Psychiatric Disorder in Women.* London: Tavistock.

Chick, J., Lloyd, G. & Chrombie, E. (1985) Counselling problem drinkers in medical wards: a controlled study. *British Medical Journal*, **290**, 965–967.

Colgan, S., Creed, F. & Klass, H. (1988) Symptom complaints, psychiatric disorder and abnormal illness behaviour in patients with upper abdominal pain. *Psychological Medicine*, **18**, 887–892.

Conway, S. C., Creed, F. H. & Symmond, D. P. M. (1994) Life events and the onset of rheumatoid arthritis. *Journal of Psychosomatic Research*, **38**, 837–848.

Craig, T. K. & Brown, G. W. (1984) Goal frustrating aspects of life event stress in the aetiology of gastrointestinal disorder. *Journal of Psychosomatic Research*, **28**, 411–421.

Crauford, D., Creed, F. H. & Jayson, M. (1990) Life events and psychological disturbance in patients with low back pain. *Spine*, **15**, 490–494.

Creed, F. H. (1985) Life events and physical illness. *Journal of Psychosomatic Research*, **29**, 113–123.

—— (1993) Stress and psychosomatic disorders. In *Handbook of Stress: Theoretical and Clinical Aspects* (eds L. Goldberger & S. Breznitz), pp. 496–510. New York: Macmillan Publishing.

——, Firth, D., Timol, M., *et al* (1990*a*) Somatisation and illness behaviour in a neurology ward. *Journal of Psychosomatic Research*, **34**, 417–437.

——, Gowishunkur, J., Russel, E., *et al* (1990*b*) General practitioner referral rates to district psychiatry and psychology services. *British Journal of General Practice*, **40**, 450–545.

——, Murphy, S. & Jayson, M. V. (1990*c*) Measurement of psychiatric disorder in rheumatoid arthritis. *Journal of Psychosomatic Research*, **34**, 79–87.

——, Guthrie, E., Black, D., *et al* (1993) Psychiatric referrals within the general hospital: comparison with referrals from general practitioners. *British Journal of Psychiatry*, **162**, 204–211.

Ebbage, J., Farr, C., Skinner, D. V., *et al* (1994) The psychosocial assessment of patients discharged from accident and emergency departments after deliberate self-poisoning. *Journal of Royal Society of Medicine,* **87**, 515–516.

Feldman, E., Mayou, R., Hawton, K., *et al* (1987) Psychiatric disorder in medical in-patients. *Quarterly Journal of Medicine*, **63**, 405–412.

Fitzpatrick, R. M. & Hopkins, A. (1981) Referrals to neurologists for headaches not due to structural disease. *Journal of Neurology, Neurosurgery and Psychiatry*, **44**, 1061–1067.

Ford, M. J., Miller, P. Mc. C., Eastwood, J., *et al* (1987) Life events, psychiatric illness and the irritable syndrome. *Gut*, **28**, 160–165.

Gilchrist, A. C. & Creed, F. (1994) Depression, cognitive impairment and social stress in multiple sclerosis. *Journal of Psychosomatic Research*, **38**, 193–201.

Goldberg, D. (1972) *The Detection of Psychiatric Illness by Questionnaire.* Oxford: Oxford University Press.

—— (1986) Use of the general health questionnaire in clinical work. *British Medical Journal*, **293**, 1188–1189.

——, Eastwood, M. R., Kedwood, H. B., *et al* (1970) A Standardised Psychiatric Interview for use in community surveys. *British Journal of Preventive and Social Medicine*, **24**, 18–23.

—— & Huxley, P. (1980) *Mental Illness in the Community.* London: Tavistock.

Graham, J. R. (1987) *The MMPI. A Practical Guide* (2nd edn). New York: Oxford University Press.

Grove, J. L., Butler, P. & Millac, P. A. H. (1980) The effect of a visit to a neurological clinic upon patients with tension headache. *The Practitioner*, **224**, 195–196.

Guthrie, E., Creed, F. & Whorwell, P. J. (1987) Severe sexual dysfunction in women with the irritable bowel syndrome: comparison with inflammatory bowel disease and duodenal ulceration. *British Medical Journal*, **296**, 577–578.

——, ——, Dawson, D., *et al* (1990) A controlled trial of psychological treatment for the irritable bowel syndrome. *Gastroenterology*, **100**, 450–457.

Hamilton, M. (1967) Development of a rating scale for primary depression. *British Journal of Clinical Psychology,* **6**, 278–296.

Hawton, K. & James, R. (1995) General hospital services for attempted suicide patients: a survey in one region. *Health Trends*, **27**, 18–21.

Hay, E. M., Black, D., Huddy, A., *et al* (1992) Psychiatric disorder and cognitive impairment activity in SLE. *Arthritis and Rheumatism*, **35**, 411–416.

House, A., Dennis, M., Mogridge, L., *et al* (1990) Life events and difficulties preceding stroke. *Journal of Neurology, Neurosurgery and Psychiatry*, **53**, 1024–1028.

Huyse, F. J., Zwaan, W. A. & Kupka, R. (1994) The applicability of antidepressant in the depressed medically ill: an open clinical trial with fluoxetine. *Journal of Psychosomatic Research*, **38**, 695–703.

Kingham, J. G. C. & Dawson, A. M. (1985) Origin of chronic right upper quadrant pain. *Gut,* **26**, 783–788.

Leonard, I., Babbs, C. & Creed, F. H. (1990) Psychiatric referrals within the general hospital – the communication process. *Journal of Royal Society of Medicine,* **83**, 241–244.

Lewis, S., Cooper, C. & Bennett, D. (1994) Psychosocial factors and chronic fatigue syndrome. *Psychological Medicine*, **24**, 661–671.

Lyons, J. S., Hammer, J. S., Larson, D. B., *et al* (1988) Treatment opportunities on a consultation/liaison service. *American Journal of Psychiatry*, **145**, 1435–1437.

MacDonald, A. J. & Bouchier, P. A. D. (1980) Non-organic gastro-intestinal illness: a medical and psychiatric study. *British Journal of Psychiatry*, **136**, 276–283.

Maguire, G. P., Julier, D. L., Hawton, K. E., *et al* (1974) Psychiatric morbidity and referral on two general medical wards. *British Medical Journal*, **1**, 268–270.

——, Lee, E. G., Bevington, D. J., *et al* (1978) Psychiatric problems in the first year after mastectomy. *British Medical Journal*, **1**, 963–965.

—— & Selwood, R. (1982) A liaison psychiatric service for mastectomy patients. In *Medicine and psychiatry. A practical approach* (eds F. Creed & J. Pfeffer), pp. 378–395. London: Pitman.

Mayou, R. & Hawton, K. E. (1986) Psychiatric disorder in the general hospital. *British Journal of Psychiatry*, **149**, 172–190.

—— & Smith, E. B. O. (1986) Hospital doctors' management of psychological problems. *British Journal of Psychiatry*, **148**, 194–197.

——, Hawton, K. E. & Feldman, E. (1988) What happens to patients with psychiatric disorder in general medical ward? *British Journal of Psychosomatic Research*, **32**, 541–549.

Meakin, C. J. (1992) Screening for depression in the medically ill. *British Journal of Psychiatry*, **160**, 212–216.

Moffic, H. S. & Paykel, E. S. (1975) Depression in medical in-patients. *British Journal of Psychiatry*, **126**, 346–353.

Murphy, S., Creed, F. H. & Jayson, M. V. (1988) Psychiatric disorder and illness behaviour in rheumatoid arthritis. *British Journal of Rheumatology*, **27**, 357–363.

Mutale, T., Creed, F., Maresh, M., *et al* (1991) Life events and low birth weight – analysis by infants perterm and small for gestational age. *British Journal of Obstetrics and Gynaecology*, **98**, 166–172.

Newman, S., Fitzpatrick, R., Lamb, R., *et al* (1990) Patterns of coping in rheumatoid arthritis. *Psychology and Health*, **4**, 187–200.

Nyren, O., Adami, H. O., Gustavsson, S., *et al* (1985) Social and economic effects of non-ulcer dyspepsia. *Scandinavian Journal of Gastroenterology*, **20** (suppl. 109), 41–45.

O'Hare, T. J. & Creed, F. H. (1995) Life events and miscarriage. *British Journal of Psychiatry*, **167**, 799–805.

Owens, D., Dennis, M., Jones, S., *et al* (1991) Self-poisoning patients discharged from accident and emergency: risk factors and outcome. *Journal of the Royal College of Physicians*, **25**, 218–222.

Pincus, T., Callahan, L. F., Bradley, L. A., *et al* (1986) Elevated MMPI scores for hypochondriasis, depression and hysteria in patterns with rheumatoid arthritis reflect disease rather than psychological status. *Arthritis and Rheumatism*, **29**, 1456–1466.

Ramirez, A. J. (1989) Liaison psychiatry in a breast cancer unit. *Journal of the Royal Society of Medicine*, **82**, 15–17.

Rime, B., Ucros, C. S., Bestgen, Y., *et al* (1989) Type A behaviour: specific coronary risk factor or general disease-prone condition. *British Journal of Medical Psychology*, **62**, 229–240.

Robins, L. W., Helzer, J. E., Croughan, J., *et al* (1981) *The NIMH Diagnostic Interview Schedule Version III.* Public Health Service (HSS) Publication. ADM-T42-3 (J–81, 8–81).

Ron, M. A. & Logsdail, S. J. (1989) Psychiatric morbidity in multiple sclerosis: a clinical and MRI study. *Psychological Medicine*, **19**, 887–895.

Seltzer, A. (1989) Prevalence, detection and referral of psychiatric morbidity in general medical patients. *Journal of the Royal Society of Medicine*, **82**, 410–412.

Sensky, T. (1986) The general hospital psychiatrist: Too many tasks and too few roles? *British Journal of Psychiatry*, **148**, 151–158.

——, Greer, S., Cundy, T., *et al* (1985) Referrals to psychiatrists in a general hospital – comparison of two methods of liaison psychiatry: preliminary communication. *Journal of Royal Society of Medicine*, **78**, 463–468.

Sharpe, M. & Bass, C. (1992) Pathophysiological mechanisms in somatization. *International Review of Psychiatry*, **4**, 81–97.

Shaw, J. & Creed, F. (1991) The cost of somatization. *Journal of Psychosomatic Research*, **35**, 307–312.

Spurrell, M. T. & Creed, F. H. (1993) Lymphocyte response in depressed patients and subjects anticipating bereavement. *British Journal of Psychiatry*, **162**, 60–64.

Strain, J. J., Lyons, J. S., Hammer, J. S., *et al* (1991) Cost offset from a psychiatric consultation–liaison intervention with elderly hip fracture patients. *American Journal of Psychiatry*, **148**, 1044–1049.

Thomas, C. (1983) Referrals to a British liaison psychiatry service. *Health Trends*, **15**, 61–64.

Toner, B. B., Garfinkel, P. E. & Jeejeebhoy, K. W. (1990) Psychological factors in irritable bowel syndrome. *Canadian Journal of Psychiatry*, **35**, 158–161.

Torem, M., Saravay, S. & Steinberg, H. (1979) Psychiatric liaison: benefits of an active approach. *Psychosomatics*, **20**, 598–611.

Van Hemert, A. M., Hengeveld, M. W., Bolk, J. H., *et al* (1993) Psychiatric disorders in relation to medical illness among patients of a general medical out-patients clinic. *Psychological Medicine*, **23**, 167–173.

Wells, K., Stewart, A., Hays, R., *et al* (1989) The functioning and well-being of depressed patients. *Journal of the American Medical Association*, **262**, 914–919.

Wilkin, D. & Smith, A. D. (1987) Variation in general practitioners' referral rates to consultants. *Journal of the Royal College of General Practitioners*, **37**, 350–535.

Wilson-Barnett, J. J. & Trimble, M. R. (1985) An investigation of hysteria using the illness behaviour questionnaire. *British Journal of Psychiatry*, **146**, 601–608.

Wing, J. K., Cooper, J. E. & Sartorius, N. (1974) *The Measurement and Classification of Psychiatric Symptoms.* London: Cambridge University Press.

Woods, T. O. & Goldberg, D. P. (1991) Psychiatric perspectives: an overview. *British Medical Bulletin*, **47**, 908–918.

Zigmond, A. & Snaith, A. (1983) The Hospital Anxiety and Depression Scale. *Acta Psychiatric Scandinavica*, **67**, 361–370.

Index

Compiled by Linda English

Page numbers in italics refer to tables, figures and/or boxes.